Infectious Diseases of the Central Nervous System

Neurologic Illness:
DIAGNOSIS & TREAMENT

EDITOR-IN-CHIEF
Michael I. Weintraub, M.D.
New York Medical College
Valhalla, NY

Hysterical Conversion Reactions
Michael I. Weintraub

Infectious Diseases of the Central Nervous System
Richard A. Thompson and John R. Green, eds.

Infectious Diseases of the Central Nervous System

Edited by
Richard A. Thompson, M.D.,
Division of Neurology,
Barrow Neurological Institute of St. Joseph's
Hospital and Medical Center,
Phoenix, Arizona

John R. Green, M.D., F.A.C.S.,
Chairman of Neurosurgery,
and Chairman, Barrow Neurological Institute
of St. Joseph's Hospital and Medical Center,
Phoenix, Arizona

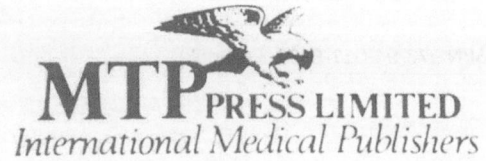
MTP PRESS LIMITED
International Medical Publishers

Published in the UK and Europe by
MTP Press Limited
Falcon House
Lancaster, England

Published in the US by
SPECTRUM PUBLICATIONS, INC.
175-20 Wexford Terrace
Jamaica, NY 11432

ISBN 978-94-011-6334-7   ISBN 978-94-011-6332-3 (eBook)
DOI 10.1007/978-94-011-6332-3

Contributors

J. Richard Baringer, MD, Professor and Chairman, Department of Neurology, University of Utah Medical Center; Acting Chief of the Neurology Service, Veterans Administration Medical Center, Salt Lake City, Utah

John L. Beggs, PhD, Department of Neuropathology, Barrow Neurological Institute of St. Joseph's Hospital and Medical Center, Phoenix, Arizona

William E. Bell, MD, Chairman, Division of Pediatric Neurology; Professor, Departments of Pediatrics and Neurology, University of Iowa College of Medicine, Iowa City, Iowa

Paul E. Bendheim, MD, Postdoctoral Fellow, Department of Neurology, University of California School of Medicine, San Francisco, California

David C. Bolton, PhD, Postdoctoral Fellow, Department of Neurology, University of California, San Francisco, California

Karen A. Bowman, BA, Staff Research Associate III, Department of Neurology, University of California, San Francisco, California

Harvey W. Buchsbaum, MD, Neurological Associates of Tucson, Tucson, Arizona

S. Patricia Cochran, BS, Staff Research Associate IV, Department of Neurology, University of California, San Francisco, California

Robert M. Crowell, MD, Professor and Head, Department of Neurological Surgery, College of Medicine, University of Illinois at Chicago, Chicago, Illinois

T. Forcht Dagi, Neurosurgical Service, Massachusetts General Hospital, Boston, Massachusetts

John O. Fleming, MD, Associate Professor, Department of Neurology, University of Southern California School of Medicine, Los Angeles, California

Peter T. Frame, MD, Associate Professor of Clinical Medicine, Assistant Professor of Pathology, Departments of Medicine and Pathology, University of Cincinnati, Cincinnati, Ohio

Darlene F. Groth, BA, Staff Research Associate III, Department of Neurology, University of California, San Francisco, California

John A. Hodak, MD, Chairman, Division of Neuroradiology, Barrow Neurological Institute of St. Joseph's Hospital and Medical Center, Phoenix, Arizona

Kenneth P. Johnson, MD, Professor and Chairman, Department of Neurology, Unviersity of Maryland Hospital, Baltimore, Maryland

Jocelyn J. Mayled, BA, Research Associate of Immunology, Advanced Genetics Research Institute, San Francisco, California

Michael P. McKinley, PhD, Adjacent Assistant Professor, Department of Neurology, University of California School of Medicine, San Francisco, California

Robert L. McLaurin, MD, Professor, Division of Neurological Surgery, University of Cincinnati Medical Center, Cincinnati, Ohio

Daniel G. Nehls, MD, Resident in Neurosurgery, Barrow Neurological Institute of St. Joseph's Hospital and Medical Center, Phoenix, Arizona

Robert G. Ojemann, MD, Professor of Surgery, Massachusetts General Hospital, Boston, Massachusetts

Stanley B. Prusiner, MD, Associate Professor, Department of Neurology, University of California School of Medicine, San Francisco, California

W. Eugene Stern, MD, Professor of Neurosurgery, University of California at Los Angeles, School of Medicine, Los Angeles, California

John D. Waggener, MD (Deceased) Department of Neuropathology, Barrow Neurological Institute of St. Joseph's Hospital and Medical Center, Phoenix, Arizona

Leslie P. Weiner, MD, Chairman, Department of Neurology, Professor, Neurology and Microbiology, University of Southern California School of Medicine, Los Angeles, California

Jerry S. Wolinsky, MD, Professor, Department of Neurology, The University of Texas Health Science Center at Houston, Houston, Texas

Nicholas T. Zervas, MD, Chief of Neurosurgical Service, Massachusetts General Hospital; Professor of Surgery, Harvard Medical School, Boston, Massachusetts

Preface

The contents of this volume are based upon the proceedings of a Symposium entitled "Infectious Diseases of the Central Nervous System" held in Phoenix, Arizona, and sponsored by the Barrow Neurological Institute and Foundation during its Ninth Annual Symposium. The purpose of the Symposium was to bring together knowledgeable experts in this field to review information that is available and to enhance our knowledge of new developments in the field of infectious diseases in the central nervous system. Because the subject could not be covered in its entirety by this volume, we have placed particular emphasis on recent developments and new information.

The volume includes a remarkably fresh and interesting discussion of viral diseases as they affect the nervous system, including conventional and unconventional virus agents, and in addition, discussions of pathophysiology and epidemiology and postinfectious diseases of the nervous system.

A similar approach is taken to the treatment of bacterial infection. Discussions of pathophysiology are intertwined with discussions of diagnostic techniques, prevention techniques and treatment of bacterial infections.

Additional surgical problems are discussed regarding prevention and management of perioperative infection and brain abscess. Special consideration was given to coccidioidomycosis which is prevalent in the western states; also, there is a discussion of parasitic infections.

This volume will be of interest to neurologists and neurosurgeons and any physician dealing with infectious disease.

RICHARD A. THOMPSON, M.D.
JOHN R. GREEN, M.D.
Editors

Contents

Acknowledgments

We are indebted to the internationally recognized authors who have contributed to this volume and given such an excellent Symposium on which the volume is based. Appreciation is also expressed to the Symposium Committee consisting of Richard A. Thompson, M.D., Chairman; William B. Helme, M.D.; John A. Hodak, M.D.; Daniel Pollen, M.D.; John D. Waggener, M.D.; Joseph C. White, M.D.; and Elizabeth Wilkinson-Fannin, M.D.

1

Pathophysiology and Epidemiology
of Acute Viral Infections

Leslie P. Weiner and John O. Fleming

INTRODUCTION

The diseases which result from acute viral infections of the central nervous system (CNS) are dependent on the nature of the invading microorganism, the response of the host, and the CNS cells that are infected. The clinical and pathological features of acute viral infections are diverse and include meningitis, encephalitis, poliomyelitis, and immune mediated postinfectious demyelinating syndromes. In this report we review neurotropic viruses, their epidemiology, viral entry and spread, host factors involved in susceptibility including the host immune response, invasion of the brain, clinical syndromes, and the outcome of acute infections. Each topic could be the subject of a lengthy review; it is our intention here to give an overview.

VIRUSES

Viruses have certain characteristic features such as a well-defined structure (protein and only one type of nucleic acid), the lack of metabolic apparatus for energy production, the necessity to replicate inside cells, and the capacity to induce an immune response when inoculated into a suitable host. They have been called parasites at the genetic level.[1] These

1

classic or "conventional" viruses, as exemplified by herpes simplex or poliovirus, are easily seen by electron microscopy and may be quantitated and analyzed by well-established laboratory methods.

Recently it has been shown that diseases may be caused by agents which resemble conventional viruses in some respects but differ significantly from viruses in other ways. For example, Creutzfeldt-Jakob disease, which results in CNS degeneration, is initiated by an ultrafiltrable agent which is extremely resistant to usual viral inactivators such as formalin and ultraviolet light, has not been visualized by electronmicroscopy, and appears not to stimulate the host immune system. This and similar agents have been categorized as unconventional viruses.

We will limit our discussion to conventional viruses affecting the human CNS. Conceptually, it is important to distinguish disease caused by classic viruses from those caused by the relatively uncharacterized unconventional agents.

Conventional viruses carry their genetic material as a single or double strand of nucleic acid. This can be either DNA or RNA, but not both in one type of virus. The nucleic acid is entwined and/or surrounded with protein; together, they form the nucleocapsid. The surrounding protein is called the capsid protein. In the "naked" viruses the virion, or virus particle, is complete when it contains its nucleic acid and protein. The naked RNA viruses include the picornaviruses (e.g., poliovirus) and the naked DNA viruses include adenoviruses, parvoviruses, and papovavirus (e.g., JC virus, the progressive multifocal leukoencephalopathy agent).

In the enveloped viruses the capsid proteins are surrounded by an envelope of virus-coded proteins in host cell lipid. The envelope is acquired as the nucleocapsid buds from cellular membranes. Herpes viruses bud through nuclear membranes, coronaviruses bud through vesicles comprising membranes of the endoplasmic reticulum, and paramyxoviruses, measles, and many other viruses bud from the plasma membranes, and thus acquire their envelopes as they leave the cell.

Viruses have a variety of sizes and shapes. The parvovirus are as small as 20 nm and the poxviruses reach a size of 300 nm. The rhabdoviruses (rabies) are bullet shaped, the coronaviruses (respiratory viruses) are pleomorphic, the poxviruses are brick shaped, and the adenovirus resemble a crystal with protein projections.

The replication cycle of each viral type is unique. The virus must attach itself to the plasma membrane. Viral receptors on the cell surface are the major factor in determining cell susceptibility to infection and viral tropism, that is, the propensity of a virus to infect a specific cell type. Wild-type poliovirus selectively damages anterior horn cells, but attenuated polioviruses which make up the vaccine strain do not have

CNS tropism nor are they receptors for these strains present for the most part on CNS cells. Viral receptors are glycoproteins. In experimental studies it has been suggested that viral receptors might be part of the H-2 complex[2] or a neurotransmitter receptor.[3]

Following attachment, the virus must penetrate the plasma membrane. Viral penetration is affected by structures at the cell surface such as viral receptors, glycoproteins on the surface of the virus, and the environment in which the contact between the cell and virus takes place. Most viruses enter the cell by a phagocytic mechanism called viropexis.[4] Paramyxoviruses, measles, respiratory syncytial virus, and vaccinia are viruses with evidence of penetration by fusion of viral envelope with cell membrane. In herpes simplex infection viropexis is the primary mechanism with fusion being an auxillary process.

After penetration, the capsid protein is "uncoated." The viral nucleic acid is then ready for two processes: (1) replication, in which copies of the viral genome are produced for incorporation into progeny virions, and (2) transcription, in which messenger RNA (mRNA) coding for viral proteins is made. Obviously, different viruses must use different replication–transcription strategies depending on whether their nucleic acid is DNA or RNA, single or double stranded, and of negative or positive sense polarity. Baltimore has classified animal viruses into six general classes on this basis.[5]

Viral mRNA is translated into proteins in ribosomes in the cytoplasm. Viral proteins are either structural or nonstructural. Structural protein is morphologically part of the mature viral particle or virion. Nonstructural proteins, usually enzymes such as nucleic acid polymerases, are essential for the viral multiplication cycle but are not part of the virion released extracellularly. These nonstructural proteins are important in replication, transcription, control of host cell macromolecular synthesis, viral assembly, and virion release from cells.

The assembly of viral proteins and nucleic acid into the viral particle takes place in the nucleus for most DNA viruses and in the cytoplasm for most RNA viruses. The virus is released by a variety of mechanisms. The naked viruses such as poliovirus are released by lysis of the cell.[6] Enveloped viruses pick up their lipid coats by budding through membranes. Measles and mumps bud through the plasma membrane; herpes viruses attain their envelope by budding through nuclear membranes and then diffusing through the plasma surface membrane to reach the extracellular environment. Coronaviruses and arboviruses bud from cytoplasmic membranes and make their way out either by passage through surface membrane or by membrane channels.

EPIDEMIOLOGY AND RISK FACTORS

The epidemiology of viral infection is influenced by a number of factors. Infections can be spread directly from man to man by respiratory or salivary airborne routes (paramyxoviruses), by fecal-oral ingestion (enteroviruses, e.g., poliovirus), or by venereal spread (herpes simplex II). Infections can be acquired from animals (zoonoses) or via vectors such as mosquitos or ticks. In the insect-borne viral infections such as Eastern equine (EEE), Western equine (WEE), or St. Louis encephalitides, the vector–vertebrate reservoir includes mosquitoes and birds. This type of spread has accounted for regional epidemics in the southwestern U.S. and Texas.[7]

Seasonal variations of viral infections occur with a limited number of viruses, and these outbreaks can affect massive numbers of people. The variation often depends on reproductive cycles of the vector and the social habits of the vertebrate reservoir, such as migration patterns. In man-to-man spread, such as occurs with the enteroviruses, infection occurs in late summer or early fall. Spread is dependent on social contacts, crowds, flies, and the outdoor activity of children, who are the source and the target of fecal contamination.

Exposure is but one element of the pathogenesis of disease produced by viruses. In an epidemic of St. Louis encephalitis or even poliovirus, hundreds of thousands of may be infected but only a handful will be victim to CNS disease. Multiple factors become critical in determining the outcome of infection. Most relate to the immune response, but some may involve the presence of viral receptors and cellular molecular processes which have yet to be defined. Genetic factors are most critical, but certainly nutrition plays an important part in host-defense. Malnourished individuals, particularly those with low protein, cannot mount an effective immune response. Sex of the individual also plays a role. Through most of life, males are more susceptible to viral infections. However, during pregnancy when immune mechanisms are depressed in general, women are more susceptible.[8]

Age also plays a role. Before birth, diseases related to cytomegalovirus and rubella are most common. At birth herpes simplex type II is devastating, producing systemic disease and marked cerebral necrosis. In infants, parainfluenza viruses, adenovirus, polio, and other enteroviruses are most common. In the young child, rhinoviruses, coronaviruses, measles, rubella, mumps, influenza, polio, and chicken pox are the most common, and many of these viruses are associated with CNS invasion. In adolescence, infectious mononucleosis attributed to Epstein–Barr virus is common, and in the senior citizen, exacerbations of varicella zoster are a frequent occurrence.[9]

The patterns of disease often bear little relationship to incidence. Herpes simplex, varicella, Coxsackie, rhinovirus, parainfluenzea, influenza virus, adenovirus, and coronaviruses are all viruses of high incidence and low mortality. Rabies, Marburg virus, Lassa fever, EEE, and WEE viruses are viruses of low incidence, but high mortality. Severe infections may occur in small subpopulations converting low mortality to high mortality infections. Such subgroups include patients who are immunosuppressed or have defects in resistance secondary to malignancies or malnutrition.[9,10]

The host response plays the major role in both susceptibility to infection and the disease process. A brief review of the immune response cannot truly reflect the complexity of the cellular interactions and the biology of soluble substances which control these interactions. The B cells (so-called bursa or bone marrow derived cells) are primarily involved in humoral responses, consist of at least five populations which include precursor B cells, antibody forming B cell precusors, activated B cells, memory B cells, and the fully differentiated plasma cell. T cells (so-called thyumus-derived lymphocytes) include precursor T cells, helper T cells, memory T cells, cytotoxic lymphocytes, and suppressor T cells. Other immune cells include macrophages, K cells, and N cells, the granulocytes, mast cells, and monocytes which act primarily as phagocytic cells.[11]

The role of antibody in host defense against virus is complex. Antibodies can combine with the surface of the virus to prevent attachment to susceptible cells, decrease penetration, and interfere with uncoating on the initiation of replication. Cytophilic antibodies promote phagocytosis and digestion of viruses. Antibodies also react with the surface of enveloped viruses to activate the complement system and directly produce lysis of the virus or host cells bearing viral antigens in surface membranes. Finally, antibodies can combine with the virus, agglutinating them and making them more readily phagocytized.

Macrophages are a critically important group of cells in the protection of the animal from viral infection. They interact with lymphocytes and are involved in the production of interferon. They also influence the uptake of virus by phagocytizing virus–antibody complexes. Their role in antigen processing is important in augmenting lymphocyte activities, activating the complement system, and in altering general immune regulation.[11]

ENTRANCE, SPREAD, AND INVASION OF CNS

Virus may enter the host by penetration of the skin (St. Louis virus and other arboviruses), respiratory tract (measles, mumps), intestinal tract (enteroviruses, ie, poliovirus), and urogenital tract (herpes simplex II). Virus on entry can grow at the primary site in epithelial surfaces or, alternatively, they may penetrate and grow in the subepithelial tissues. Spread can be via lymphatics, blood, or, in rare instances, by nerves. In this latter case there is growth in perineural or Schwann cells, and the virus reaches the CNS by retrograde axoplasmic flow[12] (i.e., herpes simplex, varicella zoster, and rabies).[13,14]

With those viruses disseminated by the blood, the passage is often complex. Togaviruses, polioviruses, and hepatitis type B are free in the plasma. Measles, Epstein–Barr virus, cytomegalovirus, herpes simplex, and poxviruses are all associated with mononuclear peripheral white cells. Coloardo tick fever has been associated with transport in red cells.

Although viruses are ubiquitous and viral diseases are common, active infection of the CNS by viruses is uncommon. This is probably because of the blood–brain and blood–CSF barriers which largely separates the CNS from the systemic circulation.[15] The morphologic substrate for these barriers is complex and includes specialized cells and junctions between cells. For example, cerebral capillaries lack the fenestration found in the endothelial cells of the systemic vascular bed. Also, the apical ends of the choroid plexus epithelial cells are joined by tight junctions.

Viruses can enter the CNS at the choroid plexus by either direct passage into the CSF or by growth in choroid plexus cells as is seen in the rat parvovirus model.[16] The CNS can be reached through small vessels either by transportation in infected leucocytes, infection of the vascular endothelium, or by diffusion or viropexus through normal cellular membranes.[17]

The concept of the brain as an "immunologic privileged site" is undergoing some modification. There now appears to be a modified lymphatic system. There are, of course, no lymphatic vessels draining regional nodes, but ligation of lymphocytes in the neck will produce brain edema. These so-called "prelymphatics" may be the Virchow–Robin (V-R) spaces which merge into the subarchnoid space.[18] The V–R space has been found to contain lymphocytes and macrophages.[19] The blood–brain barrier, which appears to be relatively impermeable to proteins under normal circumstances, can be readily altered experimentally by changing blood pressure, pH, and osmotic pressure. Whether alterations of these factors influence the brain's immunity is not known. In the case of tumor and skin grafts, an immune reaction is elicited but it is slower than elsewhere. Local vascularization, which is part of the rejection mechanism, is delayed.[20] In experimental viral infection we have shown that in intranasal JHM virus infection (a neurotropic strain of mouse coronaviruses), blood–brain barrier defects occur 12 to 24 hours after the initial demonstration of viral antigen and correlates with the earliest presence of cellular infiltrates in the meninges and perivascular areas.[21]

There is good reason to think that most cells comprising the inflammatory response in the brain are of hematogenous origin. Phagocytes in the brain are primarily derived from the blood.[22,23] These phagocytes possess IgG and complement receptors.[24] In certain species, oligodendrocytes have been shown to posses a receptor to the Fc fragment of IgG, a function generally associated with immune cells.[25] We have recently shown the presence of Ia antigens of the major histocompatibility complex in the white matter of normal adult mouse brain. These cells are located in the interfascicular region and positive cells comprise about one percent of the total number.[26] Preliminary data from chimera studies indicate that Ia positive cells derived from the donor spleen will find the way into the brain of an x-irradiated recipient with a different Ia background.[27] Thus, in normal brain white matter, there are cells derived from the reticuloendothelial system synthesizing Ia antigen. These cells are usually associated with immune function and may be part of the brain's defense system.

OUTCOME OF INFECTION

There are many possible outcomes of viral infection.[28] The initial infection may be either asymptomatic (subclinical) or may result in acute disease (clinical). Either subclinical or clinical infections may be followed by complete clearance of the virus or by viral persistence. Viral persistence itself may be symptomatic, result in delayed symptomatology (e.g., subacute sclerosing panencephalitis), or give rise to many recurrences of acute episodes (e.g., herpes simplex). Another possibility which has not been shown in man but has been demonstrated in animals is the development of malignant transformation and tumors.[29] Finally, virus can trigger an unusual or idiosyncratic host response which results in acute disease. This is thought to be in the case in Reye's syndrome where a mild viral infection is followed in rare individuals by liver necrosis and brain edema.

On a cellular level, tissue damage can be the result of several processes both in acute disease and in chronic processes.[30] Virus may produce lysis of cells. This occurs in nonenveloped agents at the completion of replication and is related to release into the environment (e.g., poliovirus, adenovirus, and papovaviruses). There can be cell dysfunction and death by the inhibition of host macromolecular synthesis. These may be caused by viral nonstructural proteins, but in many instances the mechanisms have not been defined. Special functions may be inhibited. The so-called "luxury functions" may be involved. Impairment does not result in cell death, but in cell malfunction.[31] Disease may be due to immune-mediated processes directed against viral antigens (e.g., lymphocytic choriomeningitis). It is possible that immune-mediated disease may be directed at altered host antigens or that the immune response might not recognize a host antigen as self. Finally, disease may be due to the inflammatory response via nonspecific phagocytoxis, lysosomal release, hemorrhage, or thrombosis. These effects are difficult to sort out from direct viral–host interactions.[32]

A number of viral infections of the CNS are commonly encountered in neurology. The syndrome of *aseptic* or nonpurulent *meningitis* is often caused by viruses such as coxsackie, echoviruses, mumps, adenovirus, and lymphocytic choriomeningitis virus. This syndrome is usually associated with headache, fever, meningeal signs, and a predominance of mononuclear cells in the cerebrospinal fluid. The prognosis is generally good. It is important to rule out nonviral causes of this syndrome such as tuberculosis, cryptococcosis, syphillis, and partially treated pyogenic meningitis, all of which have specific therapies. Other viruses such as herpes simplex and many arboviruses (WEE, EEE, St. Louis encephalitis) may invade the brain parenchyma and produce *acute viral meningoencephalitis*. By contrast with aseptic meningitis, this syndrome frequently results in fulminant disease with significant mortality and residual effects. Some cases of Parkinson's syndrome have been sequelae of acute encephalitis. Another group of diseases is seen days to weeks after viral infections; these are termed *postinfectious encephalomyelitis*. Some forms may be hemorrhagic or demyelinating. The relationship of these syndromes to viral persistence and the immune system is unclear at present. Finally, some acute infections, both subclinical and clinical, have been shown to initiate viral persistence and chronic disease; conditions in this category include subacute sclerosing panencephalitis, measles virus, progressive multifocal leukoencephalopathy, JC, BK, SV-40 viruses, and progressive rubella panencephalitis. There is currently much interest in viruses in neurology in part because chronic viral infections have now been shown to cause diseases formerly thought to be "degenerative"; this raises the possibility that viruses may account for other neurologic diseases of obscure origin, such as multiple sclerosis.[33, 34]

CONCLUSIONS

The pathogenesis of acute CNS viral infections is dependent on a number of environmental and host factors. Overall, the incidence of CNS infections and subsequent disease is uncommon. The outcome depends on the virulence of the virus and such host factors as the patient's age, nutrition, sex, and genetic factors which influence the immune response and interferon productions.

REFERENCES

1. Luria, S.E., Darnell, J.E., Baltimore, D., and Campbell, A. *General Virology*. 3rd ed. New York: John Wiley and Sons, pp. 1–578, 1978.
2. Helenius, A., Morein, B., Friers, E., Simons, K., Robinson, P., Schirmacher, V. Terhorst, C., and Strominger, J.L. Human (HLA-A and HLA-B) and murine (H-2K and H-2D) histocompatibility antigens are cell surface receptors for Semliki Forest virus. *Proc. Natl. Acad. Sci.* 75:3846–3850, 1978.
3. Lentz, T.L., Burrage, T.G., Smith, A.L., Crick, J., and Tignor, G.H. Is the acetylcholine receptor a rabies virus receptor? *Science 215*:183–184, 1982.
4. Howe, C., Coward, J.E., and Genger, T.W. Viral Invasion: Morphological, Biochemical and Biophysical aspects. *Comprehensive Virology*. Vol. 16. Fraenkel-Conrat, H. and Wagner, R.R. (eds.) New York: Plenum Press, pp. 1–72, 1980.
5. Baltimore, D: Expression of animal virus genomes *Bacteriol. Rev.* 35:235–241, 1971.
6. Bablanian, R. Structural and functional alterations in cultured cells infected with cytocidal viruses. *Prog. Med. Viral.* 19:40–83, 1975.
7. Albrecht, P. Pathogenesis of neurotropic arbovirus infection. *Curr. Top. Microbiol. Immunol. 43*:44–91, 1968.
8. Ahluist, J. Hormonal influences on immunologic and related phenomena. In: Psychoneuroimmunology. New York: Academic Press, pp. 355–403, 1981.
9. Mims, C. A. *The Pathogenesis of Infectious Disease*. New York: Academic Press, London: Grune and Stratton, pp. 30, 130, 1976.
10. Johnson, R. T. Pathophysiology and epidemiology of acute viral infection of the nervous system. *Adv. Neurol.* 6:27–51, 1974.
11. Roitt, I.M. *Essential Immunology*. 3rd ed. Oxford: Blackwell, 1977.
12. Johnson, R.T. and Mims, C.A. Pathogenesis of viral infections of the nervous system. *N. Engl. J. Med. 278*:23–30, 84–92, 1968.
13. Cook, M.L., and Stevens, J.G. Pathogenesis of herpetic neuritis and ganglionitis in mice: Evidence for intra-axonal transport of infection. *Infect. Immunol.* 7:278–288, 1973.
14. Murphy, F.A. Rabies pathogenesis: Brief review. *Arch. Virol. 54*:279, 1977.
15. Rappaport, S.I. *Blood-Brain Barrier in Physiology and Medicine*. New York: Raven Press, 1975.
16. Lipton, J.L., and Johnson, R.T. The pathogenesis of rat virus infections in newborn hamster. *Lab. Invest.* 27:508–513, 1972.
17. Blinzinger, K., and Muller, W. The intercellular gaps of the neuropil as

pathways for virus spread in viral encephalomyelitides. *Acta Neuropathol.* 17:37–43, 1971.

18. Casley-Smith, J.R., Foldi-Borcsok, E., and Foldi, M. The prelymphatic pathways of the brain as revealed by cervical lymphatic obstruction and the passage of particles. *Br. J. Exp. Pathol.* 57:179–188, 1976.

19. Prineas, J.W. Multiple sclerosis: presence of lymphatic capillaries and lymphoid tissue in the brain and spinal cord. *Science* 203:1123–1125, 1979.

20. Ridley, A., and Cavanagh, J.B. Lymphocytic infiltration in gilomas: evidence of possible host resistance. *Brain* 94:117–124, 1971.

21. Henry, A., Stohlman, S.A., and Weiner, L.P. (unpublished data).

22. Fujita, S., and Kitamura, T. Origin of brain macrophages and the nature of the microglia. in Zimmerman: *Progress in Neuropathology.* vol. III. New York: Grune and Stratton, pp. 1–50, 1976.

23. Konigsmark, B., and Sidman, R.L. Origin of brain macrophages in the mouse. *J Neuropathol. Exp. Neurol.* 22:643–676, 1963.

24. Ochmichen, M. Mononuclear phagocytes in the Central Nervous System. Berlin: Springer, pp. 1–173, 1978.

25. Traugott, V., Snyder, D.S., and Raine, C.S. Oligodendrocyte staining by multiple sclerosis serum is nonspecific. *Ann. Neurol.* 6:13–20, 1979.

26. Ting, J.P.V., Shigekawa, B.L., Linthicum, D.S., Weiner, L.P., and Frelinger, J.A. Expression and synthesis of murine immune response-associated (Ia) antigens by brain cells. *Proc. Natl. Acad. Sci.* 78:3170–3174, 1981.

27. Ting J.P.V., Frelinger, J.A., and Weiner, L.P. (unpublished data).

28. Robb, J.A. Virus-cell interactions: a classification for virus-caused human disease. *Prog. Med. Virol.* 23:51–61, 1977.

29. Tamm, I. Cell injury with viruses. *Am. J. Pathololol.* 81:163–177, 1975.

30. Weiner, L.P. and Johnson, R.T. Virus-host cell interactions in "slow" virus diseases of the nervous system. Poste, G. and Nicolson, G.L. (eds.). In: Virus Infection and the Cell Surface. Amsterdam: North-Holland, 1977: 195–212.

31. Oldstone, M.B.A., Holmstoen, J., and Welsh, R.M. Alterations of acetylcholine enzymes in neuroblastoma cells persistently infected with lymphocytic choriomeningitis virus. *J. Cell Physiol.* 91:459–472, 1977.

32. Allison, A.C., and Sandelin, K. Activation of lysosomal enzymes in virus-infected cells and its possible relationship to cytopathic effects. *J. Exp. Med.* 116:879–887, 1963.

33. Brooks, B.R., Jubelt, B., Swarz, J.R., and Johnson, R.T. Slow viral infections. *Ann. Rev. Neurosci.* 2:309–340, 1979.

34. Wolinsky, J.S. and Johnson, R.T. Role of viruses in chronic neurologic disease. In: *Comprehensive Virology.* Vol. 16. Fraenkel-Conrat, H., and Wagner, R.R. (eds.) New York: Plenum Press, pp. 257–296, 1980.

2

Herpes Simplex Virus Infections
of the Nervous System

J. Richard Baringer

GENERAL CONSIDERATIONS:

Herpes simplex virus is one of the group of herpes viruses responsible for a variety of human infections.[1,2] These large enveloped DNA viruses, together comprising herpes simplex virus types I and II, cytomegalovirus, varicella zoster virus, and Epstein–Barr virus, are unique in that they all have the capability for persisting in humans for many years, though the sites and manner in which they persist appear to differ. Herpes simplex virus and varicella–zoster virus share the ability to produce segmental cutaneous disease which, in the case of herpes simplex, is probably related to its demonstrated potential to reside in sensory ganglia for many years. The same may be true for varicella zoster virus; direct proof of this is now emerging. Both herpes simplex virus and Epstein–Barr virus are suspected causes of human tumors, though the evidence for the latter is much more convincing. EB virus was first isolated from tumor tissues of patients with Burkitt's lymphoma in Africa and has since been strongly implicated by DNA reassociation studies in nasopharyngeal tumors. Though a role for herpes simplex virus infection has been suspected on the basis of serologic evidence in human cervical cancer, a direct association between the virus and cervical cancer is still lacking.

The way in which herpes simplex virus remains latent in human ganglionic tissue has continued to puzzle investigators.[3,4] Though most have presumed on the basis of experimental studies that the virus becomes latent in the ganglia by integration of the virus DNA into the host chromosomal DNA, recent evidence would suggest that some viral functions may be expressed during the course of latency.[5] These considerations have important implications for the success of antiviral agents since most of these compounds interfere with some aspect of the viral replicative cycle. Thus, if the virus is completely inactive during its latent state, antiviral compounds which have this method of action would not be expected to affect the ability of the virus to reside for prolonged periods in a cryptic fashion.

Herpes simplex virus type I and type II appear to be responsible for a widening array of recurrent cutaneous and neuralgic syndromes as a result of their predilection to localize in ganglia.[6,7] The two viruses can be unambiguously distinguished from one another by their patterns on restriction endonuclease digests, their polypeptide composition, and more recently by immunofluorescence identification of antigens using monoclonal antibodies specific for one or the other strain. In particular, the use of restriction endonuclease digests [8] has made it possible to do detailed epidemiologic studies. It has been found that unrelated individuals harbor herpes simplex viruses which appear to be unique and which can be distinguished from those of any other individual using this technique. Thus, the spread of herpes simplex virus within populations or, for example, within newborn nurseries can be assessed. Though the technique can be accomplished only in laboratories where personnel have sufficient familiarity and equipment, it promises to be a valuable tool in dissecting the pathogenesis of certain infections.

HERPES SIMPLEX VIRUS ENCEPHALITIS

This illness is a devastating affection of the nervous system which occurs sporadically in children and adults and may be seen, in addition, as a consequence of maternal genital infection with herpes simplex virus.[9] In children and adults, the encephalitic illness is virtually always the result of an infection by HSV-I; the virus appears to be confined to the parenchyma of the brain. In the neonatal situation, the infection is more frequently due to type II virus but it may be due to type I.[10] The infection is part of a generalized cutaneous and visceral process presumably acquired in passage of the infant through the birth canal. However, there are documented cases of intrauterine infection further complicating our understanding of the pathogenesis of this disease in the infant.

Herpes simplex encephalitis is much less frequent than encephalitis due to arthropod born viruses or the encephalitides associated with childhood illness.[11] The importance of disease lies in the frequency with which it produces a cerebral illness with a high mortality and the potential for treatment of this condition with a series of antiviral drugs. The availability of adenine arabinoside and the indication that it reduces mortality in this illness has stimulated a renewed interest among clinicians in attempting to establish the diagnosis of the disease.

Clinically, the disorder presents in children and adults as an abruptly evolving cerebral disorder.[12,13] It may be ushered in with a seizure but more frequently presents as change in behavior associated with a confusional state. Though in some cases a rapidly evolving and selective memory loss has been recognized, in the majority this feature of the illness, if present, has been obscured by the more generalized affection of cerebral cognitive processes. Patients frequently complain of headache and the behavioral changes and confusional state usually progress rapidly to states of stupor or coma. Frequently, these are complicated within the first days of the illness by the appearance of focal signs such as aphasias or hemipareses.

The most helpful initial diagnostic tests are examination of the cerebrospinal fluid, the EEG examination, and a computerized tomographic scan. Cerebrospinal fluid most often shows a mixed pleocytosis of up to 500 cells. Though occasionally there may be a few red cells in the fluid or even a trace of xanthochromia, this feature is not present often enough to be of help and when present is not diagnostic. In a few cases documented by biopsy, a pleocytosis has not been present in the first fluid sample that was examined but usually has appeared within the next day or two.[14] The cerebrospinal fluid sugar level is usually normal although it has occasionally been reported to be modestly depressed. A more profound depression of the cerebrospinal fluid sugar should always raise the question of some other diagnosis. Attempts to assay the cerebrospinal fluid for selective increase in complement fixing or other antibodies to herpes simplex virus or for HSV antigen has thus far not yielded evidence that these approaches will be helpful in the acute case.[15] Though the diagnosis can be supported by a rising serum titer of antibody over the course of two to three weeks, such testing is of no help in the acute situation. Virus can be recovered from the cerebrospinal fluid only in rare instances.

The electroencephalogram can be very helpful in suggesting the possibility that a patient with an appropriate illness has herpes simplex encephalitis.[16,17] It can be of additional value in determining whether one or both sides are involved. The EEG pattern is most often that of a nonspecific slowing in one or another temporal-frontal region but in many cases this slowing is combined with periodic high voltage discharges. Given the age of the patient and the general clinical features, the electroencephalographer can often hazard an educated guess about the possibility of herpes simplex encephalitis. It must be kept in mind, however, that the EEG patterns are not specific for this disease.

Computerized tomographic scanning has contributed significantly to the ability to make the diagnosis of herpes simplex virus encephalitis.[18,19] While the findings on CT scan are somewhat variable, the most common appearance is that of a low density lesion within one or both temporal lobes often with an adjacent low density lesion in the medial frontal lobe. There is frequently mottled and irregular contrast enhancement at the edge of the lesion and often sufficient edema of the surrounding structures to produce displacement of the midline structures. It is important to recognize that in many instances the CT scan has been normal at an early stage in the disease. This unfortunate circumstance restricts our ability to establish a correct diagnosis early in the disease and proceed with appropriate confirmatory studies and treatment.

The definitive diagnosis rests on obtaining a brain biopsy from the affected region which can then be examined by multiple means. The brain biopsy should be done on the side that is indicated either from EEG or CT studies and it is preferable that the biopsy sample be obtained from as low on the temporal lobe as possible since this is almost universally the site of maximal pathologic lesions. It has become apparent from the collaborative study of Whitley and associates that false-negative biopsies, which are rare, are sometimes due to obtaining tissue samples from areas of the brain which are distinct from those frequently involved in the process. These studies have revealed, in addition, that brain biopsy has a relatively low morbidity and mortality.[20] Among the patients in the combined study who turned out not to have herpes simplex encephalitis but who were subjected to brain biopsy, adverse results from the procedure were uncommon. It is of utmost importance that the biopsy material be handled in an appropriate fashion. It is not sufficient to send the material to the pathology laboratory for routine histologic studies. In the majority of cases in our experience, ordinary hemotoxylin and eosin staining, while revealing the presence of an inflammatory process, does not show inclusions when virus has been easily demonstrable by fluorescent antibody test, electron microscopy, or culture. Fluorescent antibody test is the most rapid way of establishing the diagnosis of herpes simplex virus encephalitis and it has the advantage of being specific and relatively sensitive. Electron microscopy may reveal herpes type particles. Though it does not serve to distinguish between cytomegalovirus, varicella zoster virus, and Epstein–Barr virus, in the appropriate clinical situation the appearance of herpes particles by electron microscopy would be highly suggestive of the disease. However, accomplishing the test usually takes a matter of several days. Recovery of the virus in tissue culture remains the benchmark for establishing the diagnosis. In the vast majority of cases, the virus can be identified within two to three days by its typical cytopathic effect in culture. However, occasional cases have taken as long as a week or more and in one instance in our own laboratory 18 days elapsed between the time the culture was obtained and the time the virus was detected.

Information concerning the current treatment of herpes simplex encephalitis has come largely from the efforts of Whitley and his collaborators[20,21] at the University of Alabama in Birmingham, where the national collaborative study is directed. They have demonstrated in a biopsy-controlled double-blind study of adenine arabinoside that this drug is superior to placebo in reducing the mortality from herpes simplex virus encephalitis. Subsequent data from the same study have indicated that the age and status of the patient at the time of start of treatment are important variables affecting the outcome. Patients under 30 years of age fare much better than older patients. In every category patients who are alert or only mildly lethargic at the time the treatment is instituted fare better than those who are stuporous or in coma. Efforts are currently being made to compare the efficacy of adenine arabinoside with two other antiviral drugs—adenine arabinoside monophosphate and acycloguanosine (acyclovir). Adenine arabinoside monophosphate is expected to have antiviral effects and toxicities similar to those produced by adenine arabinoside. Its advantage is that because it is more soluble, lesser volumes of intravenous fluids are required for administration, reducing the fluid load that is necessary to administer to the patient. Acyclovir[22–24] is one of an interesting new class of antiviral drugs. It is phosphorylated to its effective form by the viral thymidine kinase and is not similarly handled by cellular thymidine kinases. In addition, its activity against viral DNA polymerase is many fold greater than that against cellular DNA polymerases. It is anticipated that this selective phosphorylation and selective action may provide a much wider margin of safety for this drug than for conventional antiviral drugs.

The use of agents to minimize cerebral edema has to be seriously considered in many cases where the CT scan and clinical course indicate the potential for herniation. Mannitol may be of help because of its ability to shrink normal brain. Though steroids theoretically may be helpful in reducing edema due to normal capillary permeability, their use in herpes simplex virus encephalitis has not received carefully controlled study. Limited animal studies would suggest that there may be only slight delay in clearing of virus when potent steroids are administered[25]; whether these results can be extrapolated to the human situation is unknown.

HERPES SIMPLEX MENINGITIS AND POLYRADICULITIS

It is becoming increasingly apparent that genital herpes simplex virus infections have the potential for producing recurrent, often severe, syndromes of radiculitis usually involving the sacral segments and producing segmental pain in the distribution of the sacral dermatomes.[26] These episodes of pain usually attend or quickly follow an outbreak of primary or recurrent genital herpes. In some they have been associated with involvement of the sacral outflow to the bladder with retention of urine.[27] In a smaller number of cases, episodes of genital herpes have been associated with a meningitis. Though data are scattered and fragmentary, it is likely that this meningitis is in almost all instances a benign and self-limited process. Limited experience in a homosexual male population would suggest that herpes meningitis as a result of genital or anal herpes infections may be particularly common in this group. Whether the manifestations of the disorder may be unusual or particularly severe in this group because of their often associated acquired immunodeficiency remains a topic for further study. Recently we have recovered in our laboratory herpes simplex virus type 1 in a person during the fourth episode of recurrent benign lymphocytic meningitis of the type described by Mollaret.[28] Whether additional cases of Mollaret's meningitis will yield similar virologic findings remains to be seen.

REFERENCES

1. Nahmias, A.J., and Dowdle, W.R. Antigenic and virological differences in herpes virus hominis. *Prog. Med. Virol.10*:110, 1968.
2. Nahmias, A.F., Josey, W.E., and Naib, Z.M. Infection with herpes virus hominis types 1 and 2. *Prog. Dermatol.* 4:7, 1969.
3. Baringer, J.R. Herpes simplex virus infection of nervous tissue in animals and man. *Prog. Med. Virol.* 20:1–26, 1975.
4. Stevens, J.G. Latent herpes simplex virus and the nervous system. *Curr. Top. Microbiol. Immunol.* 70:31, 1975.
5. Tenser, R.B., and Dawson, M. Herpes simplex virus mRNA in neurons of latently infected guinea pigs. *Amn. Acad. Neurol.* April 28, 1980, p. 183.

6. Baringer, J.R., Recovery of herpes simplex virus from human sacral ganglions. *N. Engl. J. Med. 29*:828–830, 1974.

7. Baringer, J.R , and Swoveland, P. Recovery of herpes simplex virus from human trigeminal ganglia. *N. Engl. J. Med. 286*:648–650, 1973.

8. Lonsdale, D.M., Brown, S.M., Subak-Sharpe, J.H., Warren, K.G., and Koprowski, H. The polypeptide and DNA restriction enzyme profiles of spontaneous isolates of herpes simplex virus type I from explants of human trigeminal, superior cervical and vagus ganglia. *J. Gen. Virol. 43*:151–171, 1979.

9. Olson, L.C., Buescher, E.L., Arterstein, M.S., et al. Herpes virus infections of the human central nervous system. *N. Engl. J. Med. 277*:1271–1277, 1967.

10. Craig, C.P.. and Nahmias, A.J. Different patterns of neurologic involvement with herpes simplex virus types 1 and 2: Isolation of herpes simplex virus type 2 from the buffy coat of two adults with meningitis. *J. Infect. Dis. 127*:365–372, 1973.

11. Meyer, H.M. Jr., Johnson, R.T., Crawford, I.P., et al. Central nervous system syndromes of "viral etiology": A study of 773 cases. *Am. J. Med. 29* :334–347, 1960.

12. Adams, H., and Miller, D. Herpes simplex encephalitis: A clinical and pathological analysis of twenty-two cases. *Postgrad. Med. J. 49*:393–397, 1973.

13. Baringer, J.R. Herpes simplex virus infections of the nervous system. In: *Handbook of Clinical Neurology.* Vol. 34. Vinken, P.J., and Bruyn, G.W., eds. Amsterdam: North Holland, pp. 145–159, 1978.

14. Johnson, K.P., Rosenthal, M.S. and Lerner, P.I. Herpes simplex encephalitis: The course in five virologically proven cases. *Arch. Neurol. 27*:103–108, 1972.

15. Lerner, A.M., Lauter, C.B., Nolan, D.C. and Shippey, M.J. Passive hemagglutinating antibodies in cerebrospinal fluid in herpesvirus hominis encephalitis. *Proc. Soc. Exp. Biol. Med. 140*:1460–1466, 1972.

16. Illis, L.S., and Taylor, E.M. The electroencephalogram in herpes simplex encephalitis. *Lancet 1*:718–721, 1972.

17. Upton, A., and Gumpert, J. Electroencephalography in the diagnosis of herpes simplex encephalitis. *Lancet 1*:650–652, 1970.

18. Thompson, J.L.G. The computed axial tomography in acute herpes simplex encephalitis. *Br. J. Radiol. 49*:86–87, 1976.

19. Zimmerman, R.D., Russell, E.J., Leeds, N.E., and Kaufman, D. CT in the early diagnosis of herpes simplex encephalitis. *Am. J. Radiol. 134*:61–66, 1980.

20. Whitley, R.J., Soong, S.J., Hirsch, M.S., Karchmer, A.W., Dolin, R., Galasso, G., Dunnick, J.K., and Alford, C.A. Herpes simplex encephalitis. Vidarabine therapy and diagnostic problems. *N. Engl. J. Med. 304*:313–318, 1981.

21. Whitley, R.J., Soong, S.J., Dolin, R., Galasso, G.J., Ch'ien, L.T., and Alford, C.A. Adenine arabinoside therapy of biopsy-proved herpes simplex encephalitis. *N. Engl. J. Med. 297*:289–294, 1977.

22. Selby, P.J., Jameston, B., Watson, J.G., Morgenstern, G., Powles, R.L., Kay, H.E.M., Thornton, R., and Clink, H.M. Parenteral acyclovir therapy for herpesvirus infections in man. *Lancet 2*:1267–1270, 1979.

23. Mitchell, C.D., Gentry, S.R., Boen, J.R., Bean, B., Groth, K.E., and Balfour, H.H. Acyclovir therapy for mucocutaneous herpes simplex infections in immunocompromised patients. *Lancet 1*:1289–1394, 1981.

24. Saral, R., Burns, W.H., Laskin, O.L. Santos, G.W., and Leitman PS. Acyclovir prophylaxis of herpes-simplex-virus infections. *N. Engl. J. Med.* *305*:63–68, 1981.
25. Baringer, J.R., Klassen, T., and Grumm, F. Experimental herpes simplex virus encephalitis: Effect of corticosteroids and pyrimidine nucleoside. *Arch. Neurol. 33*:442–446, 1976.
26. Olmstead, C.B. Genital herpes: The newest veneral disease. *Cutis 20*:113–127, 1977.
27. Steel, J.G., Dix, R.D., and Baringer, J.R. Isolation of herpes simplex virus type 1 in recurrent (Mollaret) meningitis. *Ann. Neurol. 11*:17–21, 1982.
28. Oats, J.K. and Greenhouse, P.R.D.H. Retention of urine in anogenital herpetic infection. *Lancet 1*:691–692, 1978.

3

Slow Virus Infection by Conventional Virus Agents

Jerry S. Wolinsky

Eight years have elapsed since the First Annual Symposium of the Barrow Neurologic Institute. Several sessions at that symposium, which was also devoted to infectious diseases of the central nervous system, concerned slow viral infections of the central nervous system (CNS). Detailed attention was given to three major diseases of human and veterinary medicine caused by conventional viral agents: visna,[1] subacute sclerosing panencephalitis,[2] and progressive multifocal leukoencephalopathy.[3] Since that symposium several additional subacute or chronic viral infections of the human CNS have been delineated and considerable progress has been made toward a more molecular understanding of the mechanisms which underlie some of these disorders. In this chapter we consider only those diseases which are caused by conventional viruses; that is, infectious agents whose genomes consist of nucleic acids which are replicated intracellularly utilizing host cellular synthetic machinery and which direct the synthesis of proteins necessary for their continued efficient transfer to other uninfected cells or hosts. Such a definition would exclude from consideration viriods, infectious agents of plants with very small ribonucleic acids (RNA) which lack any associated protein,[4] and the physicochemically incompletely defined transmissible agents of the subacute spongiform encephalopathies of animals (scrapie) and man (kuru, Creutzfeldt–Jakob disease).[5] The latter agents, recently refered to as prions, are discussed in detail in the next chapter.

INFECTIONS OF IMMUNE COMPROMISED HOSTS

Altered Primary Infections

In man, the slow virus diseases of the CNS caused by conventional viral agents often arise and evolve in a host whose ability to mount an immune response has been significantly impaired. This is particularly evident for the chronic enterovirus dermatomyositis, meningitis, and meningoencephalitis syndromes which complicate congenital hypogammaglobulinemic states, and subacute measles encephalitis which occurs in a clinical setting of intensive chemotherapy for childhood leukemia and other systemic malignancies. In the former, it is the lack of an effective humoral immune response which appears to result in defective viral clearance.[6,7] As a result, viral replication is continuous within the CNS and in some cases at a limited number of systemic sites. The chronicity of the CNS infection, which can last from months to years, suggests that ongoing viral induced cytopathology is modest, however the cumulative effects are devastating.[8-10] This human infection parallels laboratory models in which immunosuppression at the time of viral infection may convert an acute illness into a more protracted one in which viral clearance is delayed until the compromised host finally mounts a measurable humoral response.[11]

Patients with subacute measles encephalitis (SME) appear to have major defects in cellular immunity and show limited cellular and variable humoral responses to primary infection with measles virus.[12-18] Several months after viral exposure and presumed subclinical infection, CNS symptoms arise and usually progress rapidly over several months to death. Epilepsia partialis continuum has been a striking feature of most cases. The neural symptoms are otherwise similar to those cases of subacute sclerosing panencephalitis (SSPE) with very acute clinical courses. However, the cerebrospinal fluid (CSF) is usually normal and there may be no serologic evidence of measles infection.[18] The pathology in brain generally lacks intraparenchymal and perivascular inflammatory infiltrates. The failure to mount an adequate humoral immune response is believed to be due to defective thymus dependent-helper lymphocyte functions. One might anticipate complete virus replication in the CNS of such patients who have variable humoral and defective cellular immune mechanisms available with which to establish viral containment. Cell-free measles virus has been isolated from brain biopsy cells after rather briefly co-cultivation and passage with indicator cells in culture.[12] However, it is of interest that most attempts at virus recovery have not been successful; this is also usually the case in SSPE (see below). These observations imply that measles virus replication in the cells of human CNS may be defective, even in the absence of an immune response.

A clear parallel to SME is found in the experimental literature. Mature hamsters are rather refractory to infection by measles virus. However, mature animals previously thymectomized at birth are fully susceptible to measles infection, develop noninflammatory neural pathology, and fail to generate antiviral antibody. Virus is not readily recovered from homogenates of the brains of these animals.[19]

The passive transfer of hyperimmune sera has been advocated for both SME and chronic enterovirus infections. However, this would seem to be of limited value for SME as one might anticipate that antimeasles antibody alone could do little more than slow the tempo of the disease, perhaps effectively converting the course to that of typical SSPE. The success of attempts to treat chronic enterovirus meningoencephalitis with human hyperimmune sera appear to be dependent on the quality and amount of viral specific antibody.[6] This suggests that treatment with viral type specific neutralizing monoclonal antibodies might hold considerable promise in the future. However, the development of specific antiviral agents to supplement humoral therapy is clearly needed.

Infections of Uncertain Origin

Often it is difficult to be sure in a given patient whether the primary exposure to a specific virus preceded the development of a slow viral disease by weeks, months, years, or decades. This is because the responsible virus is often one to which the entire population is exposed and for which subclinical or banal infection at an early age is the rule. Presentation of the slow viral infection, often during an interval of acquired immunodeficiency, could therefore represent either atypical primary infection in the compromised host, or activation of persistent or latent virus in a previously normal host immune suppressed by an underlying disease process, its treatment, or both. Slow virus infections of the CNS in this category include focal adenovirus encephalitis, cytomegalovirus encephalitis, and progressive multifocal leukoencephalopathy. The reported case of focal adenovirus encephalitis[20,21] could represent renewed replication and dissemination of an agent known to persist in man at systemic sites or a more protracted course of adenovirus encephalitis in a compromised host. Similarly cytomegalovirus encephalitis, which is usually an incidental neuropathologic finding,[22] could represent activation of an asymptomatic persistent infection present for decades[23] or introduction or reintroduction of virus during renal transplantation.[24] In any event, viral replication cannot be adequately contained by the immune compromised host and viral dissemination results.[25]

Progressive multifocal leukoencephalopathy (PML) was first described as a clinicopathologic entity slightly more than two decades ago.[26] Careful fine morphologic studies[27,28] supported the early suggestion based on histopathologic change that this was a viral disease.[29] Subsequently, two distinct papovaviruses, JC virus[30] and SV40-like virus were isolated and the viral nature of the disease is now well established.

Seroepidemiologic studies using the JC virus isolate, which has proven to be the most important causative agent,[31] suggest that it is a common human pathogen. Sixty-five percent of a midwest population had acquired specific serum hemagglutination inhibition (HAI) antibody to JC virus by age 14 and over 80% of this population was seropositive by the eighth decade.[32] The nature of the primary infection remains uncertain but may well be a banal upper respiratory infection when not entirely subclinical. The seroepidemiologic evidence leaves open the question as to whether PML represents atypical primary infection in the compromised host or reactivated infection. A recent report of PML in an 11-year-old child with severe combined immunodeficiency[33] does not further elucidate the issue. It is of interest, however, that young mice infected with a related mouse papovavirus, K virus, evidence asymptomatic infection with viral replication in lung and brain.[34] All evidence of the infection disappears with time. Virus is no longer recoverable but selected tissues can remain positive for viral antigen by immunofluorescence for prolonged intervals; the ability to detect viral antigen in brain is, however, eventually lost. Yet, viral antigens will reappear in brains of previously infected animals challenged by immunosuppressive doses of corticosteroids.[35] Further, nude mice inoculated with K virus will develop both central and peripheral demyelinative lesions after extended observation intervals (D. Sheffield, personal communication). A perhaps related finding is the observation that renal transplant recipients shed BK virus, another human papovavirus, in their urine after transplantation.[36]

These observations in mice and man suggest that PML may reflect reactivation of persistent infection. Simian virus 40 (SV40) is a related and much studied papovavirus.[37] This virus is known to establish latent infection by integration of its double stranded deoxyribonucleic acid (DNA) genome into host cell nuclear chromosomal material. Integration of the viral DNA is not, however, an integral step in the lytic replicative cycle of the virus during permissive infection. Integration of the genome into nonpermissive cells would form a reservoir of viral information which might be unleashed by as yet unknown mechanisms under the selective pressure of chemotherapy.

Whether JC virus is acquired or latent in the host destined to develop PML, once viral replication is initiated in the CNS of such patients, an almost invariably progressive and certainly fatal CNS disease ensues.[38] Virus is actively replicated by and lytic for oligodendroglia. Viral particles in paracrystalline array are seen in the nuclei of enlarged and bizzare-appearing oligodendroglia. The infected cell cannot maintain its myelin-forming cytoplasmic extensions and microscopic demyelination ensues. Lysis of the infected cell releases large numbers of apparently intact virions[39] and the lytic infection of oligodendroglia spreads contiguously. The course of this expanding demyelinating process is clinically reflected in the multifocal, stepwise deterioration of the patient and can be graphically followed by serial computed tomography scanning.[40]

The oligodendroglial cell does not, however, appear to be the only target cell of this infection. The astroglia are hypertrophed in the miniplaque-like lesions and have bizzare nuclear patterns suggesting malignant transformation. The astrocytes do not, however, appear to be lytically infected and even in culture, only very immature glial cell precursors—spongioblasts—support lytic viral replication. The oncogenic potential of JC virus is readily demonstrated in laboratory animals including primates[41] and the concurrance of PML and multicentric astrocytic tumors has been reported.[42]

Histopathologic change in PML tissue is usually but not invariably. unaccompanied by inflammation and the CSF is almost invariably acellular. The lack of evidence of a host cellular response to the ongoing viral infection may in part reflect the generalized impairment of cell-mediated immune (CMI) responses typical of patients with lymphoreticular malignancy, collagen vascular disorders, sarcoidosis or the concomittant therapy of such underlying diseases. Further, lymphocytes from patients with PML have been shown to fail to secrete a lymphokine (leukocyte migration inhibition factor) when specifically stimulated by JC viral antigens in vitro.[43] A similar defect in vivo might explain the usual failure of hosts with PML to initiate and augument an appropriate inflammatory response within the CNS.

At present there is no effective therapy for PML. Several nucleoside analogs have been tried without success.[44] Withholding immunosuppressant therapy, if possible, appears prudent.

Reactivated Infections

Herpes varicella zoster (HVZ) virus, like herpes simplex virus, (HSV) appears to remain latent in dorsal root and sensory trigeminal ganglia after primary childhood infection. Reactivation of virus results in segmental vesicular skin erruptions. The frequency of shingles as a recurrent manifestation of HVZ virus is by no means that of recurrent labialis or progenitalis due to HSV. In contradistinction to recurrent HSV infections, radicular HVZ infections are more frequent among the aging population. This may, in part, be a reflection of both waning general cell-mediated immune responses and specific HVZ antigen driven in vitro cellular responses seen with aging.[45] The incidence of shingles is clearly higher in the immunocompromised host at any age and may result in a generalized systemic illness, more widespread CNS involvement, or both.[46,47] The most common major CNS complication is segmental central spread of the virus to cause myelitis, a more diffuse meningoencephalitis is less common. Both syndromes likely reflect inadequate containment of the reactivated infection to establish a new latent state. Fortunately, even in the compromised host, dissemination is relatively infrequent and fatal CNS infections are uncommon. Unfortunately, adequate predictive factors of those patients at greatest risk of CNS dissemination who might benefit from expectant therapy with adenine arabinoside[48] are not yet available.

Patients with HVZ ophthalmicus appear to be at additional risk for developing contralateral hemiplegia, frequently with evidence of more widespread CNS dysfunction. Current evidence suggests that this syndrome is due to a vasculitis[49–52] possibly related to direct viral invasion of the vessel wall via trigeminal pathways innervating these structures.[53,54] If substantiated, this would clearly implicate a common human viral pathogen for at least some forms of so-called granulomatous angiitis. The nucleoside analogs adenine arabinoside and acyclovir might eventually play some role in the management of such cases.

Recently, HVZ has been implicated in causing a PML-like disorder in three patients with underlying malignancies receiving immunosuppressant treatment.[55,56] Multifocal neurologic symptoms evolved over time and correlated with both low density PML-like and hemorrhagic lesions on computed tomography. The pathology, however, differed from that of PML in being more consistent with multiple areas of tissue necrosis and small plaque-like areas of focal demyelination with relative axonal sparing. Inclusion-bearing cells were found and HVZ viral antigens were localized to regions of tissue necrosis in deparaffinized tissue sections by immunocytochemical means.[55] Biopsy for confirmation of diagnosis should be attempted in suspected cases, as antiviral chemotherapy might well prove efficacious and should be considered.

INFECTIONS OF IMMUNOLOGICALLY INTACT HOSTS

Subacute and chronically evolving neurologic syndromes have been directly related to ongoing viral infection by measles and rubella viruses of man and visna and goat leukoencephalitis viruses of animals. In these conditions, no major defects of host cellular or humoral immunity have been consistently demonstrated. The animal diseases have been more amenable to experimental manipulation and study, have important economic implications, and share features in common with both SSPE and progressive rubella panencephalitis (PRP); they may therefore aid in understanding some aspects of their human counterparts.

Visna and Goat Leukoencephalitis

Both visna, a disease of sheep, and goat leukoencephalitis, a more recently recognized naturally occurring disease of goats, are due to closely related viruses of the lentivirus group. Visna was first reported in Iceland and its study lead Sigurdsson[57] to his pioneering concepts of slow viral infection. It is now clear that the disease is world-wide in distribution. The initial natural spread of the infection remains uncertain though the virus can be transmitted through infected colostrum. After an incubation period of months to years, affected sheep develop either a progressive pneumonitis (Maedi) or a neurologic syndrome characterized by listlessness, wasting, and often hindquarter paralysis (visna) which progresses to death in a matter of months. Goat leukoencephalitis-arthritis complex has only recently been shown to be of viral origin.[58] It can present either as a polyarthralgia and arthropathy or as a visna-like neurologic disorder. The neuropathology is similar in both visna and goat leukoencephalitis and consists of prominent choroiditis with germinal follicle-like formation, ventriculitis, and scattered intraparenchymal and perivascular inflammation often with associated demyelination.[59,60]

Lentiviruses are enveloped RNA viruses which carry a RNA-dependent DNA-polymerase (reverse transcriptase) that allows the transcription of the viral genome into a complementary DNA (cDNA) copy capable of integration into the host chromosomal pool.[61-63] The production of a cDNA copy is an obligate step in the replication of the viral genome and production of progeny virions. Viral replication in nonpermissive cells can be blocked at a number of steps. In the majority of CNS cells viral replication appears to be highly restricted. Using in situ hybridization techniques on brain tissues of sheep infected with a highly laboratory adapted strain of visna (1514), Haase and co-workers[64] have shown that several orders of magnitude more brain cells contain multiple copies of the viral cDNA than express viral antigens. Further, after experimental infection, virus is only transiently recovered from homogenates of brain, but can readily be recovered from explants of brain. These observations demonstrate a restriction of viral replication in vivo which can be relieved in vitro.[65] However, while readily explaining persistence of the viral genome, they do not readily explain the progressive nature of the disease and the apparent variation in the age of individual CNS lesions.

The development of humoral and cellular immune responses in experimental animals follows a time course which is typical for other acute and chronic viral infections.[66,67] Abrogation of early inflammatory pathology by immunosuppression suggests that a component of the pathology is immune-mediated[68] and probably reflects an appropriate host response to the initial viral replication in brain.

The observation that virus could be consistently isolated from cultures of blood-borne mononuclear cells from experimentally infected American lambs with serologic evidence of humoral immunity has lead to a number of important studies which bear on the progressive nature of visna. Serial viral isolates from individual animals differ antigenically from the parent strains used to initiate the infections; serial serologic evaluations of the same animal show an evolving spectra of neutralizing antibody responses.[69] Parallel studies in tissue culture suggest that these findings reflect ordered selection of random viral mutants under the pressure of the host neutralizing antibody responses.[70,71] Such drift of viral antigens could result in recurrent bouts of active viral replication and concomitant waves of viral induced immune-mediated cytopathology. Each episode would proceed unabated until the host could mount effective specific humoral responses to the new viral antigen. The emergence of further mutants would result in additional disease cycles.

Recently, a number of isolates from naturally infected sheep and goats have been found to differ in their biologic properties from the laboratory standard 1514 virus. These viruses were isolated from pulmonary macrophages and synovial membrane cells which have phagocytic properties. They replicate nonlytically in macrophages, budding into vacuoles rather than at the cell's surface as is more typical of visna virus maturation from fibroblasts. While by themselves noncytopathic for fibroblasts, in the presence of macrophages these field isolates induce fusion of fibroblasts in vitro.[72] They also often fail to induce measurable immune responses during the course of experimental infections. It is possible that these natural isolates may prove useful in unlocking the details of the pathogenesis of the lentivirus slow viral diseases.

Subacute Sclerosing Panencephalitis

A half century has passed since the inclusion cell pathology of SSPE suggested to Dawson that a filterable agent might be responsible for the pathogenesis of the disease.[73] However, it is only in the last several decades that evidence has been amassed to show measles virus to be the specific offender.[74–79] The typical patient with SSPE is a rural male with a known history of otherwise uncomplicated measles before age two years, who in the second decade of life develops behavioral abnormalities followed by a progressive and relentless neurologic syndrome characterized by dementia, myoclonus, and motor impairment.[80] Numerous exceptions to every element of this stereotyped pattern are encountered.[81–85] Perhaps of greatest importance is the variation in disease progression. Recent studies suggest that for most patients the clinical disease follows a characteristic subacute course with a survival half-life following first symptoms of 12 months.[86] However, five percent or more of all cases follow a protracted course lasting six or more years.[87] Extended remissions are well documented but the disease appears to eventually be universally fatal.

Diagnosis is straightforward once entertained. The overwhelming majority of patients show remarkably elevated levels of CSF immunoglobulins,[88] a reflection, in large part, of intrathecal synthesis of large quantities of antibodies with specificity for the antigenic components of measles virus.[89] A clinical diagnosis can therefore be established with confidence based on typical clinical symptomatology, elevated CSF gammaglobulin levels as a percentage of total protein, markedly depressed serum to CSF ratios of measles antibody titers, the absence of focal structural lesions by computed tomographic scanning,[90] and often a distinctive burst-suppression pattern on electroencephalograms. Cerebral biopsy for direct confirmation of diagnosis by histologic, viral-specific immunofluorescent or virus isolation technique is seldom justified as a routine.

Current concepts of the pathogenesis of SSPE remain incomplete but have been considerably refined in recent years by several lines of investigation. Measles virus is a paramyxovirus which belong to the morbillivirus group.[91] It has a negative sense, single-stranded RNA genome which together with repeated nucleocapsid proteins, and several RNA dependent-RNA polymerase and probable replicase proteins form a helically arranged tubular structure, the nucleocapsid core of the virus. The nucleocapsid core is enveloped by a lipid membrane derived from the host but from which most host proteins have been replaced by two transmembrane proteins: a glycosylated hemagglutinin protein which initiates adsorption of virions to host cells and a fusion protein or hemolysin which initiates penetration of the virus into host cells and is critical in inducing the fusion of adjacent infected and uninfected cell membranes. The remaining major structural protein of measles virus is the matrix protein. This protein is located on the inner surface of the viral envelope and may serve both to stabilize the configuration of the transmembrane envelope proteins and as a recognition site for the nucleocapsid protein. The latter interaction appears to be critical for the initiation of the release of progeny virions from infected cells by the process of budding.[92]

The replicative strategy of paramyxoviruses requires that their negative sense genome be transcribed into a family of messenger RNAs (mRNAs) which in turn then direct the translation of the major structural and one or more nonstructural viral proteins. The genome must also be transcribed into complete complementary copies which serve as templates for the replication of progeny genomes. The mRNAs associate with host polysomes, translation of these messages being dependent on host synthetic mechanisms. These viral mRNAs presumably have finite life spans, being readily degraded by ubiquitous cellular ribonucleases (RNAse). The parental genomic RNA, replicative templates, and progeny genomes are all always associated with the nucleocapsid protein, even during replication.[93] Presumably the nucleocapsid protein protects the genomic RNA from cellular RNAse. This may be an important component mechanism for the persistence of both viral genomes and antigenomes within large nucleocapsid core inclusions frequently found in cells persistently infected with measles virus.

Acute infection of tissue culture cells usually results in their lytic destruction, with cytopathic effects characteristically including the formation of multinucleate giant cells. The pressure of antiviral antibody in the media of such cultures limits the spread of infection by release of the virus into the media, but infection can continue to spread from cell to cell through the formation of increasingly large syncytia.

Persistently infected cell lines have been established both with and without the use of antibody.[94,95] Both paramyxoviruses and normal mammalian cells lack reverse transcriptases, therefore integration of the measles viral genome through a cDNA intermediate mechanism into host chromosomal DNA cannot explain such persistent infections. Analysis of cell lines persistently infected with paramyxoviruses usually implicates the presence of defective interfering (DI) particles, temperature sensitive.

mutants (ts), or both in the maintenance of such model infections.[96] However, it remains unclear whether the generation of either DI particles or ts mutants is critical for the establishment of persistent infections or is a consequence of them. Further, no role for either DI particles or ts mutants has yet been clearly established in the initiation of slow virus infections of animals or man. Of interest is the observations that at least some neurons in culture are nonpermissive for measles virus replication yet accumulate masses of viral nucleocapsid core.[97]

In man, exposure to measles virus invariably results in infection.[98] While generally considered a banal childhood infection, measles remains one of the leading worldwide causes of childhood death. Acute measles is associated with a transient, cell-associated viremia and dissemination of virus to a number of systemic sites. Circumstantial evidence suggests that subclinical invasion of the CNS is frequent. This is based on the common findings of CSF pleocytosis and diffuse EEG abnormalities in otherwise uncomplicated cases. However, frank encephalitis complicates measles in only 0.1% of all cases. This form of CNS complication is felt to be para-infectious or immune-mediated with virus or viral footprints not being regularly found in brain except in exceptional cases.[99]

Despite depression of in vivo and in vitro markers of general cellular immunity, measles-specific host cellular responses are found during acute measles[100] and a typical temporal development of antiviral antibodies is seen. Initially, antibodies to all of the major structural proteins of measles can be demonstrated in convalescent sera using immunoprecipitation techniques; however, antibodies to the M protein as a rule disappear rapidly except from sera of patients with atypical measles.[101] The latter syndrome follows natural infection in individuals previously immunized with now antiquated killed virus vaccines. Once established, immunity to reinfection is life-long. Apart from SSPE, late progressive sequalae of measles are unknown. Presumably, all measles viral genetic material is cleared after recovery from measles; however, the existence of a potential persistent reservoir of genetic information remains possible. With the sole exception that patients destined to develop SSPE tend to have had measles earlier than those who do not develop SSPE, there is no known difference in the way these two groups respond to the acute infection.

Current dogma holds that SSPE is not the result of reinfection with measles. The most important unanswered question in understanding the pathogenesis of SSPE therefore is, "What is the state of the viral genome during the long latent interval from acute measles to the appearance of the first behavioral manifestations of CNS disease?" Is virus maintained in a population of systemic, perhaps lymphoid-derived cells, where productive viral expression is modulated by humoral antibodies[102] during the latent phase until a nonneutralizable mutation evolves capable of inciting neural infection? Or, is the viral genome maintained in a select population of nonpermissive neural cells to which it had disseminated during the original infection with late release of the restriction to complete viral replication under as yet unrecognized stimuli such as endocrine changes at puberty or perhaps infection with Epstein–Barr virus?[103] Finally, is it possible that measles viral replication in brain is continuous after limited dissemination of virus to the CNS during measles, but generally is maintained at a negligible or low level through life for all but a few for whom the presence of rather nonpermissive cell types in brain, adequate humoral and cellular immune responses, and anatomic barriers to viral spread within the brain are inadequate to maintain asymptomatic persistent infection?

Considerable data are available concerning the clinically evident progressive phase of SSPE. Patients with SSPE do not have consistently demonstrable defects in their general cellular immune functions or in their measured responses to measles antigens.[81,85,104–106] Circulating and CSF inhibitors of in vitro measures of CMI [107–109] are neither universal nor likely to be important in a disease in which there is histologic evidence of an appropriate inflammatory response in the target organ. Relatively low levels of circulating immune complexes have been reported in serum samples from some cases of SSPE[85,110–112] but these do not appear to play any convincing role in immunopathogenesis.

The humoral immune response is extremely well developed with high titers of antibody in both serum samples and CSF. Careful dissection of these immunoglobulins clearly demonstrate that they are synthesized in large part within the CNS.[89, 113] The restricted patterns of these immunoglobulins on electrophoretic, immunoelectrophoretic, and immunofixation analysis confirm both their oligoclonal nature and the fact that they are in large part directed against antigenic determinants of measles virus.[113–116] As is typical of late convalescent sera, little or no antibody is found to the matrix (M) protein of measles,[117–119] an observation which probably further argues against reinfection. Reinfection might be anticipated to result in renewed production of anti-M antibodies or even apparent over production of anti-M antibodies as is seen with atypical measles.

Pathologically, there is widespread evidence of at least nonpermissive infection of all major neural cell types. Intracytoplasmic and intranuclear inclusions are seen in both glial and neuronal cells and even more widespread dissemination of viral antigens is evident using immunocytochemical methods. Demyelination presumably is the result of lytic effects of the virus on oligodendroglia; however, significant plaque-like areas of primary demyelination with relative sparing of axons are the exception. More acute destructive changes are accompanied by mononuclear cell inflammation and lipid laden macrophages. Microglial rod cells are particularly prominent, especially in cortex. Perivascular cuffs of mononuclear cells are diffusely scattered and are often rich with plasma cells, the probable sources of the viral specific immunoglobulins found in the CSF. Proliferation of astrocytes and gliosis is often pronounced as the diseases' name would imply. Smooth nucleocapsid core profiles are readily encountered in nuclear inclusions and sometimes in the cytoplasm of cells by electron microscopy. However, even in very well-preserved biopsy specimens, so-called fuzzy nucleocapsid cores in cytoplasm are rarely encountered and intact virions or budding viral particles have not been convincingly demonstrated.[120]

Viral isolation from SSPE brain specimens requires serial co-cultivation or fusion and co-cultivation of dispersed brain cells with an appropriate indicator cell line (usually monkey kidney derived). Despite refinement of techniques the percentage of cases from which virus is eventually isolated remains small.[121] It is now clear that at least in some cases of SSPE virus is not limited to the CNS. Measles virus has been recovered by co-cultivation techniques from both lymphatic tissues[122] and more recently low numbers of circulating blood cells have been shown to harbor measles antigens.[123] The latter finding, however, requires confirmation as the binding of the fluorescein conjugated antibody via Fc receptors was not controlled for in these studies.

The early morphologic and viral isolation findings suggested that while viral antigens and genome or at least genome fragments were widely distributed in the SSPE brain samples, free virus was not present and viral replication was markedly restricted. However, some intact viral genome had to be present in SSPE brain cells which could eventually be expressed and amplified by indicator cell lines after successful co-cultivation experiments. Direct confirmation of the presence of measles viral genomes in SSPE brain cells has recently been shown by in situ hybridization,[124,125] and the viral mRNA which codes for the nucleocapsid protein has also been directly demonstrated in brain homogenates.[126] The early notion that specific SSPE mutants existed no longer seems tenable as biochemical analysis of isolates from various SSPE brain specimens and comparison with the "standard" Edmonston strain have failed to show consistent important structural differences.[127]

A number of indirect lines of evidence have suggested a central role for the M protein in measles virus persistence.[128] Recent direct studies confirm this. Explant cultures of SSPE brain cells fail to synthesize detectable levels of M protein or release free virus.[129] Further, while the major nucleocapsid-associated protein (NP) can be detected in extracts of SSPE brain samples, levels of envelope proteins (H, F) often appear reduced and the M protein cannot be detected.[130] These studies clearly demonstrate that for the large populations of cells sampled by these techniques, M protein is either not synthesized, or is synthesized but very rapidly degraded. They do not, however, exclude the normal synthesis and function of M protein within a limited number of cells. This final caveat is important for if M protein is never present in infected brain cells the viral genome presumably could not be transferred from infected to uninfected cells by the budding process. However, the progressive clinical course of SSPE implies spread of infection with new symptoms reflecting destruction of additional cells or at least cessation of the so-called "luxury" functions of neurons.[131]

A number of animal models have been developed in attempts to understand persistent paramyxoviral infections of brain. The hamster model originally described by Byington, Johnson, and their colleagues has proved particularly helpful.[132,133] In this system, the level of maturation of the animal at the time of initial infection critically determines outcome, development of humoral antibody responses marks the transition from an acute productive infection to a chronic cell-associated infection of brain, and both in situ hybridization and immunohistochemical studies show progressive restriction of replication of the viral genome as measured by fewer gene copies per infected cell[124] and reduced translation of viral mRNAs as measured by disappearance of nonnucleocapsid-associated structural proteins.[134] However, just as in SSPE, most chronically infected hamsters eventually die of progressive disease, suggesting at least low level ongoing or intermittent permissive infection.

Unfortunately, despite improved understanding of disease pathogenesis, treatment of SSPE remains only supportive. Chemotherapeutic, immunosuppressive, and immunoadjuvant therapy have not favorably affected outcome of reported cases. Conflicting claims for the antiviral-immunoadjuvant isoprinosine[135] are difficult to interpret in the absence of adequate controls.[136–138] Fortunately, the risk of SSPE after live attenuated measles virus vaccine appears to be substantially lower than after natural measles.[139] Therefore, the near elimination of measles from the United States should be paralleled by an eventual marked reduction in new cases of SSPE.

Progressive Rubella panencephalitis

Progressive rubella panencephalitis was first described less than a decade ago.[140,141] It appears to be a late complication of both congenital and postnatally acquired rubella virus infections.[142] The small number of cases in the literature suggests that it is indeed rare. Reported cases have been males, often but not always with variable stigmata or handicaps of the congenital rubella syndrome, who had otherwise been normal. Cognitive defects and gait ataxia appear in the second decade and neurologic impairment slowly but inexorably increases, progressing to severe dementia, spastic quadriparesis, and death. The course is remarkably protracted over many years. Myoclonus is not a significant clinical feature. Diagnosis is established by the demonstration of a striking elevation of CSF immunoglobulin content and markedly depressed serum to CSF rubella antibody titer ratios in the appropriate clinical setting. Computed tomography may show generalized cerebral atrophy with disproportionate enlargement of the fourth ventricle and cisternal magna reflecting early severe cerebellar involvement. Changes on EEG are not distinctive. Cerebral biopsy, while confirming an ongoing inflammatory process and possibly showing distinctive vascular deposits, would not be expected to demonstrate any inclusion cell pathology nor have immunofluorescent technique disclosed viral antigens. Virus has been recovered from brain biopsy cells co-cultivated with indicator cells,[143] but culture of biopsies would not be expected to routinely yield positive results.

Rubella virus is a togavirus which is the only member of the rubivirus group. It contains a single-stranded, positive sense RNA genome which is associated with multiple 38,000 dalton core proteins to form a nucleocapsid core which has icosahedral symmetry.[144,145] The nucleocapsid core is enveloped by host membrane modified to contain two types of viral glycoprotein: a 62,000 dalton protein (E_1) which has recently been shown to be the viral hemagglutinin and a 47,000–54,000 dalton glycoprotein complex (E_2) which probably represents a variably glycosylated single protein.[146] Rubella does possess a hemolysin or fusion function[147] which could conceivably reside on E_2 and be important in viral penetration of host cells to initiate infection. The virus matures from infected cells either by budding from the cells' surface or into intracytoplasmic vacuoles. Rubella virus lacks the equivalent of a M protein; presumably a transmembrane portion of either E_1 or E_2 serves as a recognition site for C to initiate viral budding.

The positive sense genome of rubella can serve directly as both a mRNA for translation of viral proteins and as a template for primary transcription. The genome presumably codes for one or more nonstructural proteins such as a RNA-dependent RNA-polymerase and other enzymes critical for the replication process. Whether or not the C protein remains tightly associated with the genome during replication is unknown. Collections of nucleocapsid cores do not accumulate in morphologically recognizable form during the course or rubella infections either in tissue culture or in man.

Rubella virus is a poor cytopathic agent and does not significantly perturb gross measurements of host cell synthetic functions.[148] It is therefore not surprising that it readily establishes persistent steady-state infections in a variety of tissue culture cell lines, including brain cells.[149] After first trimester intrauterine infection, virus is consistently shed for up to six to eight months by the newborn and can be recovered from affected tissues for as long as three years.[150] Initially, infected host cells or their progeny thus appear to harbor the virus continuously for protracted intervals, often in the face of apparently adequate levels of neutralizing antibody. The state of the viral genome during persistent infections is unclear but, as with measles, it is not likely to be maintained via a cDNA intermediate.

Several recent observations suggest that the establishment of persistent rubella infections of man need not be restrictd to intrauterine life. Rubella virus has been serially recovered over several years from fluids from involved joints of a subset of patients with rheumatoid factor negative arthritis.[151] Some of these patients recalled clinical rubella, others prior vaccination with live attenuated virus. Virus has also been recovered from peripheral blood leukocytes from a patient with rubella vaccine-associated arthritis two years after vaccination.[152] Our own studies suggest that unusually prolonged but asymptomatic replication of virus after vaccination may be the rule rather than the exception.[153] In this context, it is perhaps surprising that PRP is as rare as it appears to be.

As with SSPE, it is unclear whether patients destined to develop PRP are different from other congenital rubella patients or children with German measles who eventually appear to clear their infections entirely without developing late sequalae. No major defects of humoral or cellular immunity have been noted in patients with PRP though they do have a circulating substance which inhibits the ability of previously sensitized cells of normal donors to respond to challenge with rubella virus antigens in vitro by secreting the lymphokine interferon.[154]

Three of four patients with PRP so examined have had rubella-specific immune complexes in their serum samples. In two of these, longitudinal studies demonstrated that they were always present in sera. Further analysis of the complexes showed that in addition to rubella antibody the complexes appeared to contain at least one antigen with immunoreactivity consistent with the E_1 glycoprotein and of a density compatible with its being a fragment of the virus or of an infected cell membrane.[155] Virus has been recovered from circulating mononuclear cells of one patient with PRP.[154] These two observations suggest that virus replicates at sites outside of brain and that a more or less continuous supply of viral antigen is available for the formation of soluble immune complexes with antirubella antibody.

The humoral responses of patients with PRP have been studied in some detail. Oligoclonal bands are present in both serum samples and CSF and can be absorbed from CSF by rubella-infected cell pack antigens.[156] Both serum and CSF selectively immunoprecipitate all of the known structural antigens of rubella virus.[157] Calculated intrathecal synthetic rates for IgG are markedly elevated with intrathecal rubella specific IgG rates as high as 77 mg/day. Despite high synthetic rates, rubella-specific IgG only accounts for a relatively small proportion (16 to 20%) of the total excess of these immunoglobulins. As might be anticipated, significant amounts of rubella-specific IgG, and in one case each IgA and IgM, can be measured in neutral extracts of PRP brain samples[157] (unpublished observations).

Pathologic findings in PRP have been limited to brain and are those of a panencephalitis. Perivascular inflammation with mononuclear and plasma cells and intraparenchymal inflammation including an active microglial cell response are found in both grey and white matter of hemispheres, cerebellum, and brain stem. An irregular patchy demyelination with gliosis is a dominant feature evident on gross inspection of the sectioned hemispheric white matter. Perivascular mineralized deposits are prominent in intraparenchymal and meningeal vessels and probably reflect sites of immunoglobulin deposition.[158] No inclusion cells are evident and neither virus or viral antigens have as yet been directly demonstrated in brain tissues.

No information is as yet available on the types of brain cells harboring rubella genomes, the level of gene expression in these cells, or comparative analysis of isolates from PRP cases with standard laboratory stains. The presence of viral-specific circulating immune complexes in PRP serum samples and striking vascular deposits suggest some role for an immune complex-mediated component to the neural pathology, but the pathogenesis of this slow viral infection remains very incomplete. Attempts at treatment have not been successful.[154]

CONCLUSIONS

It is reasonable to expect that the list of subacute and chronic viral diseases of the human nervous system will continue to be expanded over the next few decades and this is especially likely for those which occur in the immunocompromised host. Fortunately, these will likely remain rather uncommon complications of immunosuppression and rare diseases of the immunologically intact host. Some of the slow viral diseases, like SSPE, can be expected to all but disappear with the application of effective immunization practices, others, like the neural complications of HVZ virus are likely to be problems of continued concern. In either case, a precise molecular delineation of the pathogenesis of these slow viral infections is imperative, for these uncommon neurologic diseases may shed light on more common and enigmatic chronic systemic and neural diseases of man of unknown cause such as rheumatoid arthritis, systemic lupus erythematosus, and multiple sclerosis.

ACKNOWLEDGMENT

The author is indebted to Linda Kelly for her help in the preparation of this manuscript. JSW is supported in part by a Research Career Development Award (NS00443) from the National Institute of Neurological and Communicative Disorders and Stroke; portions of the personal research referred to have been supported by the United Cerebral Palsy Research and Educational Foundation and awards NS15721 and AI 15721 from the National Institutes of Health.

REFERENCES

1. Johnson, R.T. Slow infections of the nervous system and the subacute spongiform encephalitis. *Adv. Neurol.* 6:69–75, 1974.
2. Johnson, K.P., Byington, D.P. and Gaddis, L. Subacute sclerosing panencephalitis. *Adv. Neurol.* 6: 77–86, 1974.
3. Weiner, L.P. and Narayan, O. Progressive multifocal leukoencephalopathy. *Adv. Neurol.* 6:87–92, 1974.
4. Diener T.O. Viroids: Structure and function. *Science* 205:859–866, 1979.
5. Gajdusek, D.C. Unconventional viruses and the origin and disappearance of kuru. *Science* 197:943–960, 1977.
6. Mease, P.J., Ochs, H.D. and Wedgewood, R.J. Successful treatment of echovirus meningoencephalitis and myositis-faciitis with intravenous immune globulin therapy in a patient with X-linked agammaglobulinemia. *N. Engl. J. Med.* 304:1278–1281, 1981.

7. Weiner, L.S., Howell J.T., Langford, M.P., Stanton, G.J., Baron, S., Goldblum, R.M., Lord R.A. and Goldman A.S. Effect of specific antibodies on chronic echovirus type 5 encephalitis in a patient with hypogammaglobulinemia. *J. Infect. Dis. 140*:858–863, 1979.

8. Davis, L.E., Bodian, D., Price, D., Butler, I.J., and Vickers, J.H. Chronic progressive poliomyelitis secondary to vaccination of an immunodeficient child. *N. Engl. J. Med. 297*:241–245, 1977.

9. Webster, A.B.D , Tripp, J.H., Hayward, A.R., Dayan A D., Doshi, R., Macintyre, E.H. and Tyrrell, A.J. Echovirus encephalitis and myositis in primary immunoglobulin deficiency. *Arch. Dis. Child. 53*:33–37, 1978.

10. Wilfert, C.M., Buckley R.H., Mokanakumar, T , Griffith, J.F., Katz, S.L., Whisnant, J.K., Eggleston, P.A., Moore, M., Treadwell, E., Oxman, M.N. and Rosen, F.S. Persistent and fatal central nervous system echovirus infections in patients with agammaglobulinemia. *N. Engl. J. Med. 296*:1485–1489, 1977.

11. Seay, A.R. and Wolinsky, J.S. Ross River virus-induced demyelination. I. Pathogenesis and histopathology. *Ann. Neurol.* in press, 1982.

12. Aicardi, J., Goutieres, F., Arsenio-Nunes, M.L., and Lebon, P. Acute measles encephalitis in children with immunodepression. *Pediatrics 59*:232–239, 1977.

13. Haltia, M., Paetau, A., Valieri, A., Erkkilä, H., Donner, M., Kaahinen, K. and Holström, T. Fatal measles encephalopathy with retinopathy during cytotoxic therapy. *J. Neurol. Sci. 32*:323–330, 1977.

14. Murphy, J.V. and Yunis, E.J. Encephalopathy following measles infection in children with chronic illness. *J. Pediatr. 88*:937–942, 1976.

15. Pullan, C.R., Noble, T.C., Scott, D.J., Wisniewski, K. and Gardner, P.S. Atypical measles infections in leukaemic children on immunosuppressive treatment. *Br. Med. J. 1*:1562–1565, 1976.

16. Roos, R.P., Graves, M.C., Wollmann, R.L., Chilcote, R.R. and Nixon, J. Immunologic and virologic studies of measles inclusion body encephalitis in an immunosuppressed host: the relationship to subacute sclerosing panencephalitis. *Neurology 31*:1263–1270, 1980.

17. Spalke, G. and Eschenbach, C. Infantile cortical measles inclusion body encephalitis during combined treatment of acute lymphoblastic leukemia. *J. Neurol. 220*:269–277, 1979.

18. Wolinsky, J.S., Swoveland, P., Johnson, K.P. and Baringer, J.R. Subacute measles encephalitis complicating Hodgkin's disease in an adult. *Ann. Neurol. 1*:452–457, 1977.

19. Johnson, K.P., Feldman, E.G. and Byington, D.P. Effect of neonatal thymectomy on experimental subacute sclerosing panencephalitis in adult hamsters. *Infect. Immun. 12*:1464–1469, 1975.

20. Chou, S.M., Roos, R., Burrell, R., Gutmann, L., and Harley, J.B. Subacute focal adenovirus encephalitis *J. Neuropathol. Exp. Neurol. 32*:34–50, 1973.

21. Roos, R., Chou, S.M., Rodgers, N.G., Basnight, M. and Gajdusek, D.C. Isolation of an adenovirus 32 strain from human brain in a case of subacute encephalitis. *Proc Soc. Exp. Biol. Med. 139*:636–640, 1972.

22. Dorfman, L.J. Cytomegalovirus encephalitis in adults. *Neurology 23*:136–144, 1973.

23. Wu, B.C., Dowling, J.N., Armstrong, J.A. and Ho, M. Enhancement of mouse cytomegalovirus infection during host-versus-graft reaction. *Science 190*:56–58, 1975.

24. Ho, M., Suwansirikul, S., Dowling, J.N., Youngblood, L.A. and Armstrong, J.A. The transplanted kidney as a source of cytomegalovirus infection. *N. Engl. J. Med. 293*:1109–1112, 1975.

25. Murray H.W., Knox, D.L., Green, W.R. and Susel, R.M. Cytomegalovirus retinitis in adults: a manifestation of disseminated viral infection. *Am. J. Med. 63*:574–583, 1977.

26. Astrom, K.E., Mancall, E.L., and Richardson, E.P. Progressive multifocal leukoencephalopathy: A hitherto unrecognized complication of chronic lymphatic leukemia and Hodgkins disease. *Brain 81*:93–111, 1958.

27. Silverman, L. and Rubenstein, L.J. Electron microscopic observations on a case of progressive multifocal leukoenephalopathy. *Acta Neuropathol. 5*:215–224, 1965.

28. ZuRhein, G.M. and Chou, S. Particles resembling papovaviruses in human cerebral demyelinating disease. *Science 148*:1477–1479, 1965.

29. Richardson, E.P. Progressive multifocal leukoencephalopathy. *N. Engl. J. Med. 265*: 815–823, 1961.

30. Padgett, B.L., Walker, D.L., ZuRhein, G.M., Eckroade, R.J. and Dessel, B.H. Cultivation of papova-like virus from human brain with progressive multifocal leucoencephalopathy. *Lancet 1*:1257–1260, 1971.

31. Padgett, B.L. and Walker, D.L. New human papovaviruses. *Prog. Med. Virol. 22*:1–35, 1976.

32. Padgett, B.L. and Walker, D.L. Prevalence of antibodies in human sera against JC virus, an isolate from a case of progressive multifocal leukoencephalopathy. *J. Infect. Dis. 127*:467–470, 1973.

33. ZuRhein, G.M., Padgett, B.L., Walker, D.L., Chun, R.W.N., Horowitz, S.D. and Hong, R. Progressive multifocal leukoenephalopathy in a child with severe combined immunodeficiency. *N. Engl. J. Med. 299*:256–257, 1978.

34. Greenlee, J.E. Effect of host age on experimental K virus infection of mice *Infect. Immun. 33*:297–303, 1981.

35. Greenlee, J.E. Protracted K virus infection in suckling mice and its reactivation by immunosuppression. Fifth International Congress of Virology, Strassbourg. 1981:118A.

36. Gardner, S.D. The new human papovaviruses: their nature and significance. *Rec. Adv. Clin. Virol. 1*:91–115, 1977.

37. Reddy V.B., Thimmappaya, B., Dhar, R., Subramanian, K.N., Zain, S., Pan, J., Ghosh, P.K., Celma, M.L. and Weissman, S.M. The genome of SV-40. *Science 200*:494–502, 1978.

38. Hedley-White, E.T., Smith, B.P., Tyler, H.R. and Peterson, W.P. Multifocal leukoencephalopathy with remission and five year survival. *J. Neuropathol. Exp. Neurol. 25*:107–116, 1966.

39. Dörries, K., Johnson, R.T., and ter Meulen, V. Detection of polyoma virus DNA in PML-brain tissue by (in situ) hybridization. *J. Gen. Virol. 42*:49–57, 1979.

40. Rand, K.H., Johnson, K.P., Rubinstein, L.J., Wolinsky, J.S., Penney, J.B., Walker, D.L., Padgett, B.L. and Merrigan, T.C. Adenine arabinoside in the treatment of progressive multifocal leukoencephalopathy. Use of urine cytology to assess response to treatment. *Ann. Neurol. 1*:458–462, 1977.

41. London, W.T., Houff, S.A., Madden, D.L., Fuccillo, D.A., Gravell, M., Wallen, W.C., Palmer, A.E. and Sever, J.L. Brain tumors in owl monkeys inoculated with a human polyomavirus (JC virus). *Science 201*:1246–1249, 1978.

42. Castaigne, P., Rondat, P., and Escourolle, R. Leucoencephalopathie multifocale progressive et 'gliomes' multiples. *Rev. Neurol. 130*:379–392, 1974.
43. Willoughby E., Price, R.W., Padgett, B.L., Walker, D.L. and Dupont, B. Progressive multifocal leukoencephalopathy (PML): in vitro cell-mediated immune responses to mitogens and JC virus. *Neurology 30*:256–262, 1980.
44. Smith, C.R., Sima, A.A.F., Salit, I.E. and Gentili, F. Progressive multifocal leukoencephalopathy: failure of cytarabine therapy. *Neurology 32*:200–203, 1982.
45. Berger, R., Florent, G., and Just, M. Decrease in the lymphoproliferative response to varicella-zoster virus antigen with age. *Infect. Immun. 32*:24–27, 1981.
46. Dolin, R., Reichman, R.C., Mazur, M.H., and Whitley, R.J. Herpes zoster-varicella infections in immunosuppressed patients. *Ann. Intern. Med. 89*:375–388, 1978.
47. McKendall, R.R. and Klawans, H.L. Nervous system complications of varicella-zoster virus. In: *Handbook of Clinical Neurology.* Vol 34. Vinken, P.J. and Bruyn, G.W. eds. Amsterdam: North Holland, pp. 161–183, 1978.
48. Whitley, R.J., Ch'ien, L.T., Dolin, R., Galasso, G.J. and Alford, C.A. Adenine arabinoside therapy of herpes zoster in the immunocompromised *N. Engl. J. Med. 294*:1193–1199, 1976.
49. Gilbert, G.J. Herpes zoster ophthalmicus and delayed contralateral hemiparesis: relationship of the syndrome to central nervous system granulomatous angiitis. *JAMA 229*:302–304, 1974.
50. Hilt, D.C., Buchholtz, D., Krumholz, A., Weiss, H., Gale, A. and Wolinsky J.S. Post-zoster ophthalmicus cerebral angiitis and contralateral hemiparesis. *Neurology,* 198A, 1982.
51. MacKenzie, R.A., Forbes, G.S. and Karnes, W.E. Angiographic findings in herpes zoster arteritis. *Ann. Neurol. 10*:458–464, 1981.
52. Pratesi, R., Freemon, F.R., Lowry, J.L. Herpes zoster ophthalmicus with contralateral hemiplegia. *Arch. Neurol. 34*:640–641, 1977.
53. Linnemann, C.C. and Alvira, M.M. Pathogenesis of varicella-zoster angiitis in the CNS. *Arch. Neurol. 37*:239–240, 1980.
54. Schwartz, J.N., Cashwell, F., Hawkins, H.K. and Klintworth, G.K. Necrotizing retinopathy with herpes zoster opthalmicus. *Arch. Pathol. Lab. Med. 100*: 386–391, 1976.
55. Horten, B., Price, R.W. and Jimenez, D. Multifocal varicella-zoster virus leukoencephalitis temporally remote from herpes zoster. *Ann. Neurol. 9*:251–266, 1980.
56. McCormich, W.F., Rodnitzky, R.L., Schochet, S.S. and McKee, A.P. Varicella-zoster encephalomyelitis: a morphologic and virologic study. *Arch. Neurol. 21*:559–570, 1969.
57. Sigurdsson, B. Observations on three slow infections of sheep. Maedi. Paratuberculosis. Rida, a chronic encephalitis of sheep with general remarks on infections, which develop slowly, and some of their special characteristics. *Br. Vet. J. 110*:255–270, 307–322, 341–354, 1954.
58. Crawford, T.B., Adams, D.S., Cheevers, W.P., and Cork, L.C. Chronic arthritis in goats caused by a retrovirus. *Science 207*:997–999, 1980.
59. Cork, L.C., and Narayan, O. The pathogenesis of viral leukoencephalitis-arthritis of goats: I. Persistent viral infection with progressive pathologic changes. *Lab. Invest. 42*:596–602, 1980.

60. Pétursson, G., Nathanson N., Georgsson, G., Pantich H. and Pálsson, P.A. Pathogenesis of visna. I. Sequential virologic, serologic and pathologic studies. *Lab. Invest.* *35*:402–412, 1976.
61. Clements, J.E., Narayan, O., Griffin, D.E., and Johnson, R.T. The synthesis and structure of visna virus DNA. *Virology 93*:377–386, 1979.
62. Haase, A.T. The slow infection caused by visna virus. *Cur. Top. Microbiol. Immunol. 72*:101–156, 1975.
63. Haase, A.T. and Varmus, H.E. Demonstration of DNA provirus in the lytic growth of visna virus. *Nature New Biol. 245*:237–239, 1973.
64. Haase, A.T., Stowring, L., Narayan, O., Griffin, D., and Price, D. Slow persistent infection caused by visna virus. *Science 195*:175–177, 1977.
65. Narayan, O, Griffin, D.E. and Silverstein, A.M. Slow virus infection: replication and mechanisms of persistence of visna virus in sheep. *J. Infect. Dis. 135*:800–806, 1977.
66. Griffin, D.E., Narayan, O. and Adams, R.J. Early immune responses in visna, a slow viral disease of sheep. *J. Infect. Dis 138*:340–350, 1978.
67. Griffin, D.E., Narayan, O., Bukowski, J.F., Adams, R.J. and Cohen, S. The cerebrospinal fluid in visna, a slow viral disease of sheep. *Ann. Neurol. 4*:212–218, 1978.
68. Nathanson, N., Pantich, H., Pálsson, P.A., Pétursson, G. and Georgsson, G. Pathogenesis of visna. II. Effect of immunosuppression upon early central nervous system lesions. *Lab Invest. 35*:444–451, 1976.
69. Narayan, O., Griffin, D.E. and Clements, J.E. Virus mutation during 'slow infection': temporal development and characterization of mutants of visna virus recovered from sheep. *J Gen. Virol. 41*:343–352, 1978.
70. Clements, J.E., Narayan, O., Pedersen, F S., and Haseltine, W.A. Mutation as a mechanism for escape from immunosuppression: The visna virus example. *Cold Spring Harbor Conference on Cellular Profileration 7*:953–967, 1980.
71. Narayan, O., Clements, J.E., Griffin, D.E. and Wolinsky, J.S. Neutralizing antibody spectrum determines the antigenic profiles of emerging mutants of visna virus. *Infect. Immun. 32*:1045–1050, 1981.
72. Narayan O., Wolinsky, J.S., Clements, J.E., Strandberg J.D., Griffin, D.E. and Cork, L.C. Slow virus replication: the role of macrophages in the persistence and expression of visna virus in sheep and goats. *J. Gen. Virol. 59*:345–356, 1982.
73. Dawson, J.R. Cellular inclusions in cerebral lesions of lethargic encephalitis. *Am. J. Pathol. 9*:7–16, 1933.
74. Bouteille, M., Fontaine, C., Vedrenne, C., and Delarue, J. Sur un cas d'encéphalite subaigüe à inclusions. Étude anatomo-clinque et ultrastructurale. *Rev. Neurol. 113*:454–458, 1965.
75. Connolly, J.H., Allen, I.V., Hurwitz, L.J., and Miller, J.H.D. Measles-virus antibody and antigen in subacute sclerosing panencephalitis. *Lancet 1*:542–544, 1967.
76. Freeman, J.M., Magoffin, R.L., Lennette, E.H. and Herndon, R.M. Additional evidence of the relation between subacute inclusion-body encephalitis and measles virus. *Lancet 2*:129–131, 1967.
77. Horta-Barbosa, L., Fuccillo, D.A., London, W.T., Jabbour, J.T., Zeman, W. and Sever J.L. Isolation of measles virus from brain cell cultures of two patients with subacute sclerosing panencephalitis. *Proc. Soc. Exp. Biol. Med. 132*:272–277, 1969.

78. Payne, F.E., Baublis, J.V. and Itabashi, H.H. Isolation of measles virus from cell cultures of brain from a patient with subacute sclerosing panencephalitis. *N. Engl. J. Med. 281*:585–589, 1969.

79. Tellez-Nagel, I. and Harter, D.H. Subacute sclerosing leukeoencephalitis: ultrastructure of intranuclear and intracytoplasmic inclusions. *Science 154*:899–901, 1966.

80. Detels, R., Brody , J.A., McNew, J., and Edgar, A.H. Further epidemiological studies of subacute sclerosing panencephalitis. *Lancet 2*:11–14, 1973.

81. Agnardsóttir, G. Subacute sclerosing panencephalitis. *Rec. Adv. Clin. Virol. 1*:21–49, 1977.

82. Risk, W.S., and Haddad, F.S. The variable natural history of SSPE. *Arch. Neurol. 36*:610–614, 1979.

83. Robertson, W.C., Clark, D.B. and Markesbery, W.R. Review of 38 cases of subacute sclerosing panencephalitis: Effect of amantadine on the natural course of the disease. *Ann. Neurol. 8*:422–425, 1980.

84. Silva, C.A., Paula-Barbosa, M.M., Pereira, S. and Cruz, C. Two cases of rapidly progressive subacute sclerosing panencephalitis: neuropathological findings. *Arch. Neurol. 38*:109–113, 1981.

85. ter Meulen, V. and Hall, W.W. Slow virus infections of the nervous system: virological, immunological and pathogenetic considerations. *J. Gen. Virol. 41*:1–25, 1978.

86. Haddad, F.S., Risk, W.S. and Jabbour J.T. Subacute sclerosing panencephalitis in the middle east: report of 99 cases. *Ann. Neurol. 1*:211–217, 1977.

87. Risk, W.S., Haddad, F.S., and Chemali, R. Substantial spontaneous improvement in subacute sclerosing panencephalitis: six cases from the middle east and review of the literature. *Arch. Neurol. 35*:494–502, 1978.

88. Mandelbaum, D.E., Hall, W.W., Paneth, N., Wolff, R.R. and De Vivo, D.C. SSPE, measles virus, and the matrix protein: report of a case with unusual immunochemical findings. *Ann. Neurol. 10*:351–354, 1981.

89. Tourtellotte, W.W., Ma, B.I., Brandes, D.B., Walsh, M.J. and Potvin, A.R. Quantification of de novo central nervous system IgG measles antibody synthesis in SSPE. *Ann. Neurol. 9*:551–556, 1981.

90. Manabe, Y., Ono, Y., Okuno, T., Ueda, T., Nakano, Y. and Akaishi, K. Serial CT scans in subacute sclerosing panencephalitis. *Comput. Tomogr. 5*:25–30, 1981.

91. Morgan, E.M. and Rapp, F. Measles virus and its associated diseases. *Bact. Rev. 41*:636–666, 1977.

92. Choppin, P.W., Richardson, C.D., Merz D.C., Hall, W.W., and Scheid, A. The functions and inhibition of the membrane glycoproteins of paramyxoviruses and myxoviruses and the role of the measles virus M protein in subacute sclerosing panencephalitis. *J. Infect. Dis. 143*:352–363, 1981.

93. Thorne, E.V., Dermott, E. Y-forms as possible intermediates in the replication of measles virus nucleocapsids. *Nature 268*:345–347, 1977.

94. Robbins, S.J. and Rapp, F. Evidence of antigenic variation in a persistent in vitro measles virus infection. In: *The Replication of Negative Strand Viruses*, Bishop, D.H.L. and Compans, R.W., eds. New York: Elsevier-North Holland, pp.589–594, 1981.

95. Rustigian, R., Winston, S.W. and Darlington, R.W. Variable infection of Vero cells and homologous interference after co-cultivation with HeLa cells with persistent defective infection by Edmonston measles virus. *Infect. Immun. 23*:775–786, 1979.

96. Younger, J.S. and Preble, O.T. Viral persistence: evolution of viral populations. In: *Comprehensive Virology*. (Vol. 16. Fraenkel-Conrat, H., Wagner, R.R.), eds. New York: Plenum Press, pp. 73–135, 1980.

97. Rentier, B., Claysmith, A., Bellini, W.J. and Dubois-Dalcq, M. Chronic measles virus infections of mouse nerve cells in vitro. In: *The Replication of Negative Strand Viruses*. Bishop, D.H.L., and Compans), R.W., eds New York: Elsevier-North Holland, pp. 595–601, 1981.

98. Black, F.L. Measles. In: A.S. Evans, ed. *Viral Infections of Humans. Epidemiology and Control*. New York: Plenum Press, pp. 297–316, 1976.

99. Johnson, K.P., Wolinsky, J.S. and Ginsberg, A.H. Immune mediated syndromes of the nervous system related to virus infections. In: Vinken, P.J., Bruyn, G.W., eds. *Handbook of Clinical Neurology*. Vol. 34, Amsterdam: North Holland, pp. 331–341, 1978.

100. Johnson, R.T., Hirsch, R.L., Griffin, D.E., Wolinsky, J.S., Roedenbeck, S., deSoriano, I.L. and Vaisberg, A. Clinical and immunological studies of measles encephalitis. *Ann. Neurol. 10*:74A, 1981.

101. Norrby, E., Örvell, C., Vandvick, B. and Cherry, J.D. Antibodies against measles virus polypeptides in different disease conditions. *Infect. Immun. 34*:718–724, 1981.

102. Fujinami,R.S. and Oldstone, M.B.A. Alterations in expression of measles virus polypeptides by antibody: molecular events in antibody-induced antigenic modulation. *J. Immunol. 125*:78–85, 1980.

103. Feorino, P.M., Humphrey, D., Hochberg, F. and Chilicote, R. Mononucleosis-associated subacute sclerosing panencephalitis *Lancet 2*:530–532, 1975.

104. Derakhshan, I., Massoud, A., Foroozanfar, N., Nikibin, B., Lofti, J., Shakib, N., and Ala, F. Subacute sclerosing panencephalitis: Clinical and immunologic study of 23 patients. *Neurology 31*:177–180, 1981.

105. Dhib-Jalbut, S.S., Abdelnoor, A.M., and Haddad, F.S. Cellular and humoral immunity in subacute sclerosing panencephalitis. *Infect. Immun. 33*:34–42, 1981.

106. Lennette, E.H. Cellular immunity and SSPE: summary of the conference. *Arch. Neurol. 32*:489–493, 1975.

107. Ahmed, A., Strong, D.M., Sell, K.W., Thurman, G.B., Knudsen, R.C., Wistar, R., and Grace, W.R. Demonstration of a blocking factor in the plasma and spinal fluid of patients with subacute sclerosing panencephalitis: I. Partial characterization. *J. Exp. Med. 139*:902–924, 1974.

108. Steele R.W., Fuccillo, D.A., Hensen, S.A., Vincent, M.M. and Bellanti, J.A. Specific inhibitory factors of cellular immunity in children with subacute sclerosing panencephalitis. *J. Pediatr. 88*:56–62, 1976.

109. Swick, H.M., Brooks, W.H., Roszman, T.L. and Caldwell, D. A heat-stable blocking factor in the plasma of patients with subacute sclerosing panencephalitis. *Neurology 26*:84–88, 1976.

110. Dayan, A.D. and Stokes, M.I. Immune complexes and visceral deposits of measles antigens in subacute sclerosing panencephalitis. *Br. Med. J. 2*:374–376, 1972.

111. Noronha, A.B.C., Antel, J.P., Roos, R.P. and Medof, M.E. Circulating immune complexes in neurologic disease. *Neurology 31*:1942–1047, 1981.

112. Theofilopoulos, A.N., Wilson, C.B. and Dixon, F.J. The raji cell radioimmune assay for detecting immune complexes in human sera. *J. Clin. Invest. 57*:169–182, 1976.

113. Ewan, P.W. and Lachmann, P.J. IgG synthesis within the brain in multiple sclerosis and subacute sclerosing panencephalitis. *Clin. Exp. Immunol.* 35:227–235, 1979.

114. Link, H., Panelius, M. and Salmi, A.A. Immunoglobulins and measles antibodies in subacute sclerosing panencephalitis: demonstration of synthesis of oligoclonal IgG with measles antibody activity within the central nervous system. *Arch. Neurol.* 28:23–30, 1973.

115. Vandvik, B. Immunopathological aspects in the pathogenesis of subacute sclerosing panencephalitis with special reference to the the significance of the immune response in the central nervous system. *Ann. Clin Res.* 5:308–315, 1973.

116. Vandvik B and Norrby, E. Oligoclonal IgG antibody response in the central nervous system to different measles virus antigens in subacute sclerosing panencephalitis. *Proc. Natl. Acad. Sci.* 70:1060–1063, 1973.

117. Hall, W.W., Lamb, R.A. and Choppin, P.W. Measles and subacute sclerosing panencephalitis virus proteins: lack of antibodies to the M protein in patients with subacute sclerosing panencephalitis. *Proc. Natl. Acad. Sci.* 76:2047–2051, 1979.

118. Trudgett, A., Bellini, W.J., Mingioli, E.S. and McFarlin, D.E. Antibodies to the structural polypeptides of measles virus following acute infection and SSPE. *Clin. Exp. Immunol.* 39:652–656, 1980.

119. Wechsler, S.L., Weiner, H. and Fields, B.N. Immune response in subacute sclerosing panencephalitis: reduced antibody response to the matrix protein of measles virus. *J. Immunol.* 123:884–889, 1979.

120. Dubois-Dalcq, M. Pathology of measles virus infection of the nervous system: comparison with multiple sclerosis. *Int. Rev. Exp. Pathol.* 19:101–135, 1979.

121. Katz, M. and Koprowski, H. The significance of failure to isolate infectious viruses in cases of subacute sclerosing panencephalitis. *Arch. Ges. Virusforsch.* 41:390–393, 1973.

122. Horta-Barbosa, L., Hamilton, R., Wittig B., Fuccillo, D.A. and Sever, J.L. Subacute sclerosing panencephalitis. Isolation of suppressed measles virus from lymph node biopsies. *Science* 173:840–841, 1971.

123. Wrzos, H., Kulczycki, J., Laskowki, Z., Matacz, D. and Brzosko, W.J. Detection of measles virus antigen(s) in peripheral lymphocytes from patients with subacute sclerosing panencephalitis. *Arch. Virol.* 60:291–297, 1979.

124. Haase, A.T., Swoveland, P., Stowring, L., Ventura, P., Johnson, K.P., Norrby, E. and Gibbs, C.J. Measles virus genome in infections of the central nervous system. *J. Infect. Dis.* 144:154–160, 1981.

125. Haase, A.T., Ventura, P., Gibbs, C.J. and Tourtellotte, W.W. Measles virus nucleotide sequence: detection by hybridization in situ. *Science* 212:672–674, 1981.

126. Gorecki, M., Rozenblatt, S. Cloning of DNA complementary to the measles virus mRNA encoding nucleocapsid protein. *Proc. Natl. Acad. Sci.* 77:3686–3690, 1980.

127. Rima, B.K., Lappin, S.A., Roberts, M.W., and Martin, S.J. *Comparison of the polypeptides of morbilli viruses.* Fifth International Congress of Virology, Strassbourg, 401A, 1981.

128. Lin, F.H. and Thormar, H. Absence of the M protein in a cell-associated subacute sclerosing panencephalitis virus. *Nature* 285:490–482, 1980.

129. Hall, W.W. and Choppin, P.W. Evidence for lack of synthesis of the M polypeptide of measles virus in brain cells in subacute sclerosing panencephalitis. *Virology 99*:443–447, 1979.

130. Hall, W.W., Choppin, P.W. Measles-virus proteins in the brain tissue of patients with subacute sclerosing panencephalitis: absence of the M protein. *N. Engl. J. Med. 304*:1152–1155, 1981.

131. Oldstone, M.B.A., Holmstoen, J. and Welsh, R.M. Alterations of acetylcholine enzymes in neuroblastoma cells persistently infected with lymphocytic choriomeningitis virus. *J. Cell. Physiol. 91*:459–472, 1977.

132. Byington, D.P., Castro, A.E., and Burnstein, T. Adaptation to hamsters of neurotropic measles virus from subacute sclerosing panencephalitis. *Nature 225*:554–555, 1970.

133. Byington, D.P., and Johnson, K.P. Experimental subacute sclerosing panencephalitis in the hamster: Correlation of age with chronic inclusion-cell encephalitis. *J. Infect. Dis. 126*:18–26, 1972.

134. Johnson, K.P., Norrby, E., Swoveland, P. and Carrigan, D.R. Experimental subacute sclerosing panencephalitis: selective disappearance of measles virus matrix protein from the central nervous system. *J. Infect. Dis. 144*:161–169, 1981.

135. Server A.C. and Wolinsky J.S. Approaches to antiviral therapy. In: *Muscular Dystrophy Association Conference on Amyotrophic Lateral Sclerosis*. Rowland L., ed. New York: Raven Press, pp. 519–545, 1982.

136. Haddad, F.S. and Risk, W.S. Isoprinosine treatment in 18 patients with subacute sclerosing panencephalitis: a controlled study. *Ann. Neurol. 7*:185–188, 1980.

137. Silverberg, R., Brenner, T. and Abramsky, O. Inosiplex in the treatment of subacute sclerosing panencephalitis. *Arch. Neurol. 36*:374–375, 1979.

138. Streletz, L.J. and Cracco, J. The effect of isoprinosine in subacute sclerosing panencephalitis (SSPE). *Ann. Neurol. 1*:183–184, 1977.

139. Modlin, J.E., Jabbour, J.T., Witte, J.J. and Halsey, N.A. Epideminolgic studies of measles, measles vaccine and subacute sclerosing panencephalitis. *Pediatrics 59*:505–512, 1977.

140. Townsend, J.J., Baringer, J.R., Wolinsky, J.S., Malamud, N., Mednick, J.P., Panitch, H.S., Scott, R.A.T., Oshiro, L.S. and Cremer, N.E. Progressive rubella panencephalitis. Late onset often congenital rubella. *N. Engl. J. Med. 292*:990–993, 1975.

141. Weil, M.L., Itabashi, H.H., Cremer, N.E., Oshiro, L.S., Lennette, E.H. and Carnay, L. Chronic progressive panencephalitis due to rubella virus simulating subacute sclerosing panencephalitis. *N. Engl. J. Med. 292*:994–998, 1975.

142. Wolinsky, J.S. Progressive rubella panencephalitis. In: Vinken, P.J. and Bruyn, G.W., eds. *Handbook of Clinical Neurology*. Vol. 34. Amsterdam: North Holland, pp. 331–339, 1978.

143. Cremer, N.E., Oshiro, L.S., Weil, M.L., Lennette, E.H., Itabashi, H.H., and Carnay, L. Isolation of rubella virus from brain in chronic progressive panencephalitis. *J. Gen. Virol. 29*:143–153, 1975.

144. Payment, P.D., Ajdukovic, D. and Povilanis, V. Le virus de la rubeole. I. Morphologic et proteines structurales. *Can. J. Microbiol. 21*:703–709, 1975.

145. Vaheri, A. and Hovi, T. Structural proteins and subunits of rubella virus. *J. Virol. 9*:10–16, 1972.

146. Waxham, M.N. and Wolinsky, J.S. Immunochemical identification of the hemagglutinin of rubella virus. *Virology* 126:194–203, 1983.
147. Väänänen, P. and Kääriäinen, L. Fusion and hemolysis of erythrocytes caused by three togaviruses: semliki forest, sindbis and rubella. *J. Gen. Virol.* 46:467–475, 1979.
148. Rawls, W.E. Viral persistence in congenital rubella. *Prog. Med. Virol.* 18:273–288, 1974.
149. Williams, M.P., Brawner, T.A., Riggs, H.G. and Roehrig, J.T. Characteristics of a persistent rubella infection in a human cell line. *J. Gen. Virol.* 52:321–328, 1981.
150. Menser, M.A., Harley, J.D., Hertzberg, R., Dorman, D.C. and Murphy, A.M. Persistence of virus in lens for three years after prenatal rubella. *Lancet* 2:387–388, 1967.
151. Grahame, R., Armstrong, R., Simmons, N.A., Mims, C.A., Wilton, J.M.A. and Laurent, R. Isolation of rubella virus from synovial fluid in five cases of seronegative arthritis. *Lancet* 2:649–651, 1981.
152. Chantler, J.K., Ford, D.K., and Tingle, A.J. Rubella-associated arthritis: Rescue of rubella virus from peripheral blood lymphocytes two years post vaccination. *Infect. Immun.* 32:1274–1280, 1981.
153. Coyle, P.K., Wolinsky, J.S., Buimovici-Klein, E., Mocha, R., and Cooper, L.Z. Rubella specific immune complexes after congenital infection and vaccination. *Infect. Immun.* 36:498–503, 1982.
154. Wolinsky J.S., Dau, P.C., Buimovici-Klein, E., Mednick, J., Berg, B.O., Lang, P.B. and Cooper, L.Z. Progressive rubella panencephalitis: immunovirologic studies and results of isoprinosine therapy. *Clin. Exp. Immunol.* 35:394–404, 1979.
155. Coyle, P.K., and Wolinsky, J.S. Characterization of immune complexes in progressive rubella panencephalitis. *Ann. Neurol.* 9:557–562, 1981.
156. Vandvik, B., Weil, M.L., Grandien, M. and Norrby, E. Progressive rubella panencephalitis: synthesis of oligoclonal virus-specific IgG antibodies and homogenous free light chains in the central nervous system. *Acta Neurol. Scand.* 57:53–64, 1978.
157. Wolinsky, J.S., Waxham, M.N., Hess, J., Townsend, J.J. and Baringer, J.R. Immunochemical features of a case of progressive rubella panencephalitis. *Clin. Exp. Immunol.* 48:359–366, 1982.
158. Townsend, J.J., Stroop, W.G., Baringer, J.R., Wolinsky, J.S., McKerrow, K.H. and Berg, B.O. Neuropathology of progressive rubella panencephalitis after childhood rubella. *Neurology* 32:185–190, 1982.

4

Scrapie Prions and Degenerative Diseases

Stanley B. Prusiner, Darlene F. Groth, David C. Bolton,
Paul E. Bendheim, Karen A. Bowman, S. Patricia Cochran,
Jocelyn J. Mayled, and Michael P. McKinley

Almost two decades ago, a flurry of excitement surrounded studies on slow infectious agents. It was a time when an eight-year search for the cause of kuru was drawing to a close.[1-3] Kuru had been classified as a degenerative neurologic disease of unknown origin that was confined to the Fore people and their neighboring tribes in the eastern highlands of Papua New Guinea. Almost every etiologic possibility for degenerative neurologic diseases had been considered with respect to kuru, but none had been identified.[4] Based on pathologic and clinical similarities between kuru and scrapie, a neurologic disease of sheep, Hadlow suggested in 1959 that kuru might be caused by a slow infectious agent.[5] Three years later, studies were begun by Gajdusek, Gibbs, and Alpers to test this hypothesis. In 1965, chimpanzees inoculated with brain tissue specimens from patients dying of kuru developed a kuru-like illness.[2]

These observations suggested the possibility that other degenerative diseases, especially those afflicting the nervous system, might be caused by similar slow transmissible agents.[6] If this were the case, then inoculation studies with brain tissue from patients dying of degenerative neurologic diseases might produce a disease in apes after a prolonged incubation period. That line of experimentation was rewarded in 1968 by the successful transmission of Creutzfeldt–Jakob disease (CJD) to chimpanzees.[7, 8] Almost ten years earlier, Klatzo and et al.[9] described the neuropathologic similarities between CJD and kuru.[9] Most exciting was the fact that CJD had been classified as a degenerative disease of un-known origin for more than half a century. This successful transmission study increased the vigor with which specimens from patients dying of numerous degenerative diseases were inoculated into apes and other animals.[6, 10–16]

During the ensuing decade, the inability to identify slow infectious agents as the cause of diseases similar to kuru and CJD greatly dimin-ished enthusiasm for such studies. We believe that these negative results have produced an unduly pessimistic view of the situation.

When the history of investigations of slow viral diseases of humans is examined, one sees that animal inoculation studies alone would not have revealed the infectious agents causing these diseases. Attempts to isolate by animal inoculation studies a paramyxovirus from brain speci-mens of patients dying of subacute sclerosing panencephalitis (SSPE) were unsuccessful; a similar experience was recorded with progressive multifocal leucoencephalopathy (PML). Only through specialized tech-niques developed for the rescue of viruses were the infectious agents causing SSPE and PML isolated.[17–19]

SLOW VIRUS AND PRION INFECTIONS

The concept of slow infectious diseases was first proposed by Bjorn Sigurdsson in 1954.[20] In Iceland, Sigurdsson studied several transmissi-ble diseases of sheep. He suggested four cardinal tenets as the major features of slow virus infections: (1) long incubation period lasting many months to years, (2) relatively short progressive clinical course lasting several weeks to a few months ending with death, (3) single species is the natural host, and (4) single organ is the site of disease. Sigurdsson's concept of slow infections is summarized in Table 1. Over the last three decades, a variety of slow infectious diseases have been found in both animals and man.

Two of the prototypic infectious agents that led Sigurdsson to the development of his slow virus infection concept cause scrapie and visna

TABLE 1.   Cardinal Features of Slow Infections[a]

1. Prolonged incubation period of many months to decades.
2. Short, progressive clinical course leading to death within several weeks to a few months.
3. Natural disease confined to a single host species.
4. One organ exhibits pathologic changes.

[a] Modified from Sigurdsson.

TABLE 2.   Slow Virus Diseases

Disease	Virus class	Natural host
Visna	Retrovirus	Sheep
Distemper	Paramyxovirus	Dogs
Subacute sclerosing panencephalitis (SSPE)	Paramyxovirus	Humans
Progressive multifocal leucoencephalopathy (PML)	Papovavirus	Humans
Progressive rubella panencephalitis (PRP)	Togavirus	Humans

in sheep. Attempts to isolate the scrapie agent and define its properties have been fraught with difficulty. As studies progressed, it became clear that there were fundamental differences between the scrapie agent and viruses.[21,22] The retrovirus causing visna has been isolated, well characterized, and shown to contain an RNA genome. Subsequently, viruses were isolated and identified as casual agents in three human slow infections: SSPE, PML, and progressive rubella panencephalitis (PRP) (Table 2).[18, 19]

To distinguish between two groups of slow infections, Gajdusek and co-workers[6,23] introduced the terms *conventional viruses* and *unconventional viruses*. The viruses causing visna, SSPE, PML, and PRP are called conventional slow viruses. The infectious agents causing scrapie, kuru, and CJD are called unconventional slow viruses according to this scheme.

Recent progress in the purification and characterization of an unconventional slow virus suggests that the scrapie agent is probably not a virus.[24] The novel properties of the scrapie agent distinguish it from other small infectious agents such as viruses, viroids, and plasmids. A new word, prion, has been introduced as an alternative to the terms unconventional viruses or unusual slow virus-like agent.[24] Prions are defined as small *proteinaceous infectious* particles which resist inactivation by most procedures that modify nucleic acids. This definition is operational and is likely to change once the details of the molecular structure of the scrapie agent become known. Not only does the term prion both clarify and simplify the nomenclature, but it provides a structural basis for organization. Transmission studies and neuropathologic observations on the kuru, CJD, and transmissible mink encephalopathy agents have shown that they are similar to the scrapie agent in many respects[25]; however, direct evidence for a proteinaceous structure, such as reduction of infectivity by protease digestion, has not been demonstrated for any of these agents (Table 3). These disorders have also been

TABLE 3.   Prion Diseases[a]

Disease	Natural host
Scrapie	Sheep and Goats
Transmissible encephalopathy (TME)[b]	Mink
Kuru[b]	Humans — Fore
Creutzfeldt–Jakob disease (CJD)[b]	Humans

[a] Alternative terminology includes unconventional slow virus diseases and subacute transmissible spongiform encephalopathies.
[b] Proteinaceous infectious particles causing these diseases not yet demonstrated.

called unconventional slow virus diseases and subacute transmissible spongiform encephalopathies. It is noteworthy that while the term *spongiform* accurately describes the pathologic hallmarks of kuru and CJD, such changes are inconspicious in natural scrapie of sheep and goats.[26–28] Little or no vacuolation of the neuropil is found; the main changes are neuronal degeneration and profound proliferation of astrocytes. Spongiform change in scrapie occurs mostly in experimental infections.

HYPOTHETICAL STRUCTURES FOR THE SCRAPIE AGENT

For nearly three decades the chemical structure of the scrapie agent has remained elusive. Numerous models or hypothetical structures have been proposed to explain the unusual properties associated with

TABLE 4.   Hypothetical Structures for the Scrapie Agent

Hypothetical structures

1. Sarcosporidia-like parasite
2. "Filterable" virus
3. Small DNA virus
4. Replicating protein
5. Replicating abnormal polysaccharide with membranes
6. DNA subvirus controlled by a transmissible linkage substance
7. Provirus consisting of recessive genes generating RNA particles
8. Naked nucleic acid similar to plant viroids
9. Unconventional virus
10. Aggregated conventional virus with unusual properties
11. Replicating polysaccharide
12. Nucleoprotein complex
13. Nucleic acid surrounded by a polysaccharide coat
14. Spiroplasma-like organism
15. Multicomponent system with one component quite small
16. Membrane-bound DNA

it (Table 4).[24] Our data, and that of other investigators, suggest two possible models for the scrapie agent: (1) a small nucleic acid surrounded by a tightly-packed protein coat, or (2) a protein devoid of nucleic acid, that is, an infectious protein. While the first model might seem the most plausible, there is no evidence for a nucleic acid within the scrapie agent. The second model is consistent with the experimental data, but is clearly heretical. Skepticism of the second model is certainly justified; only purification of the scrapie agent to homogeneity and determination of its chemical structure will prove which if either of these two models is correct.

There seems little advantage in championing one model over the other; however, several previously postulated structures for the scrapie agent can now be discarded (Table 4). The requirement for a protein for infectivity eliminates the possibility that the scrapie agent is composed entirely of a polysaccharide or a nucleic acid. Thus, the replicating polysaccharide and naked nucleic acid/viroid hypotheses are no longer tenable. The hypothetical nucleic acid surrounded by a polysaccharide coat can also be eliminated. Studies demonstrating the small size of the scrapie agent clearly distinguish it from conventional viruses, spiroplasma-like organisms, and parasites such as sarcosporidia.

PRIONS, VIRUSES, VIROIDS, AND PLASMIDS

As discussed above, the definition of prions must remain operational until the detailed molecular structure of these particles is known. Further studies are needed before purification of the scrapie agent to a homogeneous state is achieved. From investigations demonstrating its resistance to procedures attacking nucleic acids, its resistance to inactivation by heat, and its apparent small size, the scrapie agent is clearly a novel infectious entity.[24] The dominant molecular characteristics of the scrapie prion resemble those of a protein.[24, 29–32] Although several lines of evidence show that the scrapie agent contains a protein required for infectivity, all attempts to demonstrate a nucleic acid within the agent have been unsuccessful. Replication of the scrapie agent in natural and experimental hosts is well documented. For example, one infectious dose of the agent inoculated into the brain of a hamster appears to induce the production of more than 10^9 ID_{50} units during the ensuing 120-day period.[33, 34] The novel properties of the scrapie agent and the probes used to elucidate these properties are listed in Table 5. Current knowledge does not allow exclusion of a small nucleotide polymer buried within the protein shell of the prion. The apparent small size of the agent makes it

TABLE 5.   Novel Properties of the Scrapie Agent

1. Stable at 90°C for 30 minutes.
2. Low molecular weight infectious particles
   (minimum estimate 50,000 daltons).
3. Hydrophobic protein(s) is required for infectivity.
4. Resistant to RNases and DNases.
5. Resistant to UV irradiation at 254 nm.
6. Resistant to psoralen photoadduct formation.
7. Resistant to Zn^{++} catalyzed hydrolysis.
8. Resistant to NH_2OH chemical modification.

unlikely that this hypothetical nucleic acid is of sufficient size to act as a gene coding for the protein(s) of the surrounding shell.

In contrast to prions, the molecular structures of many viruses and viroids are well established.[35] With all of our knowledge about viruses, their definition remains complex.[35] Viruses are obligate intracellular infectious agents which contain no energy transducing or protein synthetic systems and multiply by replicative mechanisms not involving division. All viruses contain a nucleic acid genome of either DNA or RNA. This genome is surrounded by a capsid and/or coat composed of protein. In some instances, this proteinaceous shell may also contain lipid and/or polysaccharides. All of the information needed to produce progeny virus is contained within its nucleic acid genome. In contrast to viruses, viroids and plasmids do not contain protein.[36] These infectious naked nucleic acids do not have a capsid or coat. While plasmids contain genes that code for the biosynthesis of proteins,[37] viroids seem to be too small to encode the information required to direct the synthesis of proteins.[36] Hundreds of animal and human diseases caused by viruses have been identified; however, no animal or human disease caused by a viroid has been found.[36]

DETECTION OF INFECTIOUS AGENTS IN DEGENERATIVE DISEASES

Many human and animal diseases have been suspected of being caused by slow infectious agents. Eight of these common disorders for which a slow infectious cause has been suspected, but never identified, are listed in Table 6.[24, 38] These diseases include Alzheimer's senile dementia, multiple sclerosis, Parkinson's disease, amyotrophic lateral sclerosis, diabetes mellitus, rheumatoid arthritis, lupus erythematosus, as well as a variety of neoplastic diseases. In all of these diseases, scientists have searched for viruses or virus-like agents as a cause. With the excep-

TABLE 6. Some Degenerative Diseases Suspected of Being Caused by Slow Infectious Agents[a]

1. Alzheimer's senile dementia
2. Multiple sclerosis
3. Parkinson's disease
4. Amyotrophic lateral sclerosis
5. Diabetes mellitus
6. Rheumatoid arthritis
7. Lupus erythematosus
8. Cancer

[a] Adapted from Gajdusek[24] and Gross[38].

tion of a few lymphomas, no convincing evidence has been found to implicate a slow infectious agent as the cause of these disorders. It remains to be established whether the negative results in these studies are due to the fact that these diseases are not caused by slow infectious agents or that the proper techniques for detecting them have not been available.

Many techniques have been developed to detect viruses (Table 7). These techniques include: (1) light microscopic observation of inclusion bodies within the nucleus or cytoplasm of affected cells or an inflammatory response typical of a virus infection; (2) electron microscopic observation of virus-like particles; (3) inoculation of animals or plants and subsequent production of progeny virus and disease; (4) inoculation of cultured cells and subsequent production of progeny virus and destruction of the cells; (5) co-cultivation of infected cells with permissive cells; (6) helper viruses to induce the production of the latent, incomplete, or defective virus; (7) induction of latent virus by ultraviolet light; (8) sero-

TABLE 7. Techniques for Detection of Slow Infectious Pathogens

| | Identification of | | |
Method	Viruses	Viroids	Prions
1. Light microscopy	+[a]		
2. Electron microscopy	+		
3. Inoculation higher organisms	+	+	+
4. Inoculation cultured cells	+		
5. Co-cultivation	+		
6. Helper viruses	+		
7. Chemical or UV induction	+		
8. Serology	+		
9. cDNA hybridization	+	+	

[a] Plus signs (+) indicate method used to detect infectious pathogen.

logic tests for the presence of virus or viral proteins; and (9) complementary DNA or RNA probes to detect the presence of a viral genome. Most of these techniques have been used to search for viruses as causative agents in the diseases listed in Table 6. Using all these methods, investigators have been unable to identify viruses as the cause of any of these degenerative disorders.

While all of the aforementioned techniques have been used successfully in identifying the viruses of both animals and plants, methods for detecting viroid-like infectious molecules in plants are limited. The most widely used technique has been inoculation of susceptible plants, subsequent production of progeny viroids, and the development of disease several weeks later.[36] Cultured plant cells have been infected with viroids, but no characteristic pathology that could be used as an assay has been observed. Complementary DNA probes have recently been introduced for the routine diagnosis of viroid diseases.[39]

The only method of detecting prions is the inoculation of animals followed by production of progeny prions and development of disease many months or years later. The apparent small size of the scrapie agent makes detection of distinct particles by electron microscopy unlikely. Inoculation of cell cultures with prions may result in limited replication, but no reproducible cytopathology has been reported. There is no evidence to suggest that helper viruses are required for or enhance replication of prions either in animals or cell culture. Similarly, enhancement of prion replication by ultraviolet irradiation or chemical induction has not been observed. Although prions have not yet been demonstrated to be immunogenic in their native state, the existence of a protein component within the scrapie agent suggests that chemical or physical treatment of highly enriched preparations may render prions immunogenic. Production of an antibody specific for one or more prions would represent an important advance. Less promising is the possibility of detecting prions by nucleic acid hybridization since the small size of the scrapie agent seems to preclude a nucleic acid genome that codes for the protein(s) of its shell.

In viewing the data in Table 7, it is interesting to consider SSPE and PML in more detail. If the inoculation of experimental animals had been the only means of detecting the paramyxovirus causing SSPE or the papovavirus causing PML, then the viruses causing either of these slow infections still could not have been isolated. Inclusion bodies seen in brain sections from children dying of SSPE were the first clue that a virus might be the cause of this disorder.[40] Subsequent electron microscopic and serologic studies suggested that measles virus was present in the brains of these patients.[41–46] Inoculation of monkeys, hamsters, and mice failed to produce disease,[47, 48] but later studies with ferrets did produce a transmissible neurologic disorder.[49] Also, inoculation of many cultured cell lines failed to cause cytopathology.[47, 48] Eventually, isolation and passage of the SSPE virus was accomplished by fusion of brain cells isolated from patients with SSPE with embryonic monkey kidney or VERO cells.[50]

A similar saga surrounds the isolation and identification of the papovavirus causing PML. Early studies demonstrated changes in the nuclei of glial cells in brain sections from patients dying of PML.[51–53] These alterations were interpreted as evidence for a viral infection, especially since PML is usually found in patients with compromised immune function. Subsequent electron microscopic studies showed crystalline arrays of particles resembling viruses in these altered nuclei.[54, 55] Inoculation with brain extracts from patients with PML failed to produce disease in monkeys, hamsters, and mice.[56, 57] Also, inoculation of numerous cultured cell lines failed to produce cyopathology. Eventually isolation and passage of the JC virus causing PML was accomplished with primary cultures of human fetal glial cells, which were permissive for virus replication.[58] An SV_{40} virus causing PML was later isolated using primary cultures of African green monkey kidney cells.[59]

Numerous other examples of human viral diseases in which animal inoculation studies failed to demonstrate the disease are well documented. The history of research on the hepatitis viruses underscores the difficulties encountered in isolation and characterization of causative agents. Serology, electron microscopy, and assays of viral DNA synthesis have provided important tools for extending our understanding of hepatitis viruses.[60, 61]

Clearly, we need new techniques for detecting prions. Bioassays of prions in animals demand that the prion be in an infectious state and that the animal host be permissive for prion replication. In addition, the prion must not be destroyed during the inoculation process and it must eventually cause disease. Once new techniques become available for detecting prions, the search for novel infectious pathogens causing degenerative diseases in humans should gain new vigor and excitement.

ACKNOWLEDGMENT

The authors thank Dr. William J. Hadlow for critical review of the manuscript. The research was supported by Grants NS14069 and AG02132, from the National Institutes of Health, and a gift from R. J. Reynolds Industries. PEB is supported by a postdoctoral fellowship from the National Multiple Sclerosis Society. DCB is supported by a postdoctoral fellowship from the National Institutes of Health.

REFERENCES

1. Gajdusek, D.C. and Zigas, V. Degenerative disease of the central nervous system in New Guinea. The endemic occurence of "kuru" in the native population. *N. Engl. J. Med. 257:*974–978, 1957.
2. Gajdusek, D.C., Gibbs, C.J. Jr. and Alpers, M. Experimental transmission of a kuru-like syndrome to chimpanzees. *Nature 209:*794–796, 1966.
3. Gajdusek, D.C. Observations on the early history of kuru investigations. In: *Slow Transmissible Diseases of the Nervous System.* Vol. 1. Prusiner, S.B. and Hadlow, W.J., eds. New York: Academic Press, pp. 7–36, 1979.
4. Gajdusek, D.C. and Zigas, V. Clinical, pathological and epidemiological study of an acute progressive degenerative disease of the central nervous system among natives of the eastern highlands of New Guinea. *Am. J. Med. 26:*442–469, 1959.
5. Hadlow, W.J. Scrapie and kuru. *Lancet 2:*289–290, 1959.
6. Gajdusek, D.C. Unconventional viruses and the origin and disappearance of kuru. *Science 197:*943–960, 1977.
7. Gibbs, C.J. Jr., Gajdusek, D.C., Asher, D.M., Alpers, M.P., Beck, E., Daniel, P.M. and Matthews, W.B. Creutzfeldt-Jakob disease/spongiform encephalopathy: transmission to the chimpanzee. *Science 161:*388–389, 1968.
8. Gibbs, C.J. Jr. and Gajdusek, D.C. Infection as the etiology of spongiform encephalopathy. *Science 165:*1023–1025, 1969.
9. Klatzo, I., Gajdusek, D.C. and Zigas, V. Pathology of kuru. *Lab. Invest. 8:*799–847, 1959.
10. Gajdusek, D.C. and Gibbs, C.J. Jr. Attempts to demonstrate a transmissible agent in kuru, amyotrophic lateral sclerosis, and other sub-acute and chronic nervous system degenerations of man. *Nature 204:*257–259, 1964.
11. Gajdusek, D.C. The possible role of slow virus infection in chronic schizophrenic dementia. In: *Birth Defects: Article Series.* Vol. 14, No. 5. The National Foundation, pp. 81–87, 1978.
12. Gajdusek, D.C. Infectious agents in rheumatic disease. In: *Report of the Research Work Group of the National Commission on Arthritis and Related Musculoskeletal Diseases.* Bethseda, Maryland: N.I.H., pp. 114–127, 1978.
13. Gibbs, C.J. Jr. and Gajdusek, D.C. Kuru—a prototype subacute infectious disease of the nervous system as a model for the study of amyotrophic lateral sclerosis. In: *Motor Neuron Diseases: Research on Amyotrophic Lateral Sclerosis and Related Disorders.* Vol. 2. Norris, F.H. Jr. and Kurland, L.T., eds. New York: Grune and Stratton, pp. 269–279, 1969.
14. Gibbs, C.J. Jr., Gajdusek, D.C. and Alpers, M.P. Attempts to transmit subacute and chronic neurological diseases to animals. In: Pathogenesis and Etiology of Demyelinating Diseases. *Int. Arch. Allergy 36:* 519–552, 1969.
15. Gibbs, C.J. Jr. Search for infectious etiology in chronic and subacute degenerative diseases of the central nervous system. *Curr. Top. Microbiol. Immnol. 40:*44–58, 1967.

16. Goudsmit, J., Morrow, C.H., Asher, D.M., Yanagihara, R.T., Masters, C.L., Gibbs, C.J. Jr. and Gajdusek, D.C. Evidence for and against the transmissibility of Alzheimer's disease. *Neurology* 30:945–950, 1980.

17. Brody, J.A. and Gibbs, C.J. Jr. Chronic neurological diseases: subacute sclerosing panencephalitis, progressive multifocal leukoencephalopathy, kuru, Creutzfeldt-Jakob disease. In: *Viral Infections of Humans*. Evans, A.S., ed. New York: Plenum Press, pp. 519–537, 1976.

18. ter Meulen, V. and Hall, W.W. Slow virus infections of the nervous system: virological, immunological and pathogenetic considerations. *J. Gen. Virol.* 41:1–25, 1978.

19. Wolinsky, J.S. Slow virus infection by conventional virus agents. In: *Infectious Diseases of the Central Nervous System*. Thompson, R. A. and Green, J. R., eds. New York: Spectrum, 1983.

20. Sigurdsson, B. Rida, a chronic encephalitis of sheep with general remarks on infections which develop slowly and some of their special characteristics. *Br. Vet. J. 110*:341–354, 1954.

21. Hunter, G.D. The enigma of the scrapie agent: biochemical approaches and the involvement of membranes and nucleic acids. In: *Slow Transmissible Diseases of the Nervous System*. Vol. 2. Prusiner, S.B. and Hadlow, W.J., eds. New York: Academic Press, pp. 365–385, 1979.

22. Hunter, G.D. The enigma of the scrapie agent: biochemical approaches and the involvement of membranes and nucleic acids. In: *Slow Transmissible Diseases of the Nervous System*. Vol. 2. Prusiner, S.B. and Hadlow, W.J., eds. New York: Academic Press, pp. 365–385, 1979.

23. Gajdusek, D.C. Unconventional viruses. In: *Human Diseases Caused by Viruses: Recent Developments*. Rothschild, H., Allison, F. and Howe, C., eds. New York: Oxford University Press, pp. 233–258, 1978.

24. Prusiner, S.B. Novel proteinaceous infectious particles cause scrapie. *Science 216*:136–144, 1982.

25. Hadlow, W.J., Prusiner, S.B., Kennedy, R.C. and Race, R.E. Brain tissue from persons dying of Creutzfeldt-Jakob disease causes scrapie-like encephalopathy in goats. *Ann. Neurol.* 8:628–631, 1980.

26. Zlotnik, I. The pathology of scrapie: a comparative study of lesions in the brain of sheep and goats. *Acta Neuropathol. Suppl. I*:61–70, 1962.

27. Beck, E., Daniel, P.M. and Parry, H.B. Degeneration of the cerebellar and hypothalamo-neurohypophysical systems in sheep with scrapie, and its relationship to human system degenerations. *Brain* 87:153–176, 1964.

28. Hadlow, W.J., Kennedy, R.C., Race, R.E. and Eklund, C.M. Virologic and neurohistologic findings in dairy goats affected with natural scrapie. *Vet. Pathol. 17*:187–199, 1980.

29. Prusiner, S.B., Hadlow, W.J., Garfin, D.E., Cochran, S.P., Baringer, J.R., Race, R.E. and Eklund, C.M. Partial purification and evidence for multiple molecular forms of the scrapie agent. *Biochemistry* 17:4993–4999, 1978.

30. Prusiner, S.B., Groth, D.F., Cochran, S.P., Masiarz, F.R., McKinley, M.P. and Martinez, H.M. Molecular properties, partial purification and assay by incubation period measurements of the hamster scrapie agent. *Biochemistry 19*:4883–4891, 1980.

31. Prusiner, S.B., McKinley, M.P., Groth, D.F., Bowman, K.A., Mock, N.I., Cochran, S.P. and Masiarz, F.R. Scrapie agent contains a hydrophobic protein. *Proc. Natl. Acad. Sci.* 78:6675–6679, 1981.

32. McKinley, M.P., Masiarz, F.R. and Prusiner, S.B. Reversible chemical modification of the scrapie agent. *Science* 214:1259–1261, 1981.
33. Kimberlin, R. and Walker, C. Characteristics of a short incubation model of scrapie in the golden hamster. *J. Gen. Virol.* 34:295–304, 1977.
34. Prusiner, S.B., Cochran, S.P., Groth, D.F., Downey, D.E., Bowman, K.A. and Martinez, H.M. Measurement of the scrapie agent using an incubation time interval assay. *Ann. Neurol.* 11:353–358, 1982.
35. Luria, S.E., Darnell, J.E. Jr., Baltimore, D. and Campbell, A. *General Virology.* New York: J. Wiley, pp. 1–490, 1978.
36. Diener, T.O. *Viroids and Viroid Diseases.* New York: J. Wiley, 1979: 1–252.
37. Broda, P. Plasmids. San Francisco: W. H. Freeman, pp. 1–148, 1979.
38. Gross, L. Cancer and slow virus diseases—some common features. *N. Engl. J. Med.* 301:432–434, 1979.
39. Owens, R.A. and Diener, T.O. Sensitive and rapid diagnosis of potato spindle tuber viroid disease by nucleic acid hybridization. *Science* 213:670–672, 1981.
40. Dawson, J.R. Cellular inclusions in cerebral lesions of lethargic encephalitis. *Am. J. Pathol.* 9:7–16, 1933.
41. Tellez-Nagel, I. and Harter, D.H. Subacute sclerosing leukoencephalitis: ultrastructure of intranuclear and intracytoplasmic inclusions. *Science* 154:899–901, 1966.
42. Freeman, J.M., Magoffin, R.L., Lennette, E.H. and Herndon, R.M. Additional evidence of the relation between subacute inclusion-body encephalitis and measles virus. *Lancet* 2:129–131, 1967.
43. Dayan, A.D., Gostling, J.V.T., Greaves, J.L., Stevens, D.W. and Woodhouse, M.A. Evidence of a pseudomyxovirus in the brain in subacute sclerosing leucoencephalitis. *Lancet* 1:980–981, 1967.
44. Tellez-Nagel, I., Harter, D.H., Johnson, A.B. and Carver, D. Virus-like particles in subacute sclerosing encephalitis; electron microscopic, virological and histochemical studies. *J Neuropathol. Exp. Neurol.* 26:121–123, 1967.
45. Pelc, S., Périer, J.-O., Quersin-Thiry, L. Résultats expérimentaux obtenus dans l'encéphalite humaine, type encéphalite subaiguë a inclusions, leuco-encéphalite sclérosante subaiguë. *Rev. Neurol.* 98:3–24, 1958.
46. Bouteille, M., Fontaine C., Vendrenne C.L., Delarue, J. Sur un cas d' encéphalite subaiguë à inclusions. Etude anatomo-clinique et ultrastructurale. *Rev. Neurol.* 113:454–458, 1965.
47. Connolly, J.H., Allen, I.V., Hurwitz, L.J. and Millar, J.H.D. Measles-virus antibody and antigen in subacute sclerosing panencephalitis. *Lancet* 1:542–544, 1967.
48. Tellez-Nagel, I. and Harter, D.H. Subacute sclerosing leukoencephalitis. I. Clinico-pathological, electron microscopic and virological observations. *J. Neuropathol. Exp. Neurol.* 25:560–581, 1966.
49. Katz, M., Balian Rorke, L., Masland, W.S., Koprowski, H. and Tucker, S.H. Transmission of an encephalitogenic agent from brains of patients with subacute sclerosing panencephalitis to ferrets. *N. Engl. J. Med.* 279:793–798, 1968.
50. Chen, T.T., Wantanabe, I., Zeman, W. and Mealey, J. Jr. Subacute sclerosing panencephalitis: propagation of measles virus from brain biopsy in tissue culture. *Science* 163:1193–1194, 1969.

51. Aström, K.-E., Mancall, E.L. and Richardson, E.P. Jr. Progressive multifocal leuko-encephalopathy: hitherto unrecognized complication of chronic lymphatic leukemia and Hodgkin's disease. *Brain 81*:93–111, 1958.
52. Cavanagh, J.B., Greenbaum, D., Marshall, A.H.E. and Rubenstein, L.J. Cerebral demyelination associated with disorders of the reticuloendothelial system. *Lancet 2*:524–529, 1959.
53. Richardson, E.P. Jr. Progressive multifocal leukoencephalopathy. *N. Engl. J. Med. 265*:815–823, 1961.
54. ZuRhein, G.M. and Chou, S. M. Particles resembling papova viruses in human cerebral demyelinating disease. *Science 148*:1477–1479, 1965.
55. Silverman, L. and Rubenstein, L.J. Electron microscopic observations on a case of progressive multifocal leukoencephalopathy. *Acta Neuropathol. 5*:215–244, 1965.
56. Schwerdt, P.R., Schwerdt, C.E., Silverman, L. and Rubinstein, L.J. Virions associated with progressive multifocal leukoencephalopathy. *Virology 29*:511–514, 1966.
57. Dolman, C.L., Furesz, J. and Mackay B. Progressive multifocal leukoencephalopathy: two cases with electron microscopic and viral studies. *Can. Med. Assoc. J. 97*:8–12, 1967.
58. Padgett, B.L., Walker, D.L., ZuRhein, G.M., Eckroade, R.J. and Dessel, B.H. Cultivation of papova-like virus from human brain with multifocal leucoencephalopathy. *Lancet 1*:1257–1260, 1971.
59. Weiner, L.P., Herndon, R.M., Narayan, O., Johnson, R.T., Shah, K., Rubinstein, L.J., Preziosi, T.J. and Conley, F.K. Isolation of virus related to SV40 from patients with progressive multifocal leukoencephalopathy. *N. Engl. J. Med. 286*:385–390, 1972.
60. Blumberg, B.S. Australia antigen and the biology of hepatitis B. *Science 197*:17–25, 1977.
61. Tiollais, P., Charnay, P. and Vyas, G.N. Biology of hepatitis B virus. *Science 213*:406–411, 1981.

5

Acute Immune-Mediated Diseases of the Nervous System

Kenneth P. Johnson

INTRODUCTION

Two diseases, one affecting the peripheral nervous system (PNS) and the other affecting the central nervous system (CNS), are recognized; they are most certainly the result of an immune-mediated attack on some component of myelin. These diseases are of interest for a number of reasons. First, both may be quite severe, ending fatally in a significant number of cases and producing serious neurologic dysfunction in others. They are relatively common, although the PNS disease is recognized much more frequently. Both diseases share a relationship to a preceding infectious process, a remarkably similar time course between the infection and onset of neurologic disease, and strikingly similar pathologic features. Finally, faithful animal models for both conditions have been developed and the antigens required to produce the experimental disease have been defined in great detail.

The CNS disease has been described by a variety of terms but is most commonly noted as para or postinfectious encephalomyelitis. Several years ago, we suggested that a more appropriate term would be immune-mediated encephalomyelitis, which conveys some information about the pathogenesis of the condition. In rare cases, when the condition is hyperacute, a hemorrhagic component is observed pathologically and then the term *hemorrhagic immune-mediated encephalomyelitis* (HIME) may be used.[1]

The PNS disease is most commonly called the Guillain-Barré syndrome, although the terms idiopathic polyneuritis or postinfectious polyneuritis are also frequently used.[2] For this condition, we have suggested the term acute immune-mediated polyneuritis (AIMP), which was selected again because it provides more information about the pathogenic mechanisms producing the condition.

An intriging mystery still surrounds these conditions: how can a seemingly mild or banal infection, usually due to respiratory virus, trigger such a massive immunologic attack on a specific component of nervous tissue? Unfortunately, almost nothing is known about that stage of the disease process. On the other hand, modern vaccination procedures have markedly decreased the incidence of IME while new experimental therapies, currently undergoing evaluation, hold promise of markedly reducing the threat and morbidity of AIMP.

IMMUNE-MEDIATED ENCEPHALOMYELITIS (IME)

IME typically presents as a biphasic disease. First, the patient may develop an infection such as acute measles (rubeola) with standard features or an acute mild respiratory infection of unknown cause. As symptoms of the infection are waning, the second phase appears, heralded by headache, fever, stiff neck, and the appearance of focal neurologic signs most commonly suggestive of central white matter disease. Seizures of a variety of types may occur. This second phase of disease may progress rapidly to a fatal outcome in seven to ten days; however, the majority of patients stabilize within a week and most recover completely. A significant number of patients, perhaps 10 to 20 percent, have permanent neurologic deficits such as focal epilepsy, reduced mental capacity, personality changes, and localized signs such as ataxia or paralysis.

Rarely, this condition may proceed rapidly to death in three to five days. In such cases, it is not uncommon to find that the pathologic changes in the brain include perivascular focal hemorrhages and that both erythrocytes and neutrophils predominate in the cerebral spinal fluid (CSF). In the more typical case, the CSF shows a moderately high increase in total protein and a modest increase in leukocytes, primarily lymphocytes which may reach 500 or 1,000 per milliliter. The CSF sugar level is usually normal. Often, an increase CSF pressure is noted during the acute phase.

The pathology of IME consists primarily of focal inflammation and demyelination in a perivenular distribution in the cerebral hemispheres and brain stem.[2] Thus, the white matter is most affected where perivascular inflammatory cuffs may be several cells thick and where the zone of demyelination may be a millimeter or more across. When observed microscopically, the white matter may be speckled with many small areas of demyelination all related directly to a central vein. Specimens observed several years after the event show focal demyelination with secondary gliosis but an absence of inflammation. Occasionally, large demyelinated plagues are evident.[3]

A large variety of infectious agents have been temporally associated with IME; however, the agents most frequently noted are measles, mumps, rubella, and varicella-zoster viruses.[1] Of these, the most important agent is measles. IME was said to complicate approximately one of every 2,000 cases of acute measles before the widespread use of live rubeola vaccine. IME may also complicate mild respiratory infections in which no specific virus has yet been implicated. Of interest, IME may also occur as a complication of vaccinations employing vaccinia virus or fixed rabies virus grown in neural tissues.

The epidemiology of IME indicates that all age groups may be affected; however, children with acute infections caused by the agents listed previously most commonly develop the syndrome. It occurs throughout the world.

No specific therapy has been defined for IME and most patients are cared for supportively with anticonvulsants, measures to decrease fever, and other supportive measures. There are no adequate studies to suggest that immunosuppression is beneficial. Several measures have markedly decreased the incidence of IME, however. Of these, the most important is the widespread use of live measles (rubeola) vaccines. Conservative studies have suggested that the measles vaccination policy followed in the United States has saved several thousand lives, prevented tens of thousands of cases of mental retardation, and has saved many millions of dollars.[4] IME almost never complicates measles vaccination. The worldwide irradiation of smallpox which has lead to an abandonment of routine smallpox vaccination has also helped to reduce the number of cases of IME. Finally, the introduction of new vaccines for rabies, manufactured from human diploid cells rather than mammalian CNS tissue, has markedly reduced the chance of developing IME as a result of iatrogenic exposure to brain antigen.

ACUTE IMMUNE-MEDIATED POLYNEURITIS (AIMP)

The typical clinical course of AIMP (Guillain–Barré syndrome) is one of the most dramatic events in clinical neurology. A previously well person may develop a mild respiratory infection, then, as it is clearing or within two weeks after it ends, the patient will note paresthesias in the feet along with mild distal weakness. Commonly, ascending symmetrical weakness extends rapidly over two to five days, although occasionally it may progress in a step-wise fashion over one to two weeks. Along with the increasing weakness which may produce respiratory distress, there is almost universal facial paresis. While the motor symptoms always predominate, many patients note some sensory loss in a distal, symmetrical fashion as well. Occasional patients note deep cramping muscle pain. In addition to the hazards of respiratory paralysis, the autonomic system is frequently involved, leading to unpredictable hypertension and the risk of serious or ever fatal cardiac arhythmias. In unusual cases, there may be weakness of the extraoccular muscles or of the sphincters. Predictably, there is early loss of most or all deep tendon reflex activity.

After the period of maximum weakness, there is a short static period then slow recovery which may take weeks to many months; however, most patients who survive the acute stages of AIMP generally recover almost completely with time. Recovery is less often complete and the appearance of fatal complications is more common in patients who develop AIMP after the age of 60. Most patients with AIMP have relatively severe muscle atrophy; however, muscle size as well as strength slowly returns during the lengthy convalescence when renervation of muscle takes place.

Variants of AIMP have been recognized. Rarely, patients thought to have a chronic form of IMP follow a slowly progressive course during which they have increasing atrophy and ever more complete weakness. More often, the disease may evolve into a relapsing course where there are several episodes of increasing symmetrical weakness followed by slow recovery.[5] Finally, an unusual variant known as the Fisher-type of disease occurs in which the predominant symptoms and signs develop in the muscles innervated by cranial nerves.[6] Such patients often develop weakness of the extraoccular muscles with diplopia.

The pathology of AIMP is very similar to that of IME: the two predominant characteristics are focal demyelination and inflammation.[1] The large motor and sensory fibers of peripheral nerves show myelin loss in a patchy distribution from the roots to the peripheral extensions. The inflammatory cells are most commonly lymphocytes. After the acute stage, there is proliferation of Schwann cells followed by slow remyelination of the affected axons. The typical CSF pattern is one of very high total protein levels with an absence of a pleocytosis. After the first few days of disease, nerve conduction velocity studies show marked slowing.

AIMP may complicate a large variety of mild infections and in most instances the nature of the infecting agent is unknown. The disease has been associated with infection with the human herpes viruses, cytomegalovirus, and EB virus. However, a wide variety of other viruses including measles, mumps, and influenza have also been associated with it. In unusual cases, the syndrome may follow surgical procedures or other trauma. It may also follow various types of vaccination. In 1976 and early 1977, a well-defined epidemic of AIMP was associated with the swine influenza vaccination campaign.[7] Of interest, however, is the fact that the influenza vaccines used since that time have not been associated with an incidence of AIMP. The disease has also been associated with the rabies vaccine produced in suckling rodent brain and used in South America.

The disease occurs throughout the world with approximately the same frequency, but appears to have a slight predominance in late adolescence and early adult life and after the age of 50. It may appear throughout the year.

Therapy for AIMP consists primarily of supportive care, but this must be coordinated and applied rapidly and then maintained with great diligence over long periods of time for the patients are often extensively paralyzed and dependent on almost complete support for prolonged periods. In this disease as in few others, the quality and diligence of nursing care is often the key important element in survival.

Once the diagnosis is considered, patients must be monitored closely for increasing respiratory paralysis at two- to four-hour intervals. Arrangements must be made for a tracheostomy before it is required. At the beginning, comprehensive 24-hour plans for respiratory care, skin care, urinary tract care, and adequate nutrition must be initiated. Many patients require respiratory assistance for prolonged periods. Of special importance is the recognition of autonomic disorders which are part of the syndrome.[1] Many patients are monitored in an intensive care setting for the first two to three weeks of the disease. Great care must be exercised in manipulating or moving patients during this period for cardiac arhythmias leading to arrest and cerebral anoxia or death are not uncommon at this time. Dedicated support of many body systems must be maintained for several months; however, because the peripheral nervous system has the capacity to regenerate almost completely, such care frequently results in complete recovery. Beyond the first two to three critical weeks, an active rehabilitative program should be undertaken to preserve joint function and assist the patient during the return of muscle strength.

No specific therapy has been shown to be of benefit in AIMP. High-dose cortical steriods have been suggested; however, at least one recent report suggest that this form of therapy is detrimental. Uncontrolled reports had suggested that plasma exchange may be of benefit in AIMP. Other reports have stated that this is of little value. At least two control trials of plasma exchange are currently underway to determine the therapeutic benefit from this rather aggressive form of therapy.

EXPERIMENTAL MODELS OF IME AND AIMP

Faithful animal models which duplicate both the time sequence, clinical course, and pathology of these conditions now exist. For some time, it has been recognized that the common monophasic form of experimental allergic encephalomyelitis (EAE) may mimic IME closely. The time course from initial challenge with white matter antigen plus complete Freund's adjuvant (CFA) is approximately 10 to 14 days. A similar time course is noted in human IME complicating various vaccination programs or after influenza infection where the incubation period is usually very short. The perivascular demyelination and inflammation seen in EAE is similar to that noted in the IME, and the use of multiple adjuvants such as CFA and pertusis vaccine allows one to produce a hyperacute hemorrhagic white matter disease similar to human HIMP. Many studies have shown that the antigen responsible for EAE is myelin basic protein (MBP), the dominant protein of CNS myelin.[5] Investigation has shown that biochemical differences exist between the MBP of various species and that specific small fragments of the molecule are all that are required to produce clinically or pathologically evident EAE. Transfer studies have shown that EAE may be initiated in naive animals with cells but not with serum from involved animals indicting that the process is a cellular immune disease.

It is possible to produce AIMP with similar methods, however, using peripheral nerve myelin and CFA. The time course from challenge to clinical disease is also approximately 10 to 14 days and the pathology is highly reminiscent of human AIMP, that is, focal demyelination with inflammation. The experimental disease of peripheral nerve is frequently termed experimental allergic polyneuritis or EAN. It too may be transferred by cells but not with serum antibodies. Both EAE and EAN can be produced in a variety of animal hosts and either central or peripheral myelin from many hosts have been shown to be immunogenic in either the same species or in other species using appropriate experimental protocols. While both EAE and EAN closely mimic their human counterparts, no one has been able to consistently produce the experimental diseases with a preceding infection as noted in the human diseases. Thus, the pathogenic mechanism essential for the trigger of these immune-mediated attacks on central or peripheral myelin remains to be elucidated.

CONCLUSIONS

Two very similar human diseases—IME, which affects the CNS, and AIMP, which affects the PNS—have been described. Both frequently follow a mild infectious process or a vaccination usually by 10 to 15 days and both display common pathologic elements, focal demyelination and inflammation. The human disease affecting the peripheral nervous system (AIMP) is observed much more frequently. Animal models—EAE, which mimics IME, and EAN, which mimics AIMP—have been well studied and found to be caused by cell mediated immunologic processes resulting from sensitization to central or peripheral nerve myelin proteins. Unfortunately, the mechanism by which mild infection triggers the immune-mediated pathology is still little understood. Several vaccination procedures have markedly reduced the number of cases of IME, most importantly, the wide use of measles vaccination during infancy. The therapy for AIMP is largely supportive; however, if close attention is given to care of many organ systems, patients with this disease are likely to survive with complete recovery. Current controlled trials are underway to assess the benefit of plasma exchange in the therapy of AIMP.

ACKNOWLEDGMENT

This research was supported in part by the Veterans Administration Research Service and Grant NS18172 from the U.S. Public Health Service.

REFERENCES

1. Johnson, K.P., Wolinsky, J.S. and Ginsberg, A.H. Immune mediated syndromes of the nervous system related to virus infections. In: *Handbook of*

Clinical Neurology. Vol 34. Vinken P.J. and Bruyn G.W., eds. Amsterdam: North Holland, pp. 391–434, 1978.

2. Asbury, A.K., Arnason, B.A. and Adams, R.D. The inflammatory lesion in idiopathic polyneuritis. Its role in pathogenesis. *Medicine 48*:173–215, 1969.
3. Uchimura, I. and Shiraki, H. A. Contribution to the classification and pathogenesis of demyelinatring encephalomyelitis. *J. Neuropathol. Exp. Neurol. 16*:2139–203, 1957.
4. Witte, J.J. and Axnick, N.W. The benefits from 10 years of measles immunization in the United States. *Public Health Rep 90*:205–207, 1975.
5. Arnason, B.G.W. Inflammatory polyradiculoneuropathies. In: *Peripheral Neuropathy.* Dyck, P.J., Thomas, P.K. and Lambert, eds. Philadelphia: W.B. Saunders, pp. 1110–1148, 1975.
6. Fisher, M. An unusual variant of acute idiopathic polyneuritis (a syndrome of opthalmoplegia, ataxia and areflexia) *N. Engl. J. Med. 225*:57–65, 1956.
7. Schonberger, L.B., Bergman, D.J. Sullivan, Bolyai, J.Z., et al. Guillain-Barré syndrome following vaccination in the national influenza immunization program. United States 1976–1977. *Am. J. Epidemiol. 110*:105–123, 1979.

6

The Pathophysiology of
Bacterial Meningitis

John D. Waggener and John L. Beggs

INTRODUCTION

Bacterial meningitis is the most common type of central nervous system (CNS) infection. Most recent reviews of the subject quote an incidence of five per 100,000 with the majority of cases appearing in the pediatric age group.[1-4] Approximately 25,000 cases occur annually in the U.S. The mortality rate is 15 percent and the morbidity rate is at least twice this figure.[5]

Historically, medical science has experienced its greatest successes in the battle against pathogenic microbial invaders (this encounter is a battle in the sense that one biological creature invades and damages while the other responds defensively). As the antibiotic era emerged, CNS infections were no longer totally devastating events. From a theoretical position we had available the weaponry to master meningitis. In 1948, Adams, Kubik, and Bonner[6] were prompted to publish their now considered classic paper on *H. influenzae* meningitis because "antibiotics threatened to limit the availability of pathological material."

Yet, for 30 years we have seen little or no improvement in the overall experience. The current prognosis of bacterial meningitis is on an unimproving plateau with no significant change in sight. Statistics from our parent institution (St. Joseph's Hospital and Medical Center) are typical: in the five-year span from 1976 to 1980, there were a total of 444 cases of meningitis. The number of cases each year varied from 82 in 1979 to 99 in 1977, with 93 occurring in 1980. These statistics are also typical in that the majority of cases were caused by only three pathogens: *Hemophilus influenzae*, *Diplococcus pneumoniae*, and *Neisseria menigitidis*.

Much has been written regarding the pathogenesis, neurologic manifestations, and clinical management of meningitis; the reader is referred to recent reviews.[5,7] The purpose here is to assess the contributions of recent experimental findings to our knowledge of the pathophysiology. We include some of our own observations of experimental *E. coli meningitis* in guinea pigs.

EXPERIMENTAL MENINGITIS

During the past decade there has been renewed interest in experimental meningitis. A nontraumatic technique has been described for inducing *H. influenzae b* meningitis in infant rats.[8-11] Pneumonococcal meningitis in rabbits has been utilized by Beaty and co-workers to develop methods of: (1) quantitating the inflammatory mass;[12] (2) identifying possible mediators of CNS infections;[13] (3) evaluation of the mechanism of corticosteroid suppression of inflammation.[14] In addition, the concept that inflammation plays a significant role in the mortality and morbidity of meningitis received strong support in the *in vitro* findings of Fishman et al.[15]

Moxon et al.[8] were successful in producing *H. influenzae* meningitis in infant rats without traumatizing the CNS environs. Taking advantage of the host's inability to sneeze, the five-day old rats received an inocculum of pathogens into nasopharynx via the anterior nares. Approximately three fourths of the animals developed bacteremia and over one half developed meningitis. Bacteria invaded the nasopharyngeal mucous membrane, and an inflammatory response developed in the contiguous meninges. However, meningitis did not occur in the absence of bactereamia.

This is perhaps the first reported "naturally occurring" animal model for meningitis. The low host mortality rate provided the opportunity to study temporal progression of the disease. The reported findings support the thesis that bacteria inhabiting the nasopharynx reach the CNS via the circulation rather than by direct spread. The authors reported that organisms initially entered the CNS via the dural sinuses. This finding may be related to the widespread pachymeningitis that developed along with leptomeningeal involvement. Additional studies added credence to the long-standing impression that a focus of meningeal irritation may serve as an entry portal for blood-borne pathogens.[11]

Beaty and co-workers[12] have described a method of inducing pneumonococcal meningitis in rabbits. In a series of experiments they have used the model to evaluate a possible relationship between inflammatory mass and clinical dysfunctions. Sequential quantitative determination of inflammatory mass revealed a progressive increase to 72 hours. The mean survival time was 80 hours. Simultaneous white blood cell counts of the cerebrospinal fluid (CSF) did not correlate with the accumulating inflammatory mass. However, the increase in mass did correlate with the rise in CSF lactic acid dehydrogenase (LDH) levels. The authors concluded that LDH is an indicator of the quantity of inflammatory response. Conversely, others have related LDH levels to the bacterial population.[16] Using the model, Nolan et al.[13] found chemotactic agents in the CSF of animals with Pneumonococcal meningitis. This time sequence of appearance of chemotactic activity paralleled that of the accumulation of neutrophils in the meninges. Chemotactic activity has also been detected in the CSF of humans with meningitis.[17]

This model also provided the basis for determining how corticosteroids alter the inflammatory response.[14] Methyl prednisolone reduced the inflammatory mass without altering chemotactic activity or phagocytosis. Instead, the agent's anti-inflammatory effect resulted from inhibition of neutrophil adherence to endothelium. Margination and adherence to the endothelial wall are the initial steps in the inflammatory response. They are prerequisites for neutrophil emigration through the vessel wall to the site of injury.

Perhaps the strongest indictment of neutrophils in damaging brain parenchyma has come from an *in vitro* study by Fishman et al.[15] Incubation of brain slices with a membrane fraction derived from neutrophils resulted in cerebral edema with intracellular electrolye imbalance. The brain tissue also demonstrated increased glucose oxidation and lactate production associated with energy depletion. The authors concluded that neutrophils contain toxic factors which alter brain cell membranes. This effect probably plays a role in the development of cerebral edema and the encephalophies associated with CNS inflammatory diseases.

NEUTROPHIL EMIGRATION

In order for the inflammatory response to evolve, neutrophils must transfer from the circulation to the CSF. This crossing of the vascular wall is referred to as emigration; the event has been observed outside the CNS by students of inflammation for at least 160 years.[18] The bulk of our knowledge of emigration has been provided by *in vivo* techniques using mesenteric and ear chamber preparations. Ultrastructural studies of these preparations have shown that neutrophils cross the endothelium at inter-cellular junctions.[19,20] However, little is known concerning the route of emigration after injury to the CNS.

To study emigration in the CNS we induced meningitis in guinea pigs by intracisternal injection of *E. coli* bacteria.[21] In this model the inflammatory response in the leptomeninges is well developed at three hours after injection. The epipial veins and venules contain many neutro-phils attached to the endothelial luminal surfaces (Figures 1 and 2). The adhesive quality of the attachments is quite striking in view of the fact that tissue fixation was achieved by intra-arterial perfusion. In CNS tissues not in or near the leptomeninges, the vessel luminae were clear of all blood elements.

At sites of neutrophil attachment a bulge on the extraluminal sur-face of the endothelium is evidence that emigration is underway (Figure 2). The pathway cannot be clearly delineated by light microscopy, but the endothelial gap is apparently quite limited because the neutrophil must assume a constricted form in order to accomplish the passage. At the ultrastructural level, the intraluminal relationships between endotheli-um and the adhering neutrophil are seen in Figures 3 and 4. The intimate contacts between the opposing plasmalemmata seldom span a continu-ous area of the neutrophil surface; they occur where projections of the neutrophil form pseudopods that are capable of indenting the endotheli-al plasmalemma (Figure 4). Such contacts may represent specific adher-ence sites on the surface of both neutrophil and endothelium. Alternatively, the pattern of contacts could be interpreted as merely a manifestation of neutrophil locomotion.

Specialized junctions between the contiguous plasmalemmata are not observed. The pattern of contact sites, however, suggests a specific relationship; the paralleled leaflets are intimately associated, and the endothelial moiety exhibits increased density (Figure 4). The contact sites are usually found near an intercellular junctional complex (Figure 3).

Before initiation of emigration, the endothelial barrier remains in-tact. The tight junctions are not altered and transendothelial gaps cannot be found.

Emigration is heralded by a pseudopod of neutrophilic hyaloplasm projecting through a gap in the endothelium (Figure 5). The gap is mem-brane-bound and is invariably found in close association with a junction-al complex (Figure 5). The width remains fairly uniform and shows little tendency to further expansion, except when occupied by a segment of cytoplasm containing the nucleus (Figure 6; see also Figure 8). The entire

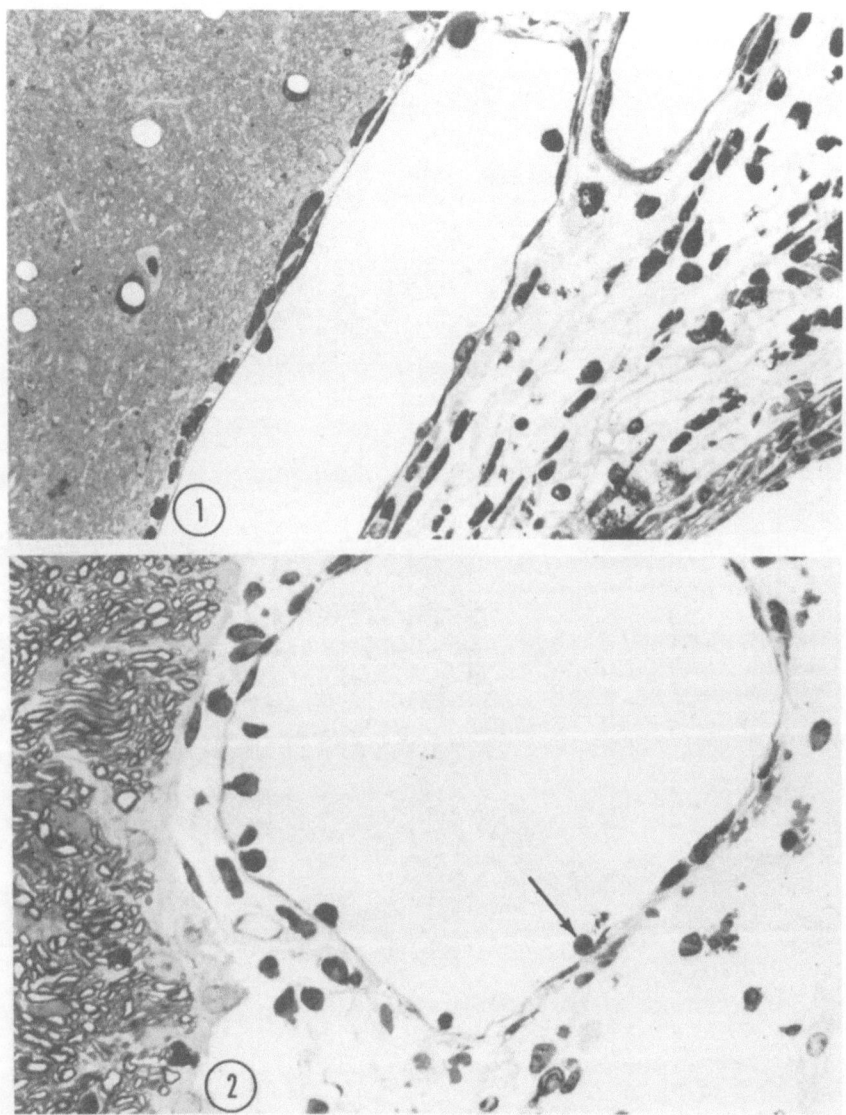

Figure 1. Acute *E. coli* meningitis. Neutrophils infiltrate the leptomeninges and cuff the thin-walled veins. One vein (left) contains three neutrophils attached to the endothelium. (Magnification, X400.)

Figure 2. Neutrophils are attached to the luminal surface of an epipial vein. The arrow identifies a neutrophil in the early stages of emigration. (Magnification, X400.)

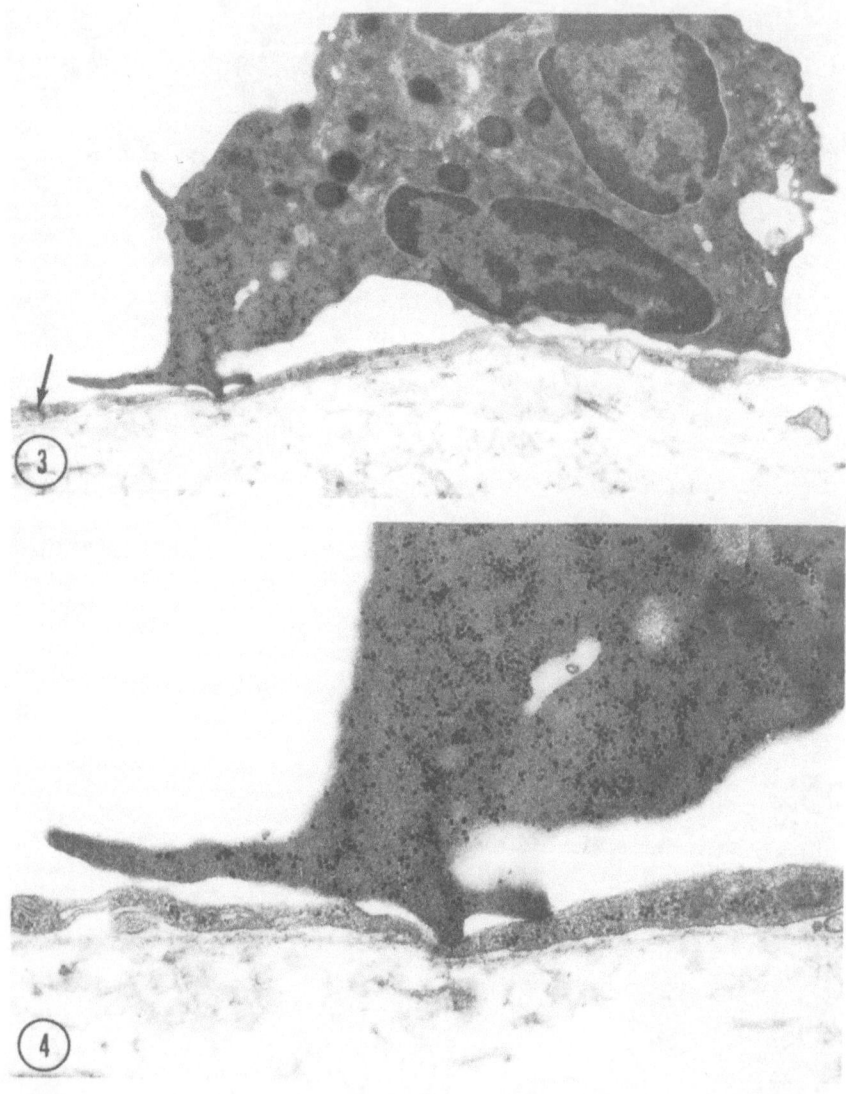

Figure 3. Neutrophil contacts on the luminal endothelium plasmalemma. A junctional complex (arrow) is identified near the contact sites. (Magnification, X10,000.)

Figure 4. Higher magnification of the contact sites shown in **Figure 3.** The subajacent endothelium is indented and compressed. The contiguous plasmalemmata are closely associated. There is increased density of the endothelial plasmalemma at the contact sites. (Magnification, X26,000.)

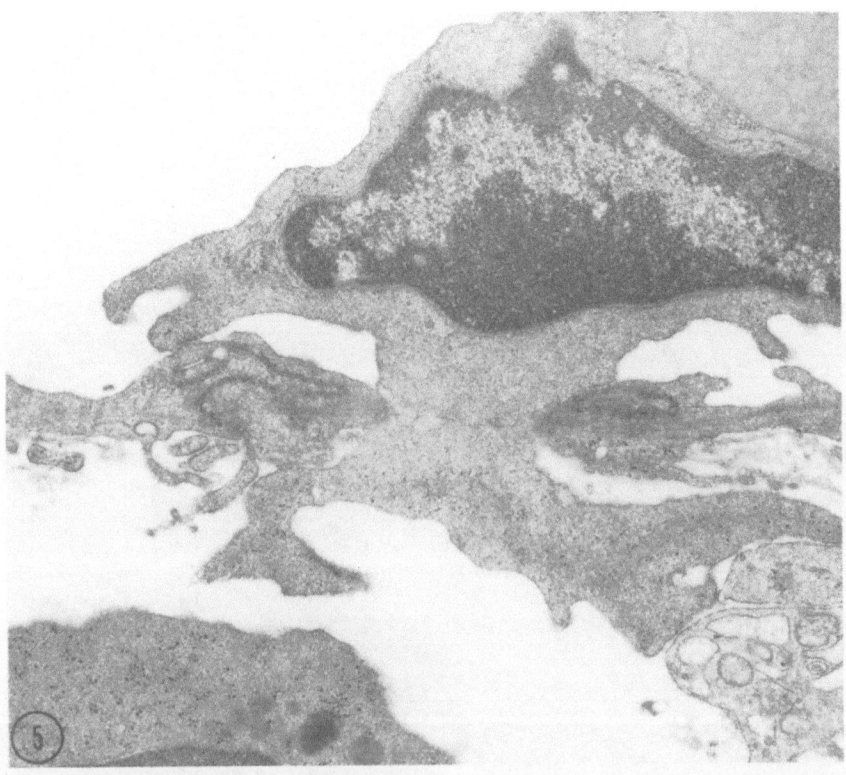

Figure 5. Emigration, early stages. A pseudopod of hyaloplasm from the intraluminal neutrophil extends through an endothelial gap. Segments of the endothelial intercellular junction can be identified on each side. At the margins the endothelial cytoplasm bears microfilaments aligned perpendicular to the gap. (Magnification, X22,000.)

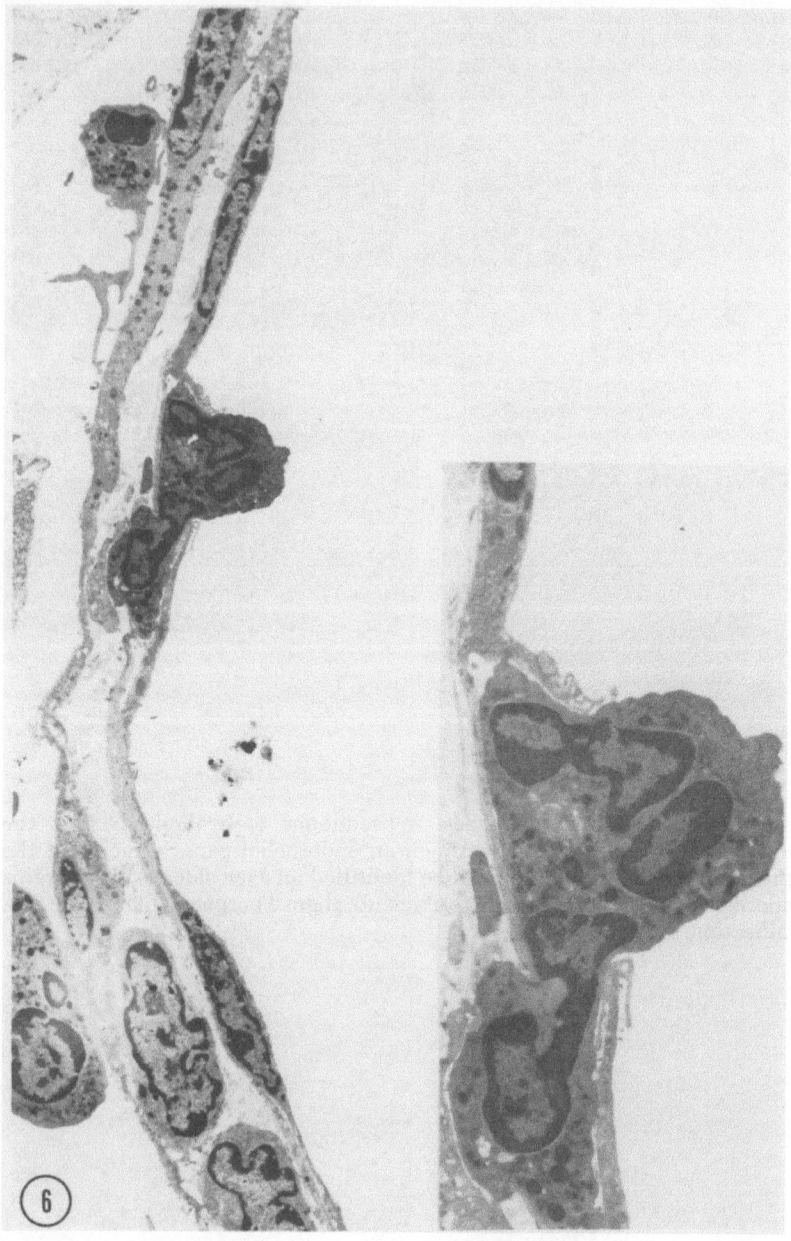

Figure 6. Emigration, midstage. The venular endothelial gap is expanded where the nucleus is in transit. Higher magnification (inset) shows the route of passage through the adventitia. (Magnification, X2,400. Inset, X5,700.)

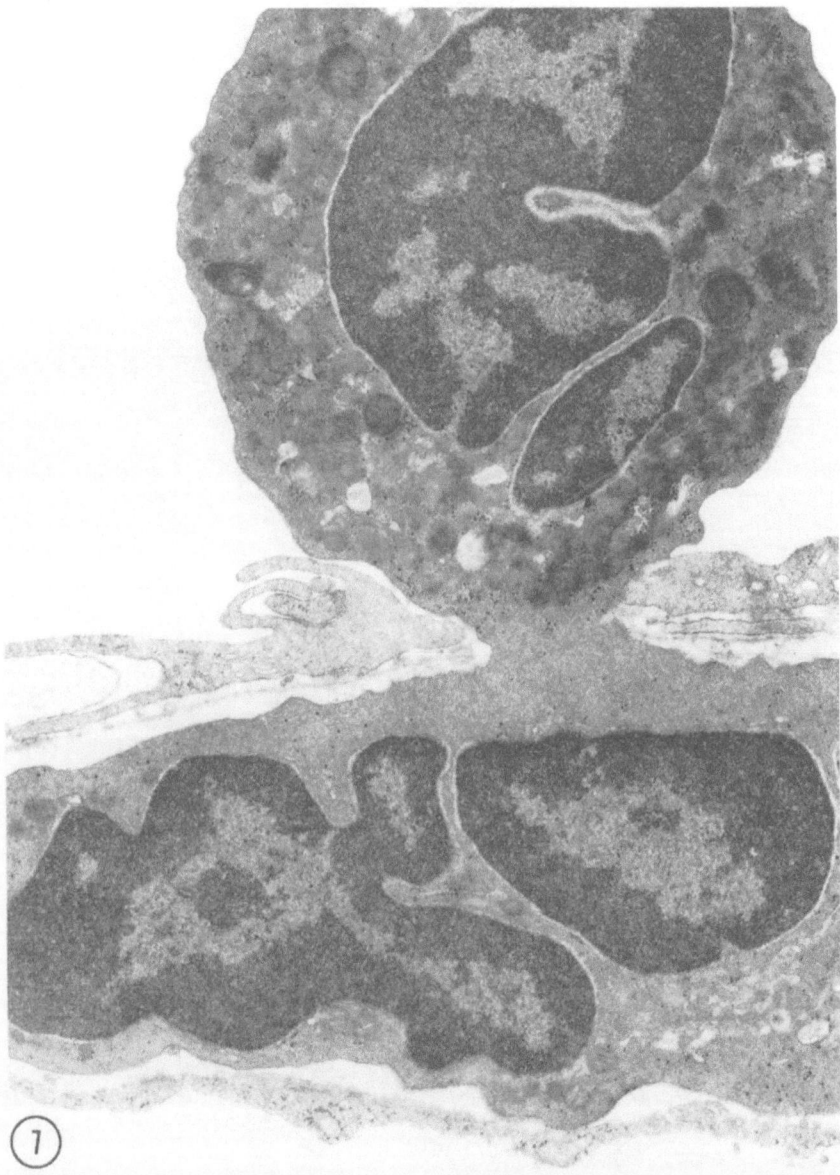

Figure 7. Emigration, midstage. The constrictive effect of the endothelial gap is evident. The portion of neutrophil within the gap contains only hyaloplasm. The nuclear segments and organelles in the extruded moiety (below) exited at a different level. Same neutrophil as shown in Figure 8; the level shown is nine serial sections from Figure 8b. (Magnification, X12,300.)

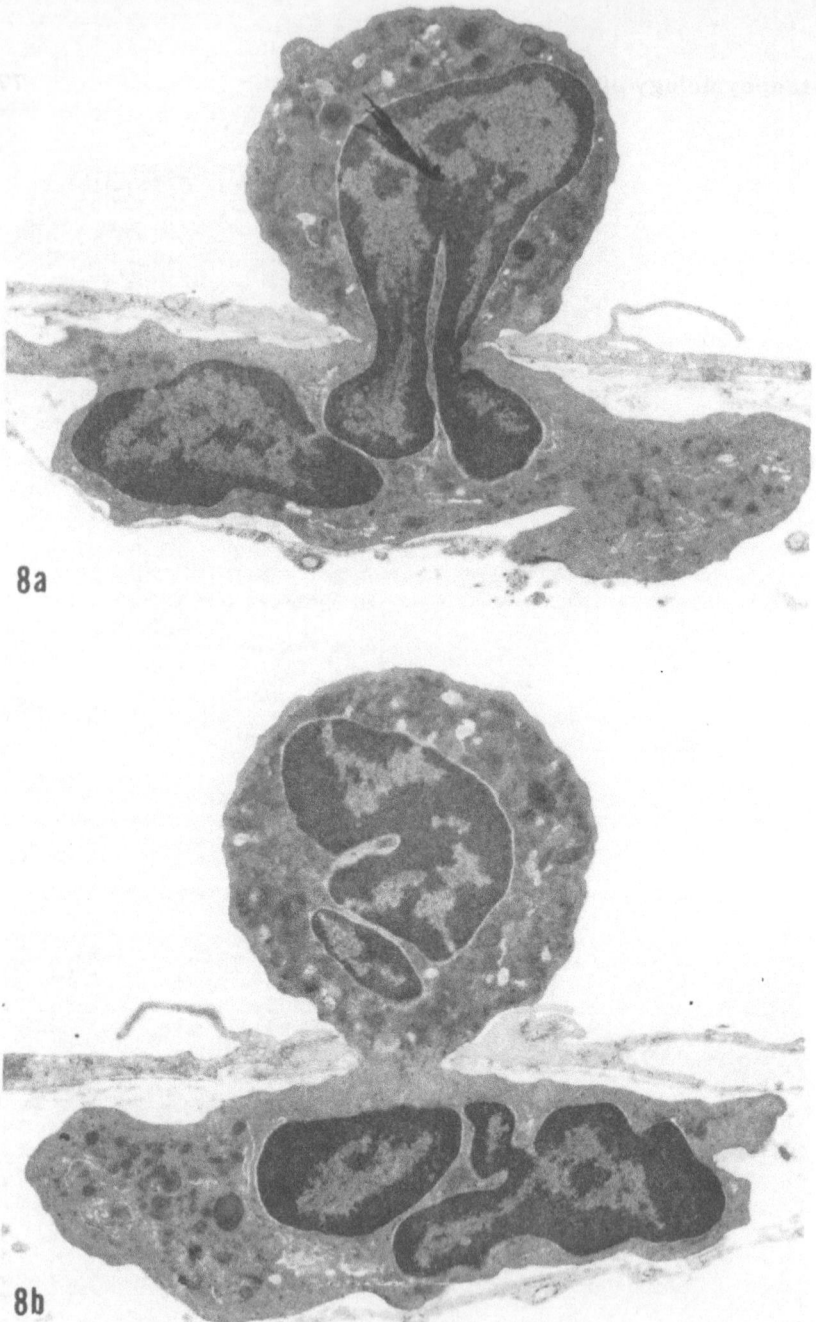

Figure 8. Serial step sections of an emigrating neutrophil. (a) Nucleus in transit. (b) Section from near the periphery of the gap. The thin adventitia does not impair the emigrative process. (c) Section immediately distal to the gap. The two segments of the neutrophil are separated by the intact endothelial junctional complex. (d) Section distal to figure c. The intraluminal and extraluminal segments appear as two separate cells. (Magnification, X5,780 for figures a through d.)

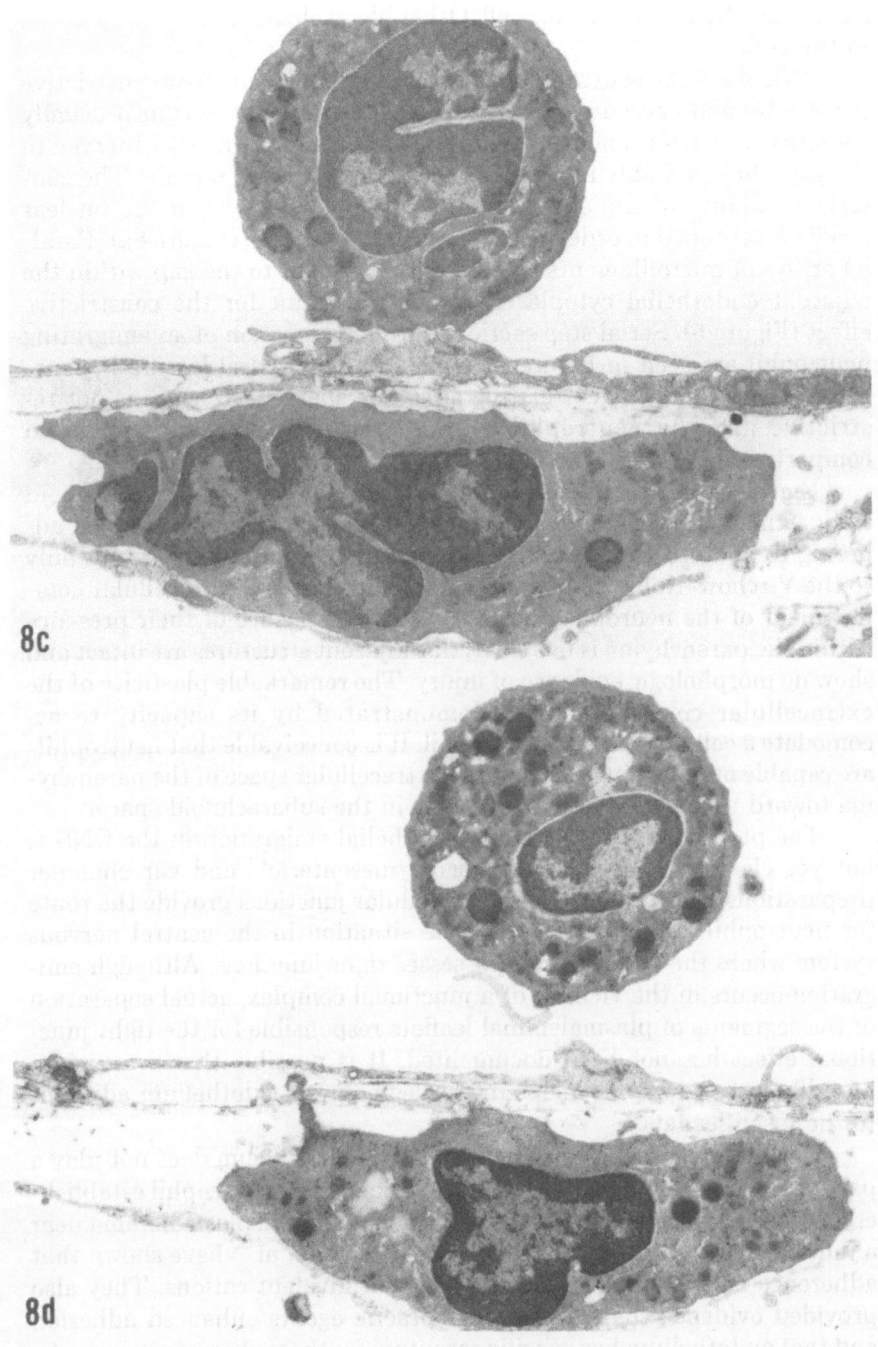

gap is filled by the emigrating cell. Other blood elements are not observed in the area.

As more of the neutrophil passes through, the hour-glass constrictive pattern becomes accentuated (Figure 7). The segment in transit usually contains only homogenous hyaloplasm. Organelles are rarely observed in the gap; they probably move in aggregates and transit rapidly. The constrictive ability of the endothelium is most evident when the nuclear profile is reshaped in order to accomplish the passage (Figure 8a). Parallel arrays of microfilaments aligned perpendicular to the gap within the adjacent endothelial cytoplasm probably account for the constrictive effect (Figure 5). Serial step sections through a portion of an emigrating neutrophil are seen in Figure 8. The endothelial basal lamina is penetrated immediately at the exiting site. The sparce adventitia is not restrictive and the neutrophil is soon free within the subarachnoid compartment.

Emigration is not limited to the vasculature within the subarachnoid compartment. In the subpial parenchyma, neutrophils are observed adhering to and crossing venular endothelium. They gain access not only to the Virchow–Robin spaces but can be found in the extracellular compartment of the neuropil (Figure 9). The significance of their presence within the parenchyma is not clear; the adjacent structures are intact and show no morphologic evidence of injury. The remarkable plasticity of the extracellular compartment is demonstrated by its capacity to accomodate a cell the size of a neutrophil. It is conceivable that neutrophils are capable of migrating through the extracellular space of the parenchyma toward the chemotactic attractions in the subarachnoid space.

The precise pathway of transendothelial emigration in the CNS is not yet clearly defined. Studies using mesenteric[19] and ear chamber preparations[20] have shown that intercellular junctions provide the route for neutrophils. This may not be the situation in the central nervous system where the endothelium possesses tight junctions. Although emigration occurs in the vicinity of a junctional complex, actual separation of the segments of plasmalemmal leaflets responsible for the tight junctional effect has not been documented. It is possible that a transient pore-like passageway develops in the segment of endothelium adjacent to the fused leaflets.

These and other findings indicate that endothelium does not play a passive role in the emigrative process. The adhering neutrophil establishes a specific relationship with the endothelial luminal plasmalemma near a junctional complex. Recent studies by Hoover et al.[22] have shown that adherence is dependent on the presence of divalent cations. They also provided evidence that certain chemotactic agents enhanced adhesion and that endothelium has specific receptors for these chemotactic agents.

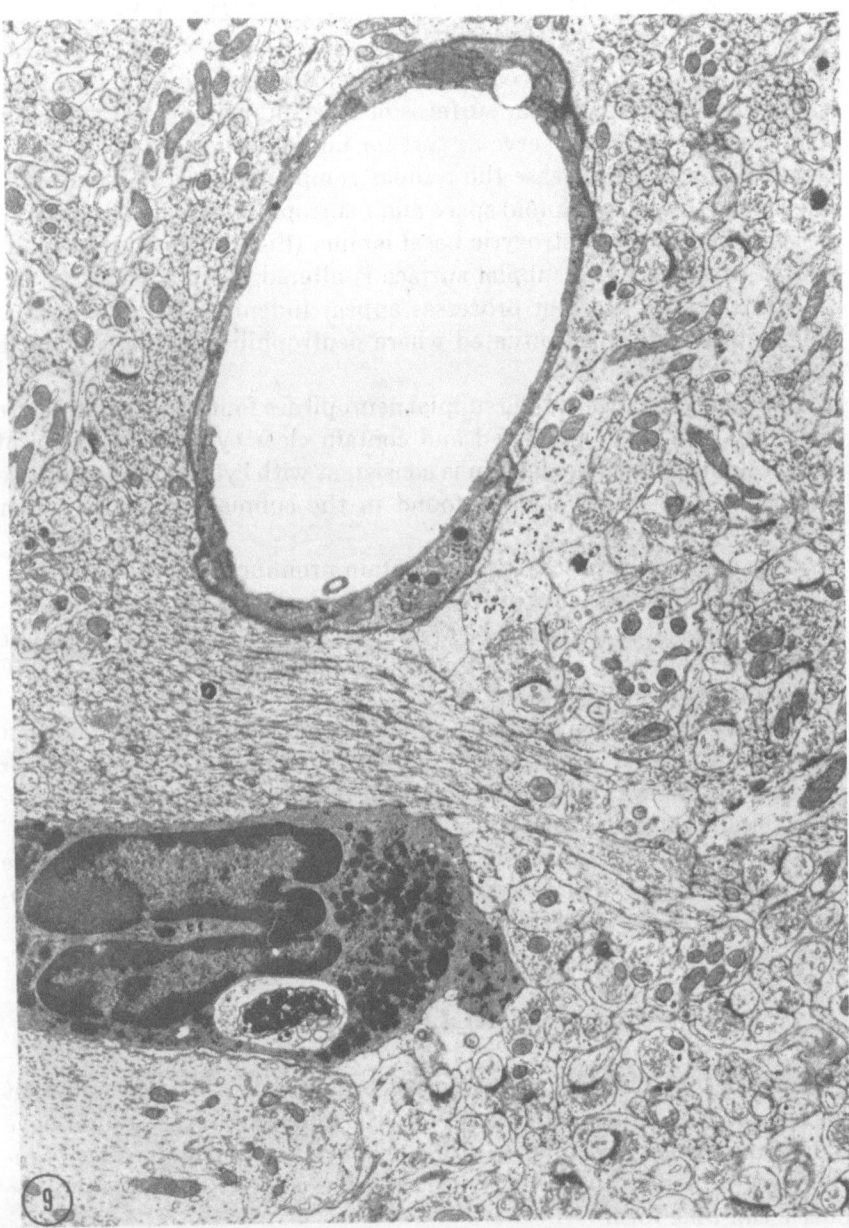

Figure 9. A neutrophil (below) occupies the extracellular space of the cerebellar molecular layer. The adjunct neurites and glial processes appear unaltered. (Magnification, X10,200.)

NEUTROPHIL–NEUROPIL RELATIONSHIPS

Once emigration is accomplished, neutrophils are found in close association with the cellular surfaces of the leptomeninges (Figure 10). Such contacts probably serve as turf for migration toward chemotactic agents. Early in the disease the cellular components of the pia are displaced into the subarachnoid space and neutrophils establish direct contact with the subpial astrocytic basal lamina (Figure 10). The normally smooth contour of the subpial surface is altered by such contacts: the contiguous astrocytic foot processes appear indented and compressed. This disfacement is accentuated where neutrophilic pseudopods touch the surface (Figure 11).

The major changes in the subpial neuropil are found in the astrocytic processes. Many are expanded and contain clear cytoplasm typical of fluid accumulation. The pattern is consistent with cytotoxic edema. The involved processes are usually found in the subpial and perivascular zones.

The edematous processes also contain prominent deposits of glycogen particles. The presence of glycogen is evidence that the normal pathway of glucose utilization has been altered. Conversion to the glycolytic pathway is thought to be at least partially responsible for depressed CSF glucose levels in meningitis.[23]

These observations provide no conclusive formation regarding what role—if any—neutrophils play in damaging brain parenchyma. Their presence within the extracellular space of the neuropil is tolerated without structural alterations in the adjacent neural and glial processes (Figure 9). However, neutrophils in the bacteria-containing CSF may not be as innocuous; once "activated" and phagocytic, they may release substances toxic to the underlying neuropil.

CONCLUSIONS

The pathophysiology of meningitis entails a cascade of events that are not yet well defined. In recent years the more rewarding studies have sought to unravel the kinetics of a single event. Many experiments involving a wide spectrum of biological expertise will be required before the puzzle can take form.

In the immediate future the endothelium should provide a fertile area for investigation. Once considered primarily as a unicellular interphase between circulation and tissue, it is now known to have multiple functions, including a major role in blood coagulation and fibrinolysis.[24]

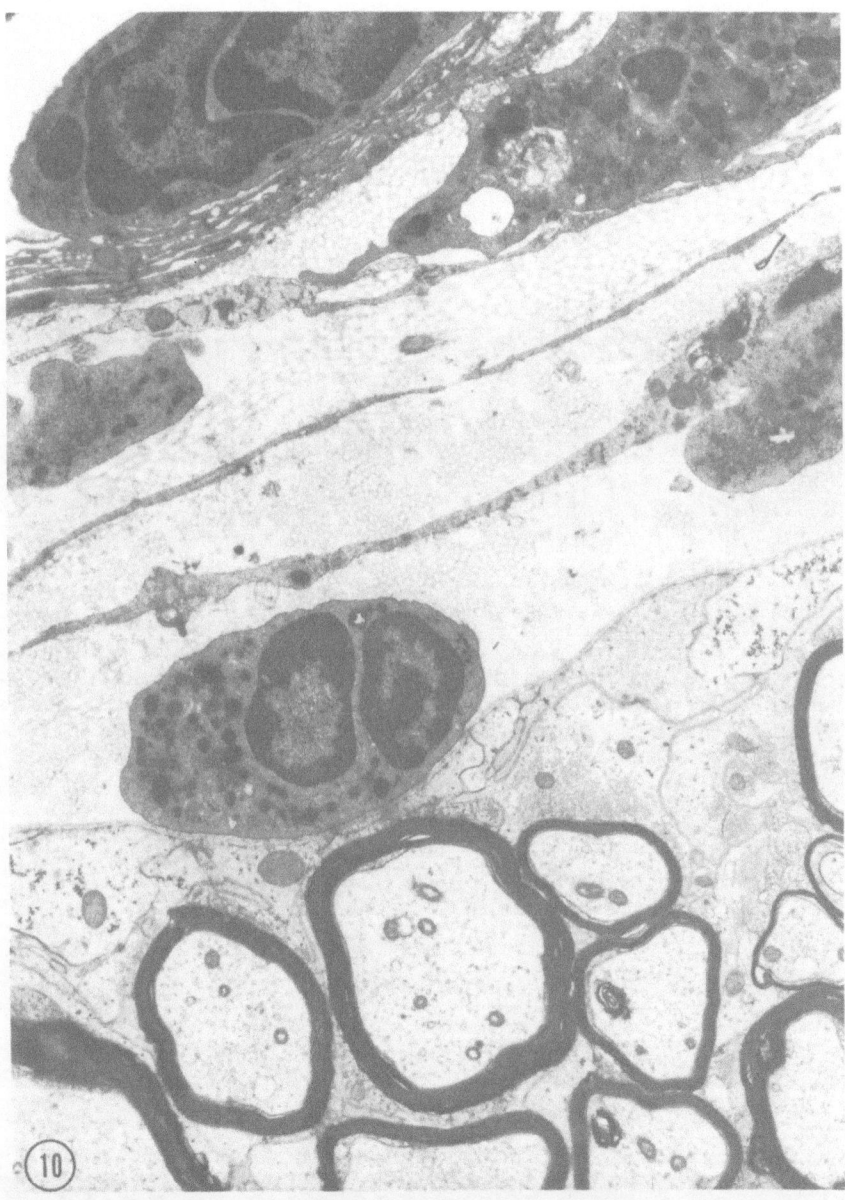

Figure 10. Neutrophils in the subarachnoid space, cervical spinal cord. One (upper left) is within a dorsal root sheath. Another (below) borders and indents the cord surface. Note the absence of pial cells along the cord's surface. (Magnification, X18,000.)

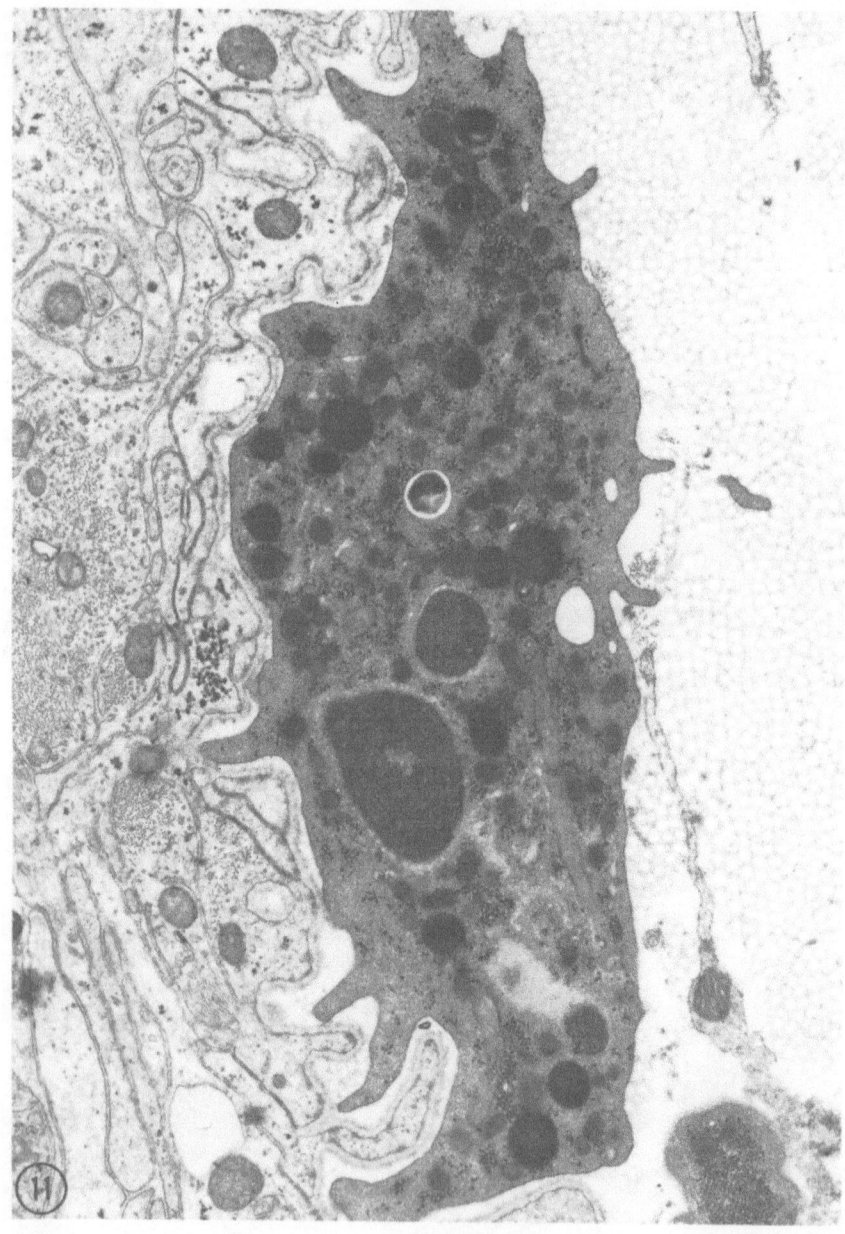

Figure 11. Pseudopods from the crab-shaped neutrophil invaginate the brain surface. Astrocytic foot processes are swollen by pale edematous cytoplasm and contain glycogen particles. (Magnification, X19,300.)

Recently developed techniques for isolation and growth in tissue culture of CNS endothelial cells now provide access to an ample quantity of tissue for study.[25,26] There is growing evidence that the functional characteristics of endothelium vary in many segments of the vascular system; this is most evident in the CNS where the unique structural features of the blood-brain barrier have been identified.[27]

The study of inflammation as a biological phenomenon has occupied many distinguished scientists and has produced a voluminous literature.[28] A recent review of the subject was published in three volumes.[29] Yet, this impressive amount of information contains virtually no mention of inflammation as related to the CNS. In the past, avoidance of neural tissue for experimentation was no doubt related to the availability of more readily attainable *in vivo* preparations elsewhere. Recent technological advances will provide an opportunity for CNS experimentation to move toward the mainstream of inflammation science.

REFERENCES

1. Cooper, R.M., and Noble, R.C. Bacterial meningitis: a review of the pathophysiology, diagnosis, and treatment. *J. Kentucky Med. Assoc.* August 1976.
2. Nankervis, G.A. Bacterial meningitis. *Med. Clin. North Am.* 58:581–592, 1974.
3. LeFrock, J.L., Prince, R.A. and Klainer, A.S. Bacterial meningitis. *J. Am. Pharm. Assoc.* 16:208–210, 216, 1976.
4. Smith, D.H., Ingram, D.L. Smith, A.L., Giles, F., and Bresnan, M.J. Diagnosis and treatment. Bacterial meningitis. A symposium. *Pediatrics* 52:586–600, 1973.
5. Underman, A.E., Overturf, G.D., and Leedom, J.M. *Bacterial Meningitis—1978.* Chicago: Year Book Medical Publishers, 1978:1–63.
6. Adams, R.D., Kubik, C.S., and Bonner, F.J. Clinical and pathological aspects of influenzal meningitis. *Arch Pediatr.* 65:408–441, 1948.
7. Swartz, M.N., and Dodge. P.R. Bacterial meningitis-a review of selected aspects. General clinical features, special problems and unusual meningeal reactions mimicking bacterial meningitis. II. Special neurological problems, postmeningitic complications and clinicopathological correlations (concluded). *N. Engl. J. Med.* 272:723–730, 779–787, 842–824, 898–902, 954–960, 1003–1009, 1965.
8. Moxon, E.R., Smith, A.L., Averill, D.R., Smith, D.H. Haemophilus influenzae meningitis in infant rats after intranasal inoculation. *J. Infect. Dis.* 129:154–162, 1974.
9. Moxon, E.R., Glode, M.P., Sutton, A. and Robbins, J.B. The infant rat as a model of bacterial meningitis. *J. Infect. Dis.* 136:186–190, 1977.
10. Moxon, E.R., and Ostrow, P.T. Haemophilus influenzae meningitis in infant rats: role of bacteremia in pathogenesis of age-dependent inflammatory responses in cerebrospinal fluid. *J. Infect. Dis.* 135:303–307, 1977.

11. Ostrow, P.T., Moxon, E.R., Vernon, N., and Kapko. R. Pathogenesis of bacterial meningitis. Studies on the route of meningeal invasion following Hemophilus influenzae inoculation of infant rats. *Lab. Invest. 40*:678–685, 1979.

12. McAllister, C.K., O'Donoghue, J.M., and Beaty, H.N. Experimental pneumococcal meningitis. II. Characterization and quantitation of the inflammatory process. *J. Infect. Dis. 132*:255–360, 1975.

13. Nolan, C.M., Clark, R.A., Beaty, H.N. Experimental pneumococcal meningitis. III. Chemotactic activity in cerebrospinal fluid[1] (38989). *Proc. Soc. Exp. Biol. Med. 150*:134–136, 1975.

14. Nolan, C.M., McAllister, C.K., Walters, B., and Beaty H.N. Experimental pneumococcal meningitis. IV. The effect of methyl prednisolone on meningeal inflammation. *J. Lab. Clin. Med. 91*:979–988, 1978.

15. Fishman, R.A., Sligar, K., and Hake, R.B. Effects of leukocytes on brain metabolism in granulocytic brain edema. *Ann. Neurol. 2*:89–94, 1977.

16. Feldman, W.E. Concentrations of bacteria in cerebrospinal fluid of patients with bacterial meningitis. *J. Pediatr. 88*:549–552, 1976.

17. Wyler, D.J., Wasserman, S.I., and Karchmer, A.W. Substances which modulate leukocyte migration are present in CSF during meningitis. *Ann. Neurol. 5*:322–326, 1979.

18. Grant, L. The sticking and emigration of white blood cells in inflammation. in: *The Inflammatory Process.* Zweifach, B.W., Grant, L., and McCluskey, R.T., eds. New York and London: Academic Press, pp. 205–249, 1973.

19. Marchesi, V.T. and Florey, H.W. Electron micrographic observations on the emigration of leucocytes. *Q. J. Exp. Physiol. Coll. Med. Sci. 45*:343, 1960.

20. Florey, H.W., and Grant, L.H. Leucocyte migration from small blood vessels stimulated by ultraviolet light: an electron microscope study. *J. Pathol. Bacteriol. 82*, 13, 1961.

21. Waggener, J.D. The pathophysiology of bacterial meningitis and cerebral abscesses: an anatomical interpretation. In: *Advances in Neurology,* Thompson, R.A. and Green, J.R., eds. New York: Raven Press, pp. 1–17, 1974.

22. Hoover, R.L., Folger, R. Haering, W.A., Ware, B.R., and Karnovsky, M.J. Adhesion of leukocytes to endothelium: roles of divalent cations, surface charge, chemotactic agents and substrate. *J. Cell. Sci. 45*:73–86, 1980.

23. Menkes, J.H. The causes for low spinal fluid sugar in bacterial meningitis: another look. *Commentary Ped. 44*:1–3 1969.

24. Mason, R.G., Mohammad, S.F., Saba, H.I., Chuang, H.Y.K., Lee, E.L., and Balis, J.U. Functions of endothelium. *Pathobiol. Annu. 9*:1–48, 1979.

25. Brendel, K., Meezan, E., and Carlson, E.C. Isolated brain microvessels: a purified, metabolically active preparation from bovine cerebral cortex. *Science 185*:953–955, 1974.

26. DeBault, L.E., Kahn, L.E., Frommes, S.P., and Cancilla, P.S. Cerebral microvessels and derived cells in tissue culture: isolation and preliminary characterization. *In Vitro 15*:473–487, 1979.

27. Reese, T.S., and Karnovsky, M.J. Fine structure localization of a blood-brain barrier to exogenous peroxidase. *J. Cell Biol. 34*:207–217, 1967.

28. Ryan, G.B., and Majno, G. Review article—acute inflammation. *Am. J. Pathol. 86*:185, 1977.

29. Zweifach, B.W., Grant, L., and McCluskey, R.T., eds. *The Inflammatory Process-Second Edition.* Vol. I, II, and III. New York and London: Academic Press, 1973, 1974.

7

Treatment of Bacterial Infections
of The Central Nervous System

William E. Bell

For optimal treatment of bacterial meningitis, it is desirable that the antibiotic chosen be bactericidal and able to achieve CSF levels in excess of the minimum bactericidal concentration for the causative organism. Combination of antimicrobials are avoided that might be antagonistic to one another relative to the organism that is isolated. For example, chloramphenicol antagonizes the bactericidal action of penicillin or ampicillin against *Streptococcus pneumoniae* and Group B Streptococcus. Chloramphenicol also interferes with the bactericidal action of gentamicin against certain Gram-negative enteric rods.

The importance of antibiotics which have bactericidal effects is partly related to the concept that CSF represents a regional site considered to be one of impaired host resistance against infection.[1,2] Immunoglobulin and complement contents are quite low in infected CSF compared with serum and, for this reason, opsonic activity which is essential for the preparation of bacteria for phagocytosis by leukocytes is impaired in CSF. This may account for the very high density of bacteria that is often found in CSF in patients with meningitis before initiation of antibiotic therapy.

Encapsulation of bacteria inhibits opsonization in serum and CSF, and most cases of sepsis-induced meningitis in previously healthy persons are caused by encapsulated organisms, including *Hemophilus influen-*

TABLE 1. Antibiotic Dosages for Bacterial Meningitis (Birth to Two Months)

Ampicillin	150–200 mg/kg/day, IV (q6-8h)
Penicillin G	
Less than one week	150,000 units/kg/day, IV (q6-8h)
One week to two months	150,000–250,000 units/kg/day, IV (q6-8h)
Group B *Streptococcus*	300,000–400,000 units/kg/day, IV (q6-8h)
Methicillin	100 mg/kg/day, IV (q6-8h)
Nafcillin	100 mg/kg/day, IV (q6-8h)
Carbenicillin	300 mg/kg/day, IV (q6-8h)
Ticarcillin	200–300 mg/kg/day, IV (q6-8h)
Kanamycin	
Less than one week	20 mg/kg/day, IM (q12h)
One week to two months	30 mg/kg/day, IM (q8h)
Gentamicin	
Less than one week	5 mg/kg/day, IM (q12h)
One week to two months	7.5 mg/kg/day, IM (q8h)
Tobramycin	
Less than one week	5 mg/kg/day, IM (q12h)
One week to two months	7.5 mg/kg/day, IM (q8h)
Amikacin	
Less than one week	15 mg/kg/day, IM (q12h)
One week to two months	22.5 mg/kg/day, IM (q8h)
Moxalactam	100 mg/kg/day, IV (q8h)
Cefotaxime	100 mg/kg/day, IV (q8h)
Chloramphenicol	
Premature (birth to 1 mth)	25 mg/kg/day, IV (q12h)
Full-term (1st 7 days)	25 mg/kg/day, IV (q12h)
Full-term (7 to 30 days)	50 mg/kg/day, IV (q8h)
Full-term (1 to 2 mths)	50-100 mg/kg/day, IV (q6h)
Intrathecal agents — administered daily or every second day (dose depends on ventricular capacity)	
Gentamicin	1–3 mg
Amikacin	2–5 mg
Methicillin	10–25 mg
Erythromycin	3–10 mg

zae type b, *Streptococcus pneumoniae*, and *Neisseria meningitidis*. Conversely, unencapsulated bacteria are much less common causes of meningitis unless secondary to an infected indwelling foreign body, such as a ventricular shunt, or a complication of a neurosurgical procedure, an open head injury, or a CSF fistula. Thus, the presence or absence of a capsule is one of the factors determining whether meningitis will develop in the immunocompetent septic patient, and the "CSF-resistance

TABLE 2. Antibiotic Dosages for Bacterial Meningitis
(Over Two Months — Up to 50 kg Body Weight)

Ampicillin	300–400 mg/kg/day, IV (q4h)
Penicillin G	250,000 units/kg/day, IV (q4h)
Methicillin	200–300 mg/kg/day, IV (q4h)
Nafcillin	200 mg/kg/day, IV (q4h)
Carbenicillin	400–600 mg/kg/day, IV (q4h)
Ticarcillin	300–400 mg/kg/day, IV (q4h)
Chloramphenicol	75–100 mg/kg/day, IV (q6h)
Gentamicin	4 mg/kg/day, IM (q8h)
Tobramycin	4 mg/kg/day, IM (q8h)
Amikacin	15 mg/kg/day, IM (q8h)
Moxalactam	150 mg/kg/day, IV (q6h)
Cefotaxime	150 mg/kg/day, IV (q4-gh)
Rifampin	15–20 mg/kg/day, PO (q8h) (up to 600 mg)
Streptomycin	20–40 mg/kg/day, IM (q12h) (not over 1g)
Vancomycin	40–60 mg/kg/day, IV (q6h)
Tetracycline	30–50 mg/kg/day, IV (q8-12h)
Sulfadiazine	150 mg/kg/day, IV (q8h)
Metronidazole	30–40 mg/kg/day, po (q6-8h)

deficiency" relative to phagocytosis contributes to the rapid progression of the suppurative process, once bacteria have gained entrance into the meninges and subarachnoid space.

In the past two decades, there have been major advances in the development of new antibiotics for the treatment of meningitis. In addition, investigative efforts have yielded a broader comprehension of the pharmacokinetics of the available drugs in various age groups (see Tables 1, 2). Relatively new additions of importance in select instances include metronidazole, moxalactam, and cefotaxime. Relatively new uses of "old" drugs have been designed for vancomycin and rifampin. Vancomycin can play a valuable role in certain cases of methicillin-resistant staphylococcal infections, enterococcal Group D *Streptococcus* infections, and *Flavobacterium meningosepticum* meningitis. Rifampin is now the drug of choice for meningococcal prophylaxis, and is used, with vancomycin, for certain cases of resistant *Staphylococcus* meningitis and for *Flavobacterium meningosepticum* meningitis.

Despite the obvious advances that have been made in recent years, there remain certain types of meningitis which create major problems in management. These include:

1. Group B *Streptococcus* meningitis in the neonate.
2. Gram-negative enteric meningitis in the neonate.
3. Gram-negative (*Escherichia coli, Klebsiella Pseudomonas, Serratia*) meningitis complicating chronic illness, craniocerebral trauma, or neurosurgical procedures in children or adults.
4. *Listeria monocytogenes* meningitis in the immunosuppressed or chronically ill adult.
5. Staphylococcal (shunt) meningitis, currently with an incidence of 50 to 60 percent caused by methicillin-resistant organisms.

One of the most perplexing problems concerning treatment is the optimal selection and route of administration of antibiotics for Gram-negative enteric meningitis in either the newborn infant or the adult. Ampicillin does not rapidly eradicate such organisms from the CSF, even when sensitive, and the aminoglycosides penetrate poorly into the CSF in doses that can be safely given. Chloramphenicol is only bacteriostatic against most members of this group and has not been shown to be consistently effective, despite its excellent penetrability into the CSF. A recent publication by Cherubin et al.[3] describes the inadequacy of chloramphenicol for treatment of *Escherichia coli* meningitis. Among 64 cases in their series, the mortality rate with ampicillin plus gentamicin was 44 percent but with chloramphenicol and an aminoglycoside it was 75 percent. Mortality rate with chloramphenicol plus ampicillin was 89 percent. While experience is still limited, the new cephalosporins and cephalosporin-like drugs, including moxalactam and cefotaxime, show promise as important drugs for these infections. Both have a high level of activity against Gram-negative enteric organisms, *Hemophilus influenzae,* and *Neisseria meningitidis,* but considerably less activity against *Pseudomonas* species, and Gram-positive organisms. Both drugs also appear to be well tolerated and penetrate well into the CSF. Moxalactam, cefotaxime, and future "third-generation" cephalosporins, alone or in combination with an aminoglycoside or one of the extended spectrum penicillins, should improve the outlook for many patients with Gram-negative bacillary meningitis and for the infrequent multiply resistant cases of *Hemophilus influenzae* meningitis.

NEONATAL MENINGITIS

For Group B *Streptococcus* meningitis in the neonate, penicillin G in a dose of 250,000 units/kg/day is the drug of choice, administered every eight hours over a 20-minute period of time. The occurrence of relapse during treatment and the difficulty with rapid eradication of the organism from the CSF in some cases has led to the need for higher doses of penicillin G in some instances.

The clinical importance of the synergism between ampicillin and gentamicin[4] against Group B *Streptococcus* remains unclear. This combination might be considered in patients who do not rapidly respond to penicillin therapy alone or when meningitis has relapsed on more than one occasion despite adequate penicillin therapy. The recent demonstration of antagonism by chloramphenicol of the bactericidal activity of ampicillin against Group B *Streptococcus* is suggestive evidence against the use of this combination for infections caused by this organism.[5] In addition to Group B *Streptococcus*, penicillin is the drug of choice for neonatal meningitis caused by *Streptococcus pneumoniae*, and the infrequent cases resulting from Group A *Streptococcus*, nonenterococcal Group D *Streptococcus*, and *Pasteurella multocida*.

Ampicillin in dosages of 150 to 200 mg/kg/day is generally optimal therapy for neonatal meningitis due to *Listeria monocytogenes*, *Proteus mirabilis*, and the rare neonatal case of β-lactamase-negative *Hemophilus influenzae*. Indole-positive *Proteus* species and *Pseudomonas* species meningitis are very difficult to overcome and require carbenicillin in combination with gentamicin or tobramycin.

Enterococcal Group D *Streptococci* are often found to exhibit multiple antibiotic resistance, including resistance to penicillin, requiring sensitivity tests for the best choice of antibiotic therapy. Because of synergism of ampicillin with gentamicin against these organisms, this combination is usually selected.[6] Most strains of *Salmonella* species are sensitive to ampicillin or chloramphenicol while staphylococcal meningitis in the newborn period is managed with a combination of methicillin or nafcillin in combination with gentamicin until the organism is specifically defined and its sensitivities are known. Should the infected infant have renal failure, nafcillin would be a more appropriate penicillinase-resistant penicillin because of its secretion via the biliary system.

Flavobacterium meningosepticum is an uncommon cause of neonatal meningitis and is usually resistant to the penicillins and the aminoglycosides but is most often sensitive to rifampin, vancomycin, and erythromycin, the latter two being drugs which gain entrance poorly into the CSF after systemic administration. Vancomycin has found its greatest value in the treatment of methicillin-resistant staphylococcal infections and has few other indications, except for its effectiveness against *Flavobacterium meningosepticum* and its occasional usefulness for enterococcal Group D *Streptococci*. Vancomycin is given intravenously for invasive infections, with a childhood, and presumably, neonatal dose of 60 mg/kg/day in divided doses every six to eight hours. Recommended treatment of *Flavobacterium meningosepticum* meningitis is oral rifampin and parenteral erythromycin with frequent CSF examinations to ascertain the response to the regimen. Lack of improvement warrants consideration of intraventricular erythromycin if the ventricular capacity permits it.

Bacteroides fragilis is another unusual cause of neonatal infection and is generally resistant to penicillin but sensitive to chloramphenicol. Suboptimal response to chloramphenicol has lead to the successful use of metronidazole in neonates with *Bacteroides fragilis* meningitis,[7] although experience with this antimicrobial in the neonate is limited. The drug has bactericidal activity against most obligatory anaerobic microorganisms including *Bacteroides fragilis* and *Fusobacterium* species. The compound diffuses well into tissues and has excellent penetration into CSF after oral administration. A dosage of metronidazole appropriate for neonates has not been established but observations in adults would suggest that an oral dose of 30 to 40 mg/kg/day in divided doses every eight hours would be expected to result in CSF levels of better than 10 μ g/ml.

The most perplexing problem is the optimal method of treatment of neonatal meningitis caused by the gram-negative members of the *Enterobacteriaceae*, particularly the most common type which is *Escherichia coli* meningitis. Systemically administered ampicillin and gentamicin is the most commonly used regimen; however, not all strains are ampicillin-sensitive, rapid eradication of bacteria in the CSF does not usually occur with ampicillin, and gentamicin penetrates CSF only in limited quantity in doses that result in peak serum levels below 10 μg/ml.

Aminoglycosides administered intrathecally into the lumbar subarachnoid space do not adequately enter the ventricular system and have not been found to improve the outcome of this illness in the neonate.[8] Intraventricular gentamicin results in much more favorable intraventricular levels relative to bacterial killing but the procedure can be very difficult in the initial stages of the illness when the ventricles are reduced in size due to cerebral swelling.

Chloramphenicol has been proposed as an alternative method of treatment of neonatal Gram-negative meningitis but the drug is claimed to be only bacteriostatic against most of the *Enterobacteriaceae*. Potential serum level-related side effects of chloramphenicol in the newborn infant make it important that blood level determinations be available if the drug is used in this age group. In addition, chloramphenicol has been found to antagonize the bactericidal effect of gentamicin against Gram-negative rods.[9]

Under the best of circumstances, therefore, treatment of neonatal Gram-negative meningitis with the currently available antimicrobials is less than optimal and there is an urgent need for new antimicrobials which are effective against Gram-negative bacilli, are relatively safe, and will penetrate into brain and CSF in adequate concentrations. There is optimism that moxalactam, a recently introduced β-lactam and β-lactamase resistant antibiotic, will fulfill these requirements. Moxalactam has been found to be effective against most of the *Enterobacteriaceae* and is active against *Bacteroides fragilis, Serratia marcescens,* and *Hemophilus influenzae.*[10,11] Studies by Schaad et al[12] have found the drug to penetrate into the CSF in quantities considerably greater than the minimum inhibitory concentration for sensitive organisms. Because of its broad spectrum of action and its ability to enter CSF, moxalactam will hopefully prove to be an excellent addition to the currently available antibiotics for treatment of neonatal Gram-negative meningitis as well as for older persons. New third-generation cephalosporins also show promise for treatment of Gram-negative neonatal meningitis. Cefotaxime is more effective against Gram-negative bacilli and penetrates CSF far better than the previously available antimicrobials in this class.

Until more effective antibiotics are available, treatment of neonatal Gram-negative bacillary meningitis in most centers is initially with ampicillin and gentamicin administered systemically with reexamination of the CSF within 24 to 48 hours after onset of therapy. If clinical and CSF improvement has not occurred after a reasonable trial with this regimen, computed tomography should be performed to ascertain if ventricular size permits intraventricular administration of gentamicin in conjunction with systemic therapy. When this method is required, the duration of daily intraventricular injections is determined by the rate of CSF improvement and when CSF sterilization occurs. Gentamicin is given by intramuscular injection in a dosage of 5 mg/kg/day at 12-hour intervals in infants less than one week of age and 7.5 mg/kg/day in divided doses every eight hours in infants from one to eight weeks of age. Dosage should be adjusted on the basis of peak and trough serum levels with peak levels optimally maintained between 5 and 10 µg/ml. With gentamicin-resistant *Escherichia coli* or *Klebsiella* species, amikacin combined with ampicillin is selected, depending on sensitivity test results. Moxalactam, cefotaxime, or other third-generation cephalosporins will hopefully replace these antimicrobials for treatment of Gram-negative meningitis in the near future.

HEMOPHILUS INFLUENZAE MENINGITIS

Treatment of *Hemophilus influenzae* meningitis, like other types of acute suppurative meningitis, requires intravenous antibiotics as well as constant attention to supportive measures. Marked hyperthermia should be prevented and adequate ventilation is mandatory to prevent hypercapnia and hypoxia which can lead precipitously to internal herniation. Intermittent intravenous doses of mannitol are sometimes indicated when intracranial hypertension is believed to be contributing to the child's downhill course and when increased pressure is not the result of subdural fluid collections. Because of the high frequency of occurrence of inappropriate antidiuretic hormone secretion in the early stages of the illness[13] flud intake should be mildly restricted for the first 48 to 72 hours unless the child is significantly dehydrated or in shock at the time of hospital admission. The presence of hypotension or shock requires immediate expansion of the blood volume by appropriate means.

Ampicillin was introduced in 1961 and within a short time it became the drug of choice for treatment of *Hemophilus influenzae* meningitis. The drug was shown to have adequate penetration into the CSF in the presence of inflamed meninges.[14] Ampicillin and chloramphenicol were found to be equally effective for treatment of *Hemophilus influenzae* meningitis but the former drug was preferable for the initial treatment of acute meningitis in children over two months of age because of its greater effectiveness against *Streptococcus pneumoniae* and *Neisseria meningitidis*. In December 1973, the first isolates of ampicillin-resistant *Hemophilus influenzae* in this country were recovered from a child with meningitis in Maryland and from a second in Georgia. The incidence of ampicillin-resistant *Hemophilus influenzae* has shown a gradual increase in recent years and varies considerably in different geographic regions. Approximately five percent of isolates nationwide are now believed to be resistant to ampicillin although much higher estimates are claimed in certain communities. The highest prevalence of resistant organisms has come from patients with meningitis and bacteremia and the lowest from those with infections of the respiratory tract. In addition, it is possible that a mixed population of bacteria can occur in CSF composed of both ampicillin-sensitive and ampicillin-resistant organisms.[15] This could conceivably lead to misinterpretation of either the Kirby-Bauer disc method or the β-lactamase determination and result in ampicillin treatment failure of meningitis which is assumed to be caused by ampicillin-sensitive *Hemophilus influenzae*.

Ampicillin resistance is the result of the production of β-lactamase by the resistant strains, the production of the enzyme being mediated by genes located on a plasmid. The enzyme rapidly hydrolyzes the β-lactam ring of penicillin and closely resembles the β-lactamase produced by enteric bacilli. Reliable laboratory methods have been developed for the rapid determination of the presence of the enzyme thus predicting from *invitro* studies the organisms resistance to ampicillin.[16] On rare occasion, ampicillin-resistant strains of *Hemophilus influenzae* have been found which are non-β -lactamase producing.[17] The mechanism of resistance in these isolates is not understood to the present date.

As a result of the emergence of ampicillin-resistant organisms, it is now recommended that ampicillin and chloramphenicol in combination should be the initial treatment of acute meningitis in the child over two months of age yet to be diagnosed etiologically, or for the child with proven *Hemophilus influenzae* meningitis. Ampicillin is administered intravenously in a dosage of 300 to 400 mg/kg/day and is given every four hours over a 20-minute period of time. The dosage of chloramphenicol is 100 mg/kg/day given every six hours. If laboratory tests prove that the organism is a non-β-lactamase former or otherwise demonstrate the organism to be sensitive to ampicillin, chloramphenicol is discontinued. If studies reveal the isolate to be β-lactamase positive (ampicillin-resistant), chloramphenicol is continued as the single drug. Chloramphenicol in concentrations that can be achieved in CSF is bactericidal for *Hemophilus influenzae* and, to this date, only a few examples of chloramphenicol-resistant *Hemophilus influenzae* have been found.

The child with *Hemophilus influenzae* meningitis who becomes severely neutropenic from chloramphenicol as well as the future prospect of an increasing prevalence of organisms resistant to both ampicillin and chloramphenicol pose major problems in regard to antibiotic therapy. Trimethoprim-sulfamethoxazole has been found to be effective against *Hemophilus influenzae* and has excellent CSF penetration.[18] The so-called third-generation cephalosporins, such as cefotaxime, have bactericidal activity against *Hemophilus influenzae* and penetrate CSF quite well. Cefotaxime is perhaps the best currently available alternative for unusual isolates of *Hemophilus influenzae* resistant to both ampicillin and chloramphenicol.

Because of the importance of the accuracy of the antimicrobial sensitivity determinations, the physician in practice who cannot be certain of the reliability of his available methods of sensitivity testing should probably depend upon chloramphenicol alone for treatment of meningitis proven to be caused by *Hemophilus influenzae*. When chloramphenicol is used, it is important to take into consideration the possible drug interaction between this antibiotic and phenobarbital or phenytoin, which are often administered to children with meningitis complicated by the occurrence of seizures. Phenobarbital can increase hepatic metabolism, resulting in a reduction of the serum chloramphenicol level, while chloramphenicol can interfere with biotransformation of phenytoin, resulting in an increase in its blood level and possible toxic effects. When chloramphenicol is given to a patient receiving phenobarbital, a child with parenchymal liver disease, or the infant under two months of age, blood level determinations of the antibiotic are valuable to arrive at the dosage required to maintain the blood level within the therapeutic range.

During the course of treatment of children with *Hemophilus influenzae* meningitis, 20 to 30 percent will experience a recurrence of fever a few days into the regimen and after fever had subsided on the second or third day of therapy.[19] Relapse of fever has many possible causes but when the organism is sensitive to the antibiotic being used and when the dosage is appropriate, recurrence of fever is not usually found to be the result of unyielding or relapsing meningitis. More common explanations include otitis media, pneumonitis, an infected cutdown or intravenous infusion site, septic arthritis, infected subdural effusions, or a hospital-acquired viral illness with a short incubation period. Drug fever is often considered and is more common with ampicillin than chloramphenicol but is probably an overestimated cause of fever. Infrequent sources of recurrent fever include pericarditis and brain abscess.

The desirability of prophylactic treatment of children less than five years of age who are household contacts of a patient with *Hemophilus influenzae* meningitis has become apparent as the result of recent observations. Nasopharyngeal carriage of *Hemophilus influenzae* type b has been shown to increase dramatically among household contacts of an infected patient and outbreaks of meningitis have been described among persons within an enclosed population. Ward et al.[20] have calculated that the risk of severe illness in the next 30 days among household contacts of a patient with *Hemophilus influenzae* meningitis is 585 times greater than the age-adjusted risk in the general population. The risk, therefore, is almost as great as that of household contacts of a patient with meningococcal disease and would warrant antimicrobial prophylaxis for young children if a safe and consistently effective drug were available. Rifampin and trimethoprim-sulfamethoxazole by the oral route have each been proposed although their degree of effectiveness remains to be established.[21] Absolute recommendations for prophylactic therapy have not yet been established and until more information is available, close medical surveillance of household contacts and of contacts in day-care centers is warranted and is acceptable in most instances.

MENINGOCOCCAL MENINGITIS

Penicillin G administered intravenously is the treatment of choice for meningococcal sepsis and meningitis. Because of the potential danger of rapid deterioration that may accompany this disease, one should achieve an effective antibiotic blood level as soon as possible when the diagnosis is suspected. This can be accomplished by administering intravenously one-half the calculated daily dosage over 30 to 60 minutes at the initiation of treatment. The relatively slower time-period for infusion of a loading dose of penicillin is because hospitals commonly stock potassium-containing penicillin which can be dangerous if a large amount is infused rapidly. The dosage of penicillin G for meningococcal meningitis is 250,000 units/kg/day, up to 20 million units per day, given intravenously every four hours over a 20-minute period. In persons allergic to penicillin, chloramphenicol provides a satisfactory alternative. Chloramphenicol has been shown to be bactericidal against most strains of *Neisseria meningitidis*[22]; however, ampicillin, and presumably penicillin, in combination with chloramphenicol may be antagonistic against certain strains of meningococci.[23] Since ampicillin in combination with chloramphenicol is now the initial regimen for treatment of meningitis in children beyond the newborn period until the causative organism is identified, it is important to discontinue the chloramphenicol as soon as possible in cases in which the meningococcus is proven to be the etiologic cause.

Treatment of fulminating meningococcemia with endotoxic shock continues to be a debatable subject. It is generally agreed that appropriate antibiotic therapy is necessary and that early initiation of therapy is more apt to be successful than that started after shock has developed. Restoration of blood volume and correction of electrolyte deficits may be necessary if vomiting or diarrhea have occurred. Intravenous fluids may suffice but in certain instances, plasma expanders or fresh whole blood may be desirable. Bicarbonate therapy in conjunction with measures to correct dehydration is useful if metabolic acidosis is present. Sodium bicarbonate, however, should not be mixed in solution with penicillin or its semi-synthetic derivatives. Central venous and arterial catheters for pressure monitoring will facilitate fluid and drug administration if hypotension or shock is present. Dopamine is the most widely used agent for treatment of septic shock and is given in an intravenous dose of 20 to 10 μg/kg/min. Because it is inactivated in alkaline solution, dopamine should not be mixed in the same intravenous bottle with sodium bicarbonate. The primary effect of this sympathomimetic amine is to increase myocardial contractility enhancing cardiac output, but it has the effect of selectively increasing renal blood flow. The value of corticosteroids in septic shock remains questionable and has been a topic of debate although they are incorporated into the regimen by most. The opponents of corticosteroid therapy for endotoxic shock argue that an experimental Shwartzman reaction can be elicited after a single dose of endotoxin in animals pretreated with cortisone.

Laboratory evidence of intravascular coagulation is considered an indication for heparin therapy by certain investigators but reports regarding its effectiveness have been quite variable.[24] Although most authors have found that laboratory abnormalities indicating intravascular coagulation revert toward normal, it is difficult to ascribe clinical improvement to heparin and death may still occur in the seriously ill patient. Corrigan[25] has recommended initial treatment with appropriate antishock measures and antibiotics without the addition of heparin. Should laboratory evidence of consumption coagulopathy persist despite these measures, and especially if accompanied by bleeding, heparin is then given in an attempt to abolish intravascular consumption. Heparin is administered intravenously in a dose of 100 units/kg and is repeated every four hours in an amount sufficient to lengthen the partial thromboplastin time or thrombin time to two to three times normal. The duration of heparin therapy required is variable and is determined by clinical judgment plus evidence of improvement of laboratory data regarding blood clotting factors and platelets. In bleeding patients it is important to replace depleted clotting factors by transfusions of platelets, cryoprecipitate, or plasma. In addition, plasma infusions will provide antithrombin III (heparin cofactor), a protein that is consumed during intravascular coagulation and which is necessary for an optimal therapeutic effect of heparin.

In certain cases of meningococcal meningitis, the course is rapidly progressive leading to deep coma in the absence of systemic hypotension or shock. Severe cerebral swelling results in high-grade increase in intracranial pressure which will eventually lead to transtentorial herniation, brain stem compression, and death. Immediate recognition of the importance of intracranial hypertension in such cases can be difficult but survival is likely to be dependent on the ability to control the intracranial pressure. The use of fluid restriction and mannitol injections may be sufficient in some instances while others require aggressive treatment. The placement of a subdural bolt or intraventricular catheter to provide a continuous measurement of the intracranial pressure greatly simplifies the development of the most appropriate treatment regimen. Methods used to control intracranial hypertension include control of hyperthermia, restriction of intravenous fluid administration, controlled ventilation to prevent hypercapnea, and intravenous injections of mannitol in doses of 0.5 to 1.0 g/kg at periodic intervals. When an intraventricular catheter is selected for pressure monitoring and can be successfully inserted into the lateral ventricle, small amounts of CSF can be aspirated at intervals. Sudden pressure spikes are controlled by intermittent hyperventilation to lower the pCO_2 to less than 30 torr, assuming that cerebral autoregulation has not been lost. The chances of success of this form of treatment in a patient with meningococcal meningitis with dramatic and progressive cerebral swelling is dependent on early recognition of the significance of increased intracranial pressure.

The importance of prophylactic treatment among household contacts and of others who have been in intimate contact with a patient with meningococcal disease has been emphasized by the recognition that such persons are at risk for an attack rate which is at least 500 to 800 times that of the general population. While penicillin has been highly successful in the treatment of meningococcal disease, it has not proven consistently effective as a prophylactic agent. The emergence of sulfadiazine-resistant meningococci has severely restricted the use of sulfa preparations for prophylaxis. Rifampin has been found to be superior to most other currently available antimicrobial agents for elimination of nasopharyngeal carriage of meningococci. It is currently recommended that rifampin be administered to all household members of an identified case of meningococcal disease, to other persons who have been in intimate contact with the patient, and to anyone directly exposed to oral secretions of the patient.[26] The latter would apply to hospital attendants who have administered mouth-to-mouth resuscitation. Other less direct contacts, such as classmates at school, are not believed to be at significant risk and need not ordinarily receive drug therapy. The dosage schedule of rifampin for meningococcal prophylaxis is 600 mg every 12 hours in four doses for adults, 20 mg/kg/day given every 12 hours in four doses for children one to 12 years of age, and 10 mg/kg/day administered every 12 hours in four doses in children less than 12 months of age. The short duration of treatment is not believed to significantly contribute to the development of meningococcal resistance to rifampin. In the unusual instance in which sulfadiazine can be used for prophylaxis, the dose is 1 g every 12 hours in adults, 500 mg every 12 hours for children one to 12 years of age, and 500 mg once per day for children less than 12 months of age. Treatment is continued for two days. In addition to chemoprophylaxis, group A or C meningococcal vaccine should be considered for household and other intimate contacts over two years of age, especially in epidemic circumstances.[27]

Meningococcal polysaccharide vaccines against disease caused by *Neisseria meningitidis* serogroups A and C were developed and licensed

after it was demonstrated that the polysaccharide antigens of these serogroups were excellent immunogens in man and that the vaccines produced
only infrequent and mild adverse effects. Both monovalent and bivalent
vaccines are now available and the vaccines are highly group-specific,
that is, group A vaccine does not provide protection against group C
meningococci. Group B polysaccharide preparations are not immunogenic in adults and a satisfactory vaccine against this serogroup has not yet
been developed. Antibody responses resulting from vaccine administration to infants under two years of age are less than in older children and
group C vaccine is not recommended in this age group. In addition, there
is concern that group C vaccine when given to young infants may give rise
to some form of immunologic tolerance resulting in less antibody response to subsequent challenge perhaps leading to greater risk of disease.

PNEUMOCOCCAL MENINGITIS

Penicillin administered intravenously is the treatment of choice for
pneumococcal meningitis. The dosage is 250,000 units/kg/day, up to 20
million units/day, given every four hours over a 20-minute time period.
Treatment is continued for a minimum of two weeks and occasionally
longer. For those who are allergic to the penicillins, chloramphenicol is
the most acceptable alternative. Because of antagonism between the two
drugs, penicillin and chloramphenicol should not be used together for
infections caused by *Streptococcus pneumoniae*. The use of corticosteroids has been advocated by some but with little established evidence of
benefit.

Streptococcus pneumoniae for many years had been considered to
be uniformly sensitive to penicillin, but in 1967 in Australia, a pneumococcal isolate from a patient with hypogammaglobulinemia was found to be
relatively resistant to penicillin.[28] Reports of poorly responding or relapsing meningitis caused by pneumococcal strains with decreased susceptibility to penicillin subsequently appeared from other countries, including
the United States. Unlike the great majority of penicillin-sensitive
pneumococcal isolates in which the minimum inhibitory concentration
of penicillin has been found to be 0.01 to 0.1 $\mu g/ml$, in these initial cases
with decreased sensitivity to penicillin, the minimum inhibitory concentrations ranged from 0.2 to 1 $\mu g/ml$. The "intermediate" sensitivity of
these organisms might still allow success with extra-neurologic infections
treated with higher than usual doses of penicillin. With meningitis, however, penicillin might be expected to be inadequate because the CSF
concentrationn of penicillin with conventional doses would only approxi-

mately equal the minimum inhibitory concentration. Pneumococcal isolates fully resistant to penicillin have more recently been identified with minimum inhibitory concentrations of 1 to 4 μg/ml.[29]

In the majority of cases, pneumococci with decreased sensitivity or absolute resistance to penicillin have come from patients who had received long-term antibiotic therapy. The mechanism accounting for decreased penicillin sensitivity is unknown and all isolates have been negative for β-lactamase production. The incidence of penicillin-resistant pneumococci in North America is uncertain but is believed to be less than three percent of isolates. Its occurrence is sufficiently common that some have proposed that invitro sensitivity testing of *Streptococcus pneumoniae* be performed when the organism causes serious infection or infection not promptly responding to therapy. Treatment of pneumococcal meningitis caused by an organism with decreased sensitivity or resistance to penicillin creates an obvious problem regarding the selection of the drug regimen and depends considerably on the minimum inhibitory concentration. Those only slightly less sensitive than customary can probably be successfully treated with increased doses of penicillin, in the range of 500,000/kg/day. When the organism is more resistant, chloramphenicol is the drug of choice, although isolates resistant to this antimicrobial have been encountered. Other antibiotics that might be considered with pencillin-insensitive pneumococcal meningitis include rifampin and vancomycin.

A polyvalent pneumococcal polysaccharide vaccine (Pneumovax ®) was commercially released in 1978. The 14-valent vaccine contains capsular polysaccharides derived from the 14 most prevalent types of pneumococci which account for approximately 80 percent of pneumococcal disease. The duration of protection provided by the vaccine is uncertain but it is believed that elevated antibody titers will persist for at least two years after immunization.

Specific indications for the use of pneumococcal vaccine have not been clearly defined although reasonable guidelines have been established. It is not recommended for children under two years of age because of the poor antibody responses in infancy to certain pneumococcal antigens within the vaccine.[30] The vaccine is recommended for children with sickle-cell disease and for patients who have had splenectomy or who have functional asplenia. Immunization is also advised for children over two years of age and adults with certain chronic diseases, including malignant disorders, immune deficiency states, diabetis mellitus, and conditions with impaired renal or hepatic function, in which there is an increased risk of pneumococcal infection. Antibody response to pneumococcal vaccine has been found to be impaired in patients with Hodgkin's disease when the vaccine is administered during or soon after treatment with irradiation and chemotherapeutic agents.[31] For this reason, it is recommended that such patients be immunized before initiation of the therapeutic regimen.

REFERENCES

1. Tofte, R.W., Peterson, P.K., Kim, Y., et al. Opsonic activity of normal human cerebrospinal fluid for selected bacterial species. *Infect. Immun.* 26:1093–1098, 1979.
2. Simberkoff, M.S., Moldover, N.H., and Rahal, J.R., Jr. Absence of detectable bactericidal and opsonic activities in normal and infected human cerebrospinal fluids. A regional host defense deficiency. *J. Lab. Clin. Med.* 95:362–372, 1980.
3. Cherubin, C.E., Marr, J.S., Sierra, M.F., et al. Listeria and Gram-negative bacillary meningitis in New York City, 1972-1979. Frequent causes of meningitis in adults. *Am. J. Med.* 71:199–209, 1981.
4. Cooper, M.D., Keeney, R.E., Lyons, S.F., et al. Synergistic effects of ampicillin-aminoglycoside combinations on Group B streptococci. *Antimicrob. Agents Chemother.* 15:484–486. 1979.
5. Weeks, J.L. Mason, E.O., Jr., and Baker, C.J. Antagonism of ampicillin and chloramphenicol for meningeal isolates of group B Streptococci. *Antimicrob. Agents Chemother.* 20:281–285, 1981.
6. Bavikatte, K., Schreiner, R.L., Lemons, J.A., et al. Group D streptococcal septicemia in the neonate. *Am. J. Dis. Child.* 133:493–496, 1979.
7. Berman, B.W., King, F.H., Jr., Rubinstein, D.S., et al. *Bacteroides fragilis* meningitis in a neonate successfully treated with metronidazole. *J. Pediatr.* 93:793–795, 1978.
8. McCracken, G.H., Jr., and Mize, S.G. A controlled study of intrathecal antibiotic therapy in Gram-Negative enteric meningitis of infancy. *J. Pediatr.* 89:66–72, 1976.
9. Paisley, J.W., and Washington, J.A. II. Susceptibility of *Escherichia coli* KI to four combinations of antimicrobial agents potentially useful for treatment of neonatal meningitis. *J. Infect. Dis.* 140:183–191, 1979.
10. Fisher, J.F., Carter, M.J., Parsons, J., et al. Moxalactam (LY 127935) in treatment of meningitis due to Gram-negative bacilli. *Antimicrob. Agents Chemother.* 19:218–221, 1981.
11. Kaplan, S.L., Mason, E.O. Jr., Garcia, H., et al. Pharmacokinetics and cerebrospinal fluid penetration of moxalactam in children with bacterial meningitis. *J. Pediatr.* 98:152–157, 1981.
12. Schaad, V.B., McCracken, G.H., Jr., Threlkeld, N., et al. Clinical evaluation of a new broad-spectrum oxa-beta-lactam antibiotic, moxalactam, in neonates and infants. *J. Pediatr.* 98:129–136, 1981.
13. Feigin, R.D., Stechenberg, B.W., Chang, M.J., et al. Prospective evaluation of treatment of *Hemophilus influenzae* meningitis. *J. Pediatr.* 88:542–548, 1976.
14. Barrett, F.F., Eardley, W.A., Yow, M.D., et al. Ampicillin in the treatment of acute suppurative meningitis. *J. Pediatr.* 69:343–353, 1966.

15. Jubelirer, D.P., and Yeager, A.S. Simultaneous recovery of ampicillin-sensitive and ampicillin-resistant organisms in Haemophilus influenzae type b meningitis. *J. Pediatr.* *95*:415–416, 1979.
16. Scheifele, D.W., Syriopoulou, V.P., Harding, A.L., et al. Evaluation of a rapid β-lactamase test for detecting ampicillin-resistant strains of *Hemophilus influenzae* type b. *Pediatrics 58*:382–387, 1976.
17. Markowitz, S.M. Isolation of an ampicillin-resistant, non-β-lactamase-producing strain of *Haemophilus influenzae. Antimicrob. Agents Chemother. 17*:80–83, 1980.
18. Pelton, S.I., Shurin, P.A., Klein, J.O., et al. Quantitative inhibition of *Haemophilus influenzae* by trimethoprim-sulfamethoxazole. *Antimicrob. Agents Chemother. 12*:649–654, 1977.
19. Balagtas, R.C., Levin, S., Nelson, K.E., et al. Secondary and prolonged fevers in bacterial meningitis. *J. Pediatr. 77*:957–964, 1970.
20. Ward, J.I., Fraser, D.W., Baraff, L.J., et al. *Haemophilus influenzae* meningitis. A national study of secondary spread in household contacts. *N. Engl. J. Med. 301*:122–126, 1979.
21. Granoff, D.M., Gilsdorf, J., Gessert, C., et al. *Hemophilus influenzae* type b disease in a day care center: eradication of carrier state by rifampin. *Pediatrics 63*:397–401, 1979.
22. Rahal, J.J., Jr., and Simberkoff, M.S. Bactericidal and bacteriostatic action of chloramphenicol against meningococcal pathogens. *Antimicrob. Agents Chemother. 16*:13–18, 1979.
23. Feldman, W.E., and Zweighaft, T. Effect of ampicillin and chloramphenicol against *Streptococcus pneumoniae* and *Neisseria meningitidis. Antimicrob. Agents Chemother. 15*:240–242, 1979.
24. Gerald, P., Moriau, M., Bachy, A., et al. Meningococcal purpura: report of 19 patients treated with heparin. *J. Pediatr. 82*:780–786, 1973.
25. Corrigan, J.J. Heparin therapy in bacterial septicemia. *J. Pediatr. 91*:695–700, 1977.
26. Jacobson, J.A., and Fraser, D.W. A simplified approach to meningococcal disease prophylaxis. *J.A.M.A. 236*:1053–1054, 1976.
27. McCormick, J.B., and Bennett, J.V. Public health considerations in the management of meningococcal disease. *Ann. Intern. Med. 83*:883–886, 1975.
28. Hansman, D., and Bullen, M.M. A resistant pneumococcus. *Lancet 2*:264–265, 1967.
29. Cates, K.L., Gerrald, J.M., Giebink, G.S., et al. A penicillin-resistant pneumococcus. *J. Pediatr. 93*:624–626, 1978.
30. Cowan, M.J., Ammann, A.J., Wara, D.W., et al. Pneumococcal polysaccharide immunization of infants and children. *Pediatrics 62*:721–727, 1978.
31. Minor, D.R., Schiffman, G., and McIntosh, L.S. Response of patients with Hodgkin's disease to pneumococcal vaccine. *Ann. Intern. Med. 90*:887–892, 1979.

8

Neuroradiologic Diagnosis of Central Nervous System Infection

John A. Hodak

The promise of computed axial tomography in the diagnosis of intracranial infections predicted by Altemus and Taveras in 1974[1] appears well supported by numerous investigators.[2-17] Early diagnosis and prompt effective treatment of CNS infections is essential to achieve lowered morbidity and mortality rates, as indicated by recent reports.[4-7] Computed tomography's revolutionary impact on the evaluation of neurologic disorders in general warrants a review of the current neuroradiologic approach to the diagnosis of CNS infection. Investigative modalities once important in diagnosis of CNS infection have either been abandoned or have assumed a secondary role since the advent of computed tomography (CT). Superior soft tissue discrimination by CT allows a more accurate assessment of the extent and location of an infective process than hitherto possible.

PLAIN FILMS AND CONVENTIONAL TOMOGRAPHY

Plain films represent an inexpensive and noninvasive technique that may provide important clues to an underlying intraspinal or intracranial infection. Osteomyelitis or disc space infection may herald the presence of a spinal extradural empyema[18] (Figure 1). Sinusitis, mastoiditis, cranial osteomyelitis, or dental caries may suggest the inflammatory origin of an expanding intracranial mass (Figures 2 and 3). Of course, classic signs such as pineal displacement or separated sutures in a child are important observations on plain radiograms of the skull. A distinctive pattern of calcifications may be a definitive finding in cases of toxoplasmosis or cytomegalic inclusion disease. Figure 4 shows an infant's skull study with the typical periventricular calcifications of cytomegalic inclusion disease.

Conventional tomography can be helpful in clarifying and documenting destructive changes hinted at on plain films. Decalcification of the vertebral endplates often with clear evidence of an accompanying osteomyelitis in cases of disc space infection may thus be demonstrated. Destructive osteitis in the paranasal sinuses will be optimally shown tomographically and in a diabetic patient should prompt a biopsy to exclude mucormycosis (Figure 5).

ANGIOGRAPHY

Angiography, once the premier diagnostic modality, now plays a secondary role, but is necessary to demonstrate the presence or absence of a mycotic aneurysm in the face of a hematoma complicating a case of intracranial suppuration (Figure 6). Cerebral angiography may be required to substantiate a clinically suspected extracerebral empyema not seen on computed tomography.[16,17] It may also help in the differential diagnosis of tumor, infarction and resolving hematoma, all of which may present with CT findings indistinguishable from a brain abscess[4,7] (Figure 7). In addition to identifying and localizing a mass effect, cerebral angiography may (20 to 50 percent)[1,4] demonstrate a distinctive rim or band of contrast outlining the capsule of a brain abscess (Figure 8). Focal zones of cerebritis and the diagnosis of multiple abscess remain difficult to determine angiographically.[9] Acute meningitis with exudate bathing the blood vessels can incite inflammatory changes or spasm in the vessel walls, either of which will be manifested angiographically as smooth or irregular arterial narrowing[19] (Figure 9). In chronic granulomatous meningitis, the basal vessels of the brain are affected in like manner[19] (Figure 10). Meningeal carcinomatosis, however, may be confused with arterial spasm and narrowing due to meningitis in an unclear clinical setting (Figure 11).

PNEUMOENCEPHALOGRAPHY, VENTRICULOGRAPHY, AND RADIONUCLIDE SCANNING

Pneumoencephalography and ventriculography and their attendant morbidity are invasive procedures largely superseded by CT. Once important in defining the sequelae of infection such as hydrocephalus, adhesive arachnoiditis, and porencephaly these findings are now easily and elegantly demonstrated by CT. Radionuclide brain scans are nonspecific and cannot differentiate cerebritis from an encapsulating lesion.[5] However, where it is urgent to arrive at a speedy diagnosis such as in Herpes simplex encephalitis, radionuclide brain scanning may play a complimentary role. Radionuclide bone scanning may be helpful in documenting osteomyelitis of the spine.

MYELOGRAPHY

Although CT scanning of the spine is gaining increasing use in the diagnosis of spinal disorders (Figure 12), myelography remains an important tool in the investigative armamentarium for the evaluation of suspected intraspinal suppuration. The presence or absence of a block can thus be expeditiously proven as well as the extent of an extra or intramedullary inflammatory process (Figure 13).

COMPUTED TOMOGRAPHY

Because of CT's superior soft tissue discrimination, analysis of CNS infection as it pertains to specific anatomic compartments is attainable. Thus, the size and extent of a lesion as well as any accompanying cerebral edema, midline displacement, distortion of adjacent anatomic structures, and/or possible herniation can be readily assessed.

Subdural and extradural empyemas are often preceded by sinusitis, mastoiditis, or introduced from direct inoculation through breaks in the skin, bone, or meninges caused by accidental or iatrogenic trauma (e.g., craniotomy, shunt procedures). Extracerebral collections with or without a definite border enhancement form the basis of a CT diagnosis (Figure 14).

While CT scanning in acute meningitis reveals no specific patterns, it is important in excluding a brain abscess.[3] Even after an adequate course of antibiotic therapy, infants and young children, especially those with hemophilus influenzae, may develop cranial enlargement due to a subdural effusion. Computed tomography is invaluable in establishing the diagnosis and monitoring its treatment (Figure 15). Occasionally, marked cortical enhancement after intravenous contrast infusion will be seen secondary to breakdown of the blood–brain barrier and apparent cortical congestion in cases of hemophilus influenzae meningitis (Figure 16). Obliteration of the basal cisterns and complicating hydrocephalus in chronic meningitis such as seen in coccidioidomycosis are readily demonstrated. Often, the accompanying marked contrast enhancement of the inflammatory tissue within the cisterns will be strikingly evident[20] (Figure 17).

Suppuration of the brain itself may be manifest as an area of cerebritis or as a frank abscess cavity. Cerebritis cannot be differentiated from an encapsulated abscess cavity angiographically,[8,9] but with some qualification can be discerned on CT. Characteristically with intravenous contrast infusion, a brain abscess presents a ring enhancing mass lesion with a central lucency often surrounded by edema (Figure 18). They may be multiple and frequently are loculated (Figure 19). The capsule of an abscess will at times be noted to be thinner on the inner or white matter surface where there are fewer fibroblasts to offer resistance to extension,[21] which explains the propensity of brain abscesses to extend toward and rupture into the ventricular system of the brain (Figure 20). The ring enhancement does not necessarily connote a well-formed capsule that will allow surgical intervention. Experimental studies[22,23] confirm what has been observed clinically in this regard.[4] Therefore, it appears that the duration of the symptoms and the patient's clinical response to antibiotic therapy are most important in deciding when to so intervene (Figure 21) Computed tomography allows careful follow-up of a lesion's progress and reports of nonsurgically treated brain abscesses can be found in the literature.[13,14]

Viral encephalitis is often a diffuse parenchymal process. However, Herpes simplex encephalitis has a predilection for temporal, orbitofrontal, and insular cortex.[21] CT scans are abnormal in approximately one half of patients with Herpes simplex encephalitis, in whom localized edema, mass effect, zones of hemorrhage, and poorly defined contrast enhancement may be seen[24] (Figure 22). Biopsy of the abnormal site is recommended as a prelude to vidarabine therapy that has resulted in an improved outcome in this still highly lethal form of encephalitis.[25,26]

Subacute sclerosing panencephalitis is a slow virus infection of the brain that most often affects children and young adults. It is caused by measles virus and is characterized clinically by slowly progressive personality change, intellectual deterioration, and seizures.[21,27] Necrosis of the white matter is a predominant feature of the pathology. This usually fatal disease has a variable appearance on CT depending upon the stage of its progression. Early in its course, CT findings are normal or only minimally abnormal. Chronic cases demonstrate cerebral atrophy, and low density lesions in the white matter and the basal ganglia[27] (Figure 23). These CT findings are not specific and diseases such as other virus infection and demyelinating and dysmyelinating diseases must be considered in the differential diagnosis.[27]

Of the fungal infections that may involve the CNS, rhinocerebral mucormycosis is among the most devastating and has a high mortality rate. Not ordinarily pathogenic, the inciting organism has a predeliction for patients in diabetic acidosis, those who have a debilitating disease, or those who are receiving therapy with anti-inflammatory or immunosuppressive drugs.[29-32] The disease begins in the nasal cavity and sinuses where the organism's propensity to invade vessels allow subsequent extension via these vessels into the orbit, meninges, brain, cavernous sinus, and carotid arteries.[29] Orbital involvement with loss of vision, periorbital swelling, and proptosis is usually ipsilateral to that side with the sinus disease or the side with the greater sinus involvement[31] if bilateral disease is present (Figure 24a). Invasion of the carotid artery and occlusion of the ophthalmic artery may be complicating findings demonstrated angiographically (Figures 25b,c). Similarly, orbital venography may reveal occlusion of the superior ophthalmic vein in the affected eye (Figure 24d).

The parisitic disease cysticerocosis may invade the CNS in parenchymal, intraventricular, leptomeningeal, or mixed forms.[2,33] The clinical features are variable depending on the number, size, anatomic location, and the pathologic stage of the lesions. Parenchymal cysticerci may have a dense CT appearance as well as a lucent cytic one, and may be surrounded by a zone of edema.[33] Homogeneous enhancement may occur after infusion of contrast. Leptomeningeal cysts are sharply marginated and the displaced brain adjacent to them may show minimal contrast enhancement[2] (Figure 25). Hydrocephalus may occur in cysticercosis as a consequence of ventricular obstruction in the ventricular form or secondary to pachymeningitis incited in the leptomeningeal form of the disease. In the chronic phase of the disease, the cysts may calcify and usually no contrast enhancement is associated with these. Calcified cysts per se do not rule out concomitant presence of living larvae.[33]

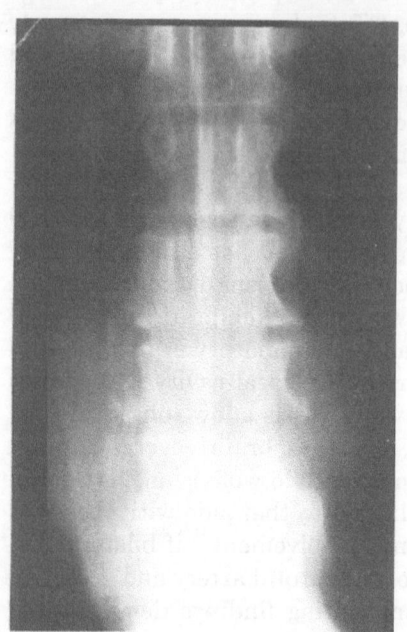

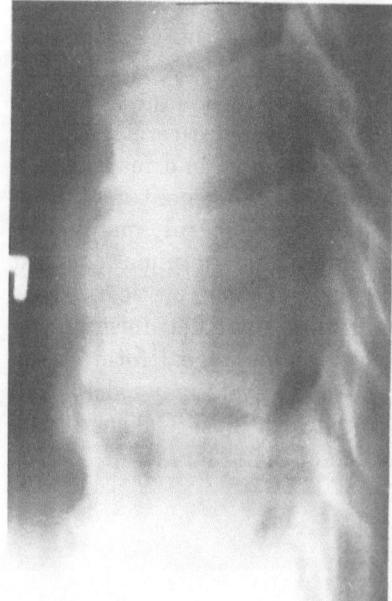

Figure 1. Thoracic disc space infection. (a) Anteroposterior tomogram. (b) Lateral tomogram. Patient with chronic pulmonary empyema presented with rapidly developing paraplegia. A paravertebral mass, disc space destruction, and vertebral body osteomyelitis were associated with a spinal extradural empyema and cord compression.

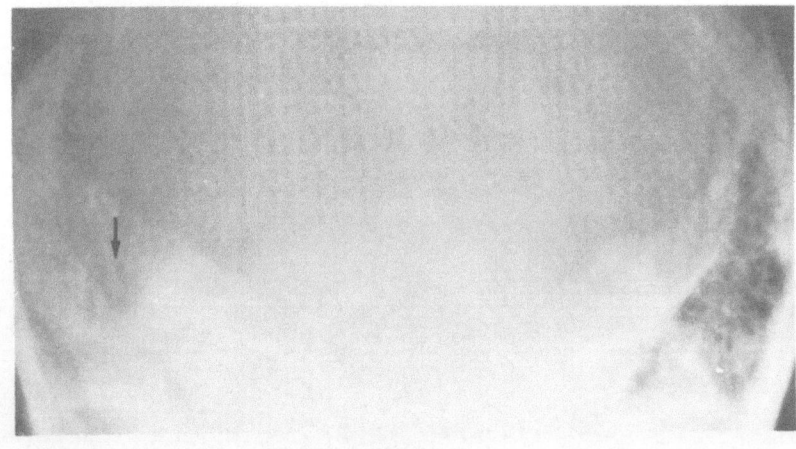

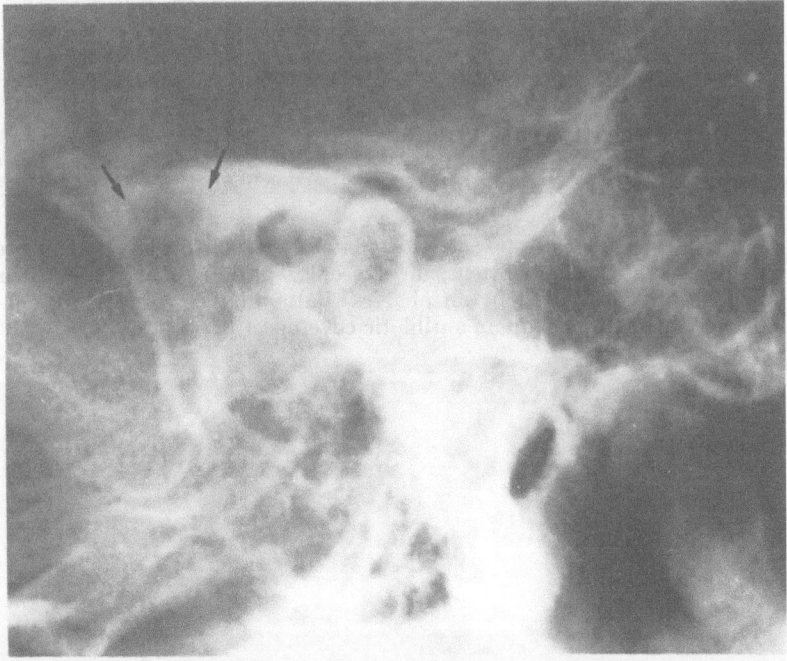

Figure 2. Chronic mastoiditis and cholesteotoma. (a) Townes view. (b) Laws view. Young male presented with fever and severe headache. Temporal lobe abscess discovered adjacent to area of bony destruction.

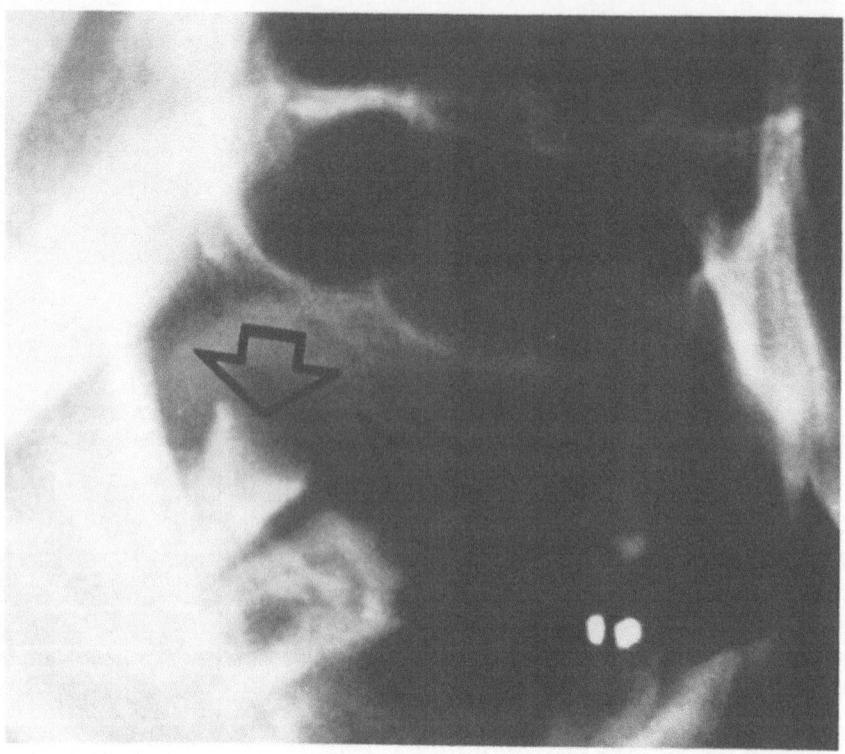

Figure 3. Dental caries. Coned down lateral view of the jaw. Patient presented afebrile in status epilepticus; an avascular parietal mass demonstrated on angiography proved to be an abscess. Later history revealed recent dental extractions with inadequate antibiotic coverage.

Figure 4 (facing page). Cytomegalic inclusion disease. (a) Lateral skull. (b) Anteroposterior skull. Infant skull study demonstrating typical periventricular calcifications.

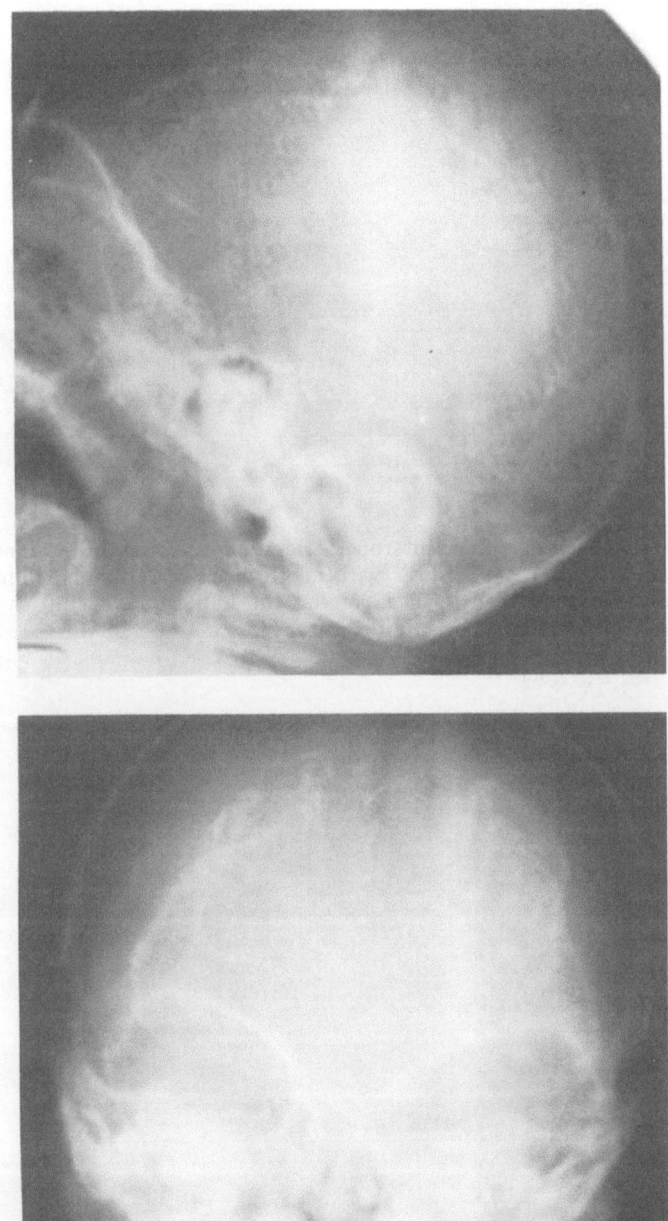

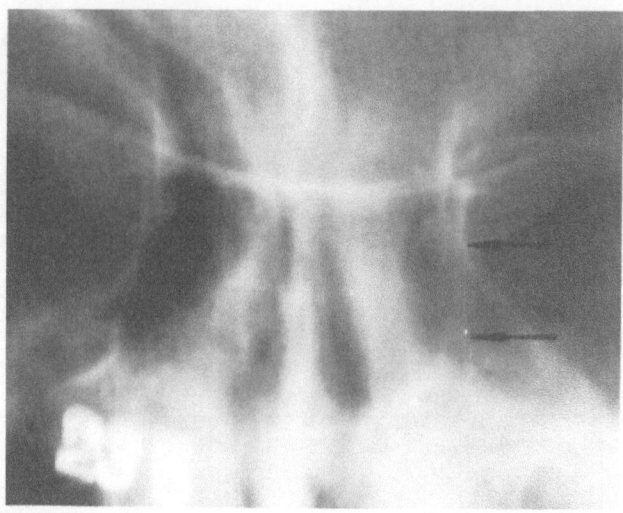

Figure 5. Mucormycosis. Anteroposterior tomogram of the ethmoid sinuses. Adult male in diabetic acidosis with acute onset of left-sided blindness and proptosis. Destructive osteitis involving the left ethmoid sinuses prompted surgical biopsy which revealed mucormycosis.

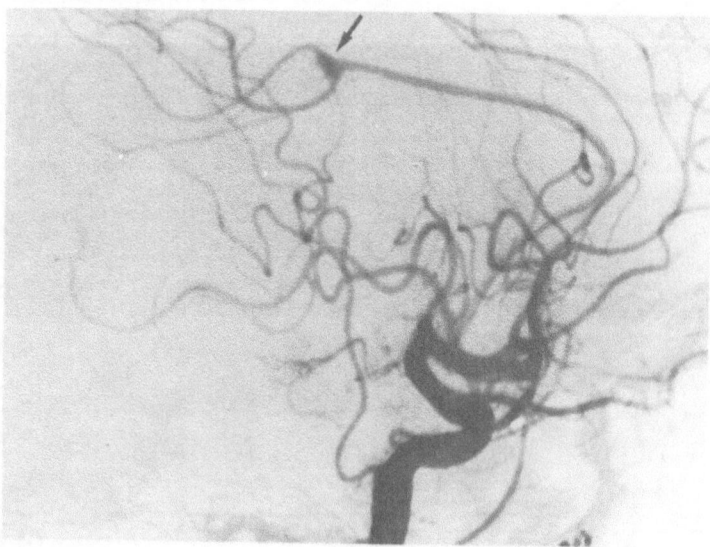

Figure 6. Mycotic aneurysm. Lateral cerebral angiogram. Mycotic aneurysm discovered incidentally in association with a deep parietal brain abscess. It had not bled.

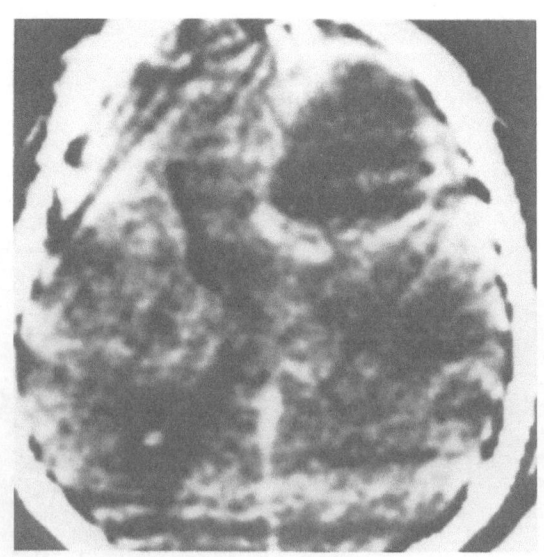

Figure 7. Glioblastoma multiforme. 55-year-old male with fever and marked obtundation. CT reveals a large ring-enhancing lesion with surrounding edema and midline shift. The mass was avascular on angiography and no tumor vessels were identified. The tumor was found to be necrotic at surgery.

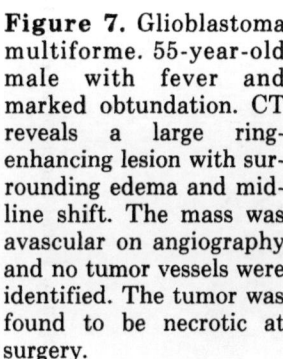

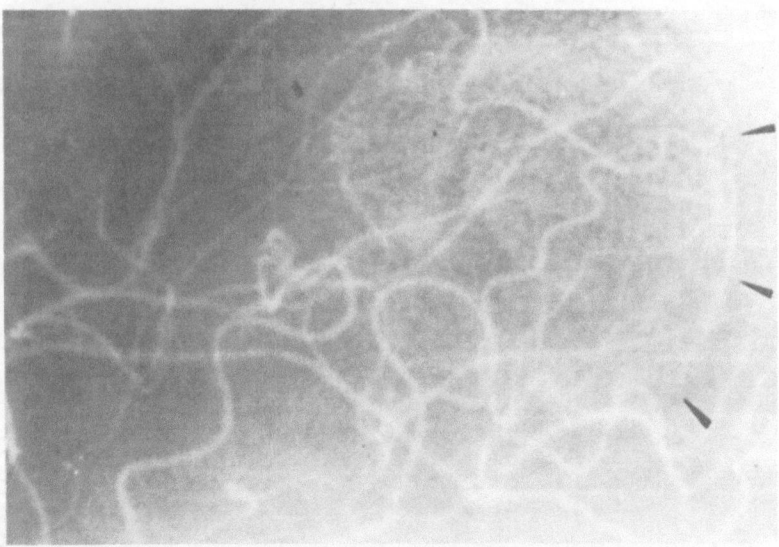

Figure 8. Rim sign. Coned down lateral view of cerebral angiogram. Parietal lobe abscess with stain along capsule resulting in a curvilinear ring-like appearance at its edge (arrowheads).

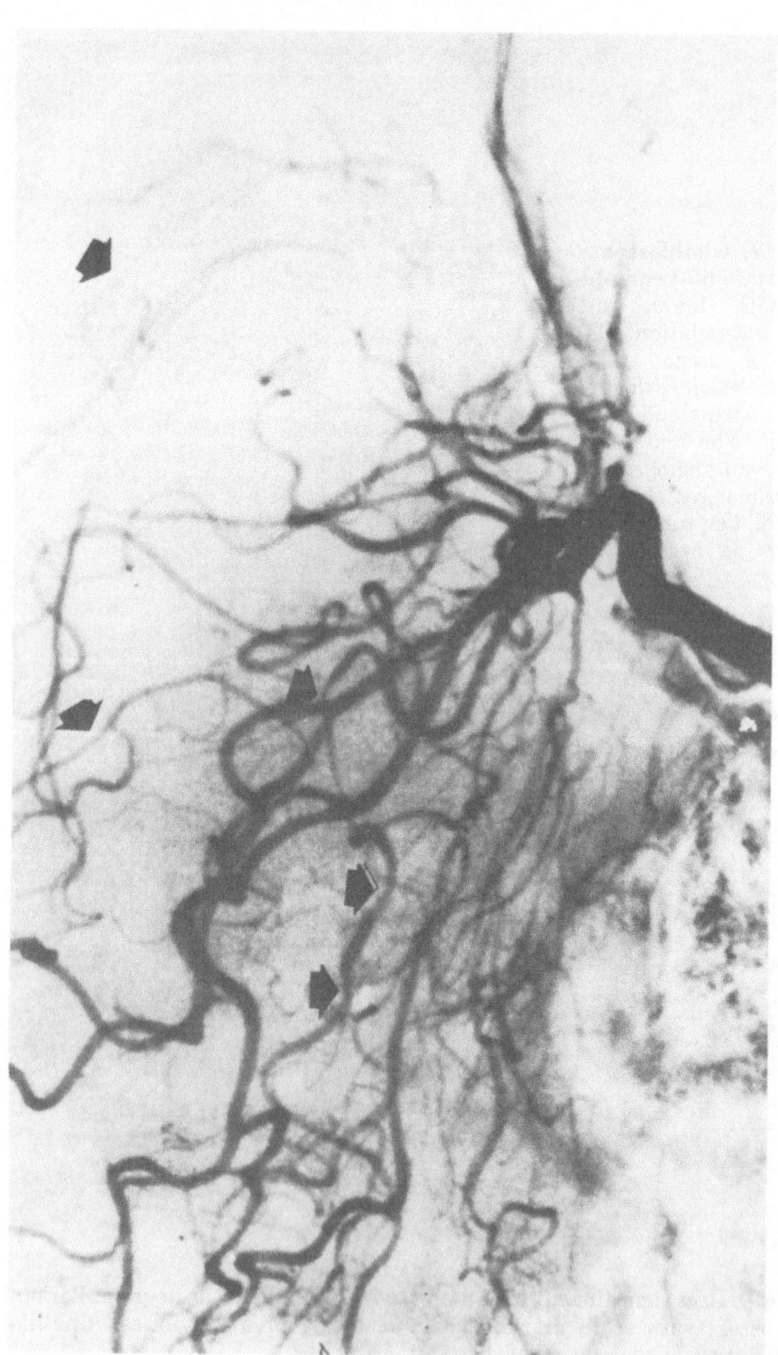

Figure 9. Coccidioidomycosis meningitis. Lateral view of cerebral angiogram. Focal zones of arterial narrowing indicating spasm or local vascular inflammatory change (arrowheads).

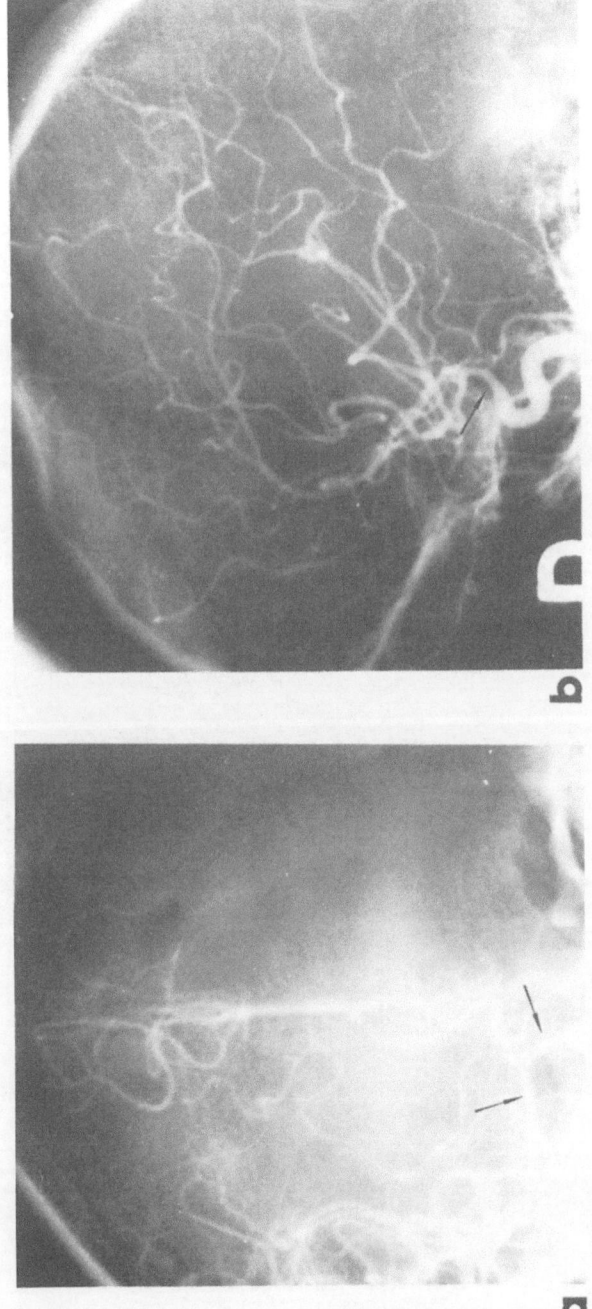

Figure 10. Tuberculous meningitis. (a) Anteroposterior and (b) lateral cerebral angiograms. Narrowing of the supraclinoid internal carotid artery and the proximal middle cerebral artery.

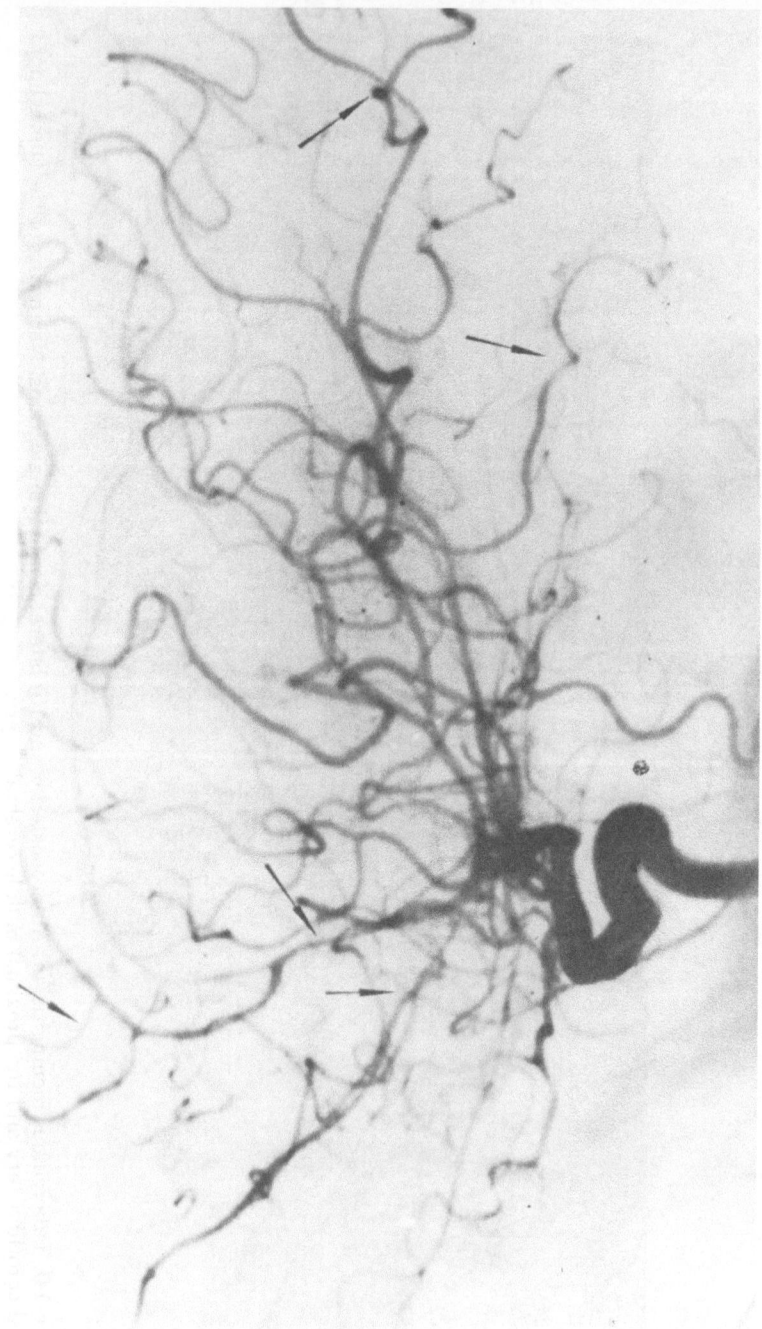

Figure 11. Meningeal carcinomatosis. Lateral cerebral angiogram. Patient with squamous carcinoma of the lung with arterial narrowing indistinguishable from that due to purulent or tuberculous meningitis.

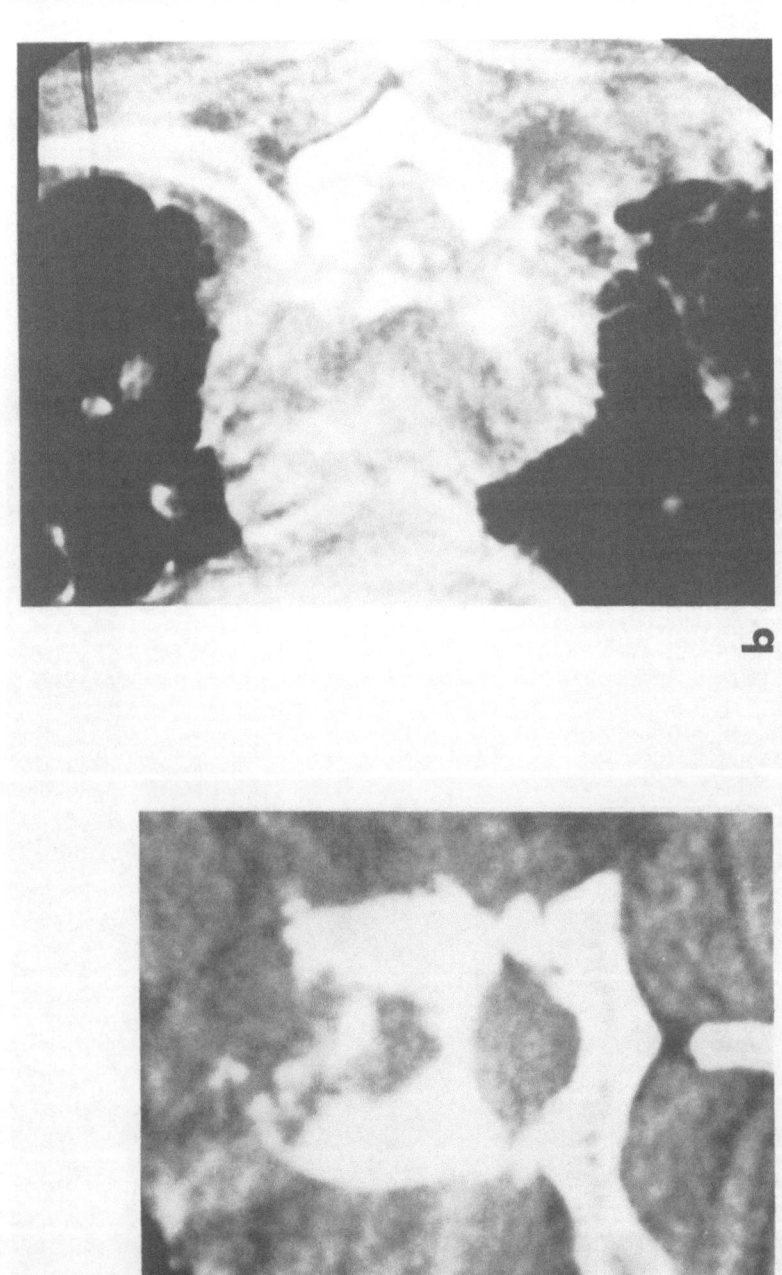

Figure 12. (a) Osteomyelitis and (b) spinal epidural abscess. Spinal CT scan demonstrates a destructive lesion of a thoracic vertebral body with extension into the spinal canal with an associated paravertebral inflammatory mass.

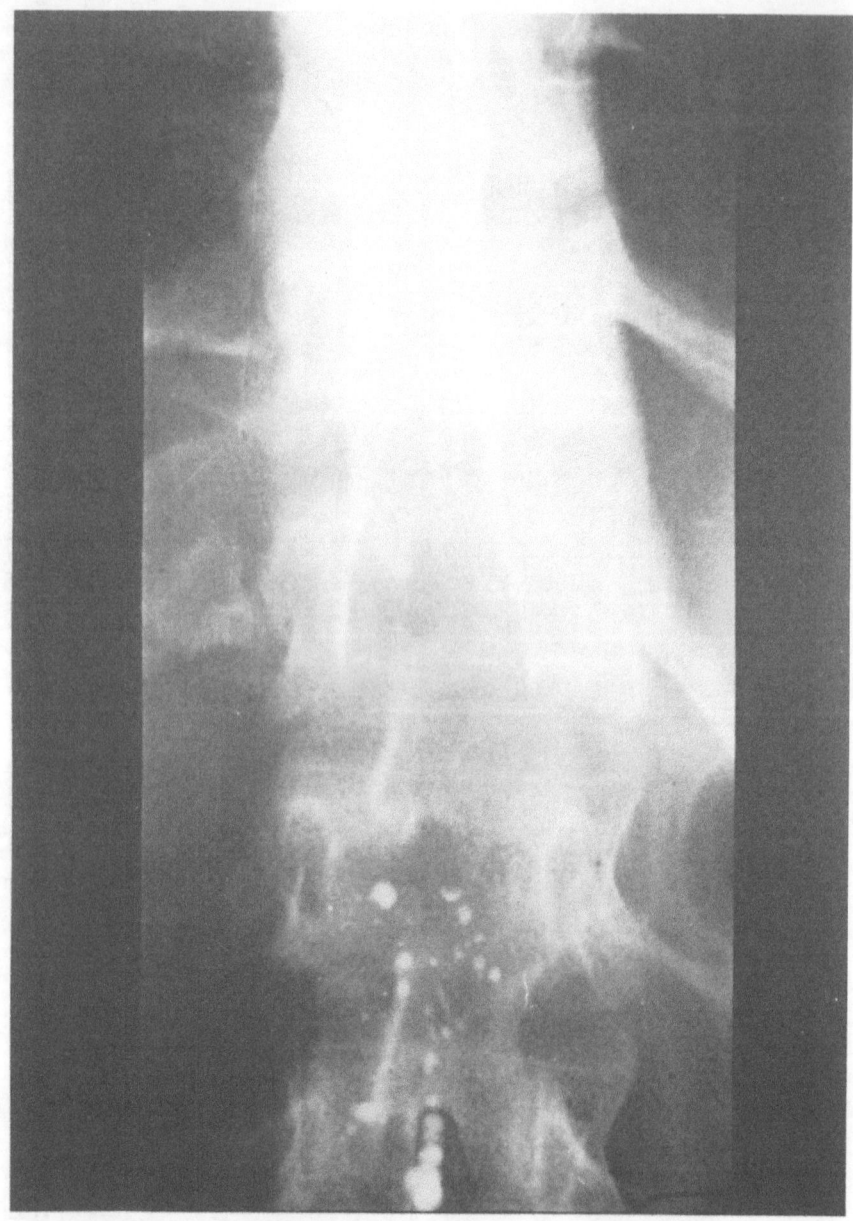

Figure 13. Tuberculoma. Pantopaque myelogram. Teenage American Indian girl with progressive paraplegia. Myelography via high lateral cervical approach demonstrates an expanding intramedullary mass of the conus medullaris which proved to be a tuberculoma at exploration.

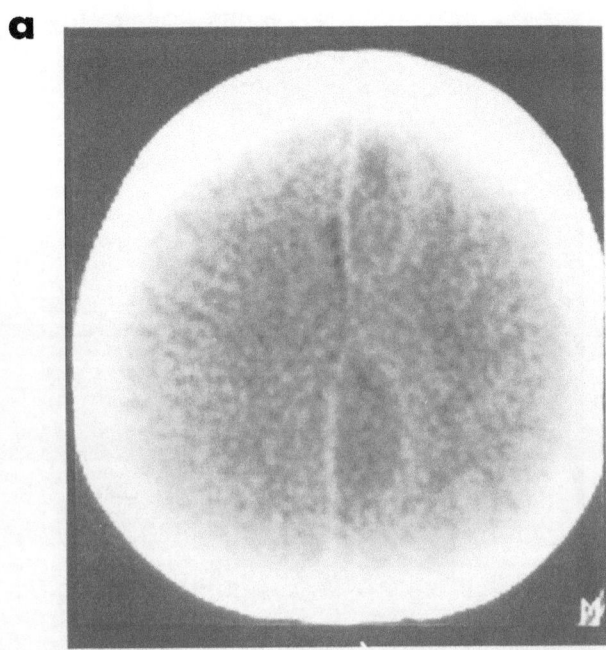

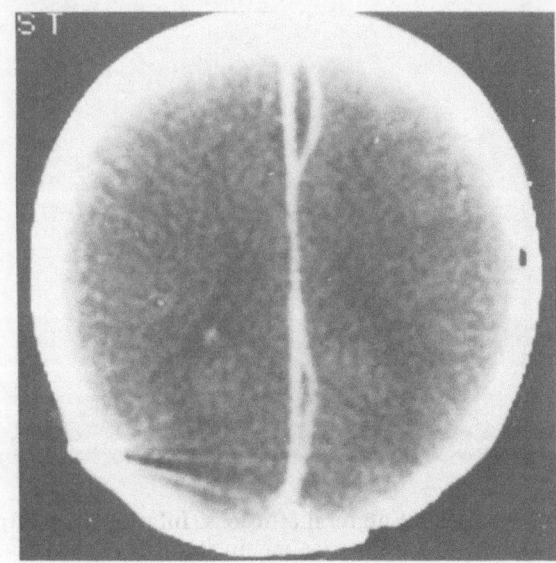

Figure 14. Subdural empyema. (a) unenhanced CT. (b) Contrast-enhanced CT performed 24 hours after initial evacuation of pus. Parafacine location of a subdural empyema is well seen and was a complication of an intraventricular shunt tube placement.

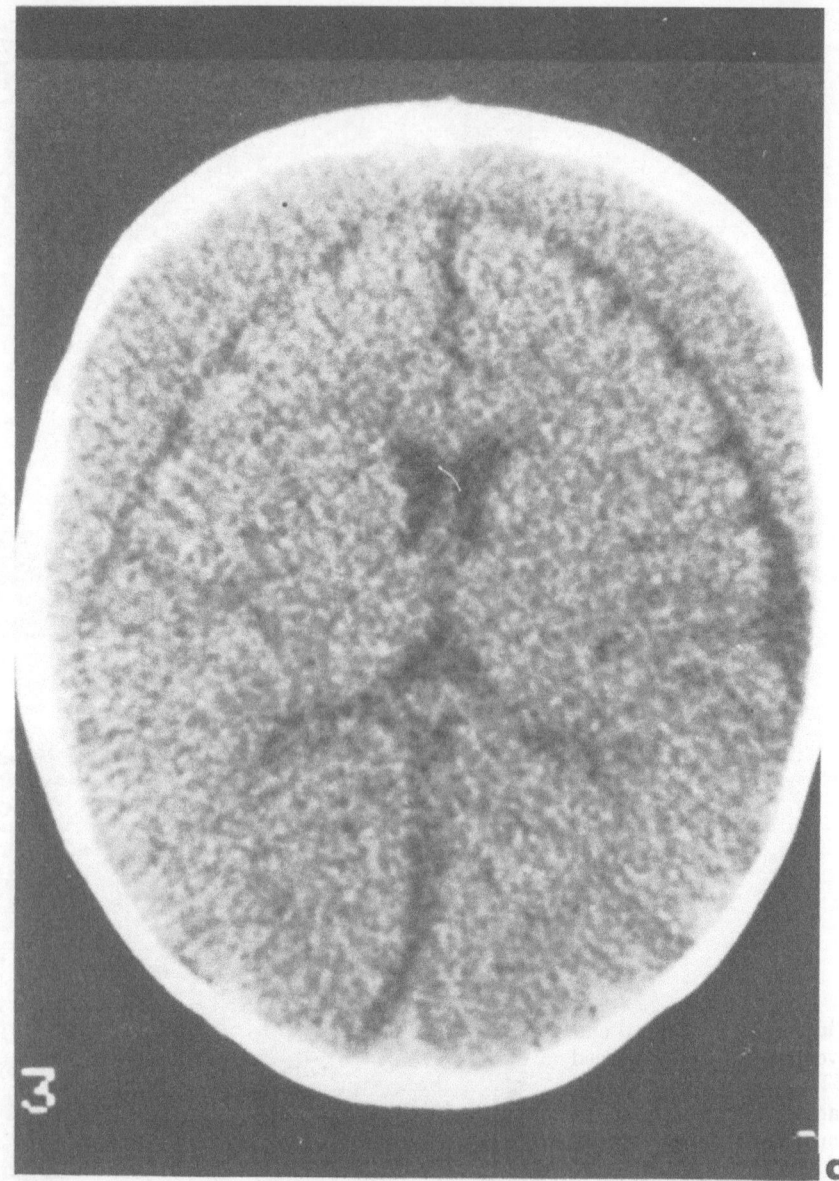

Figure 15. Subdural effusions. Infant with enlarging head following a bout of hemophilus influenzae meningitis. Noncontrast CT scan reveals large bilateral isodense subdural effusions with a sharp interface with the underlying cerebral cortex. Note the prominent frontal bossing.

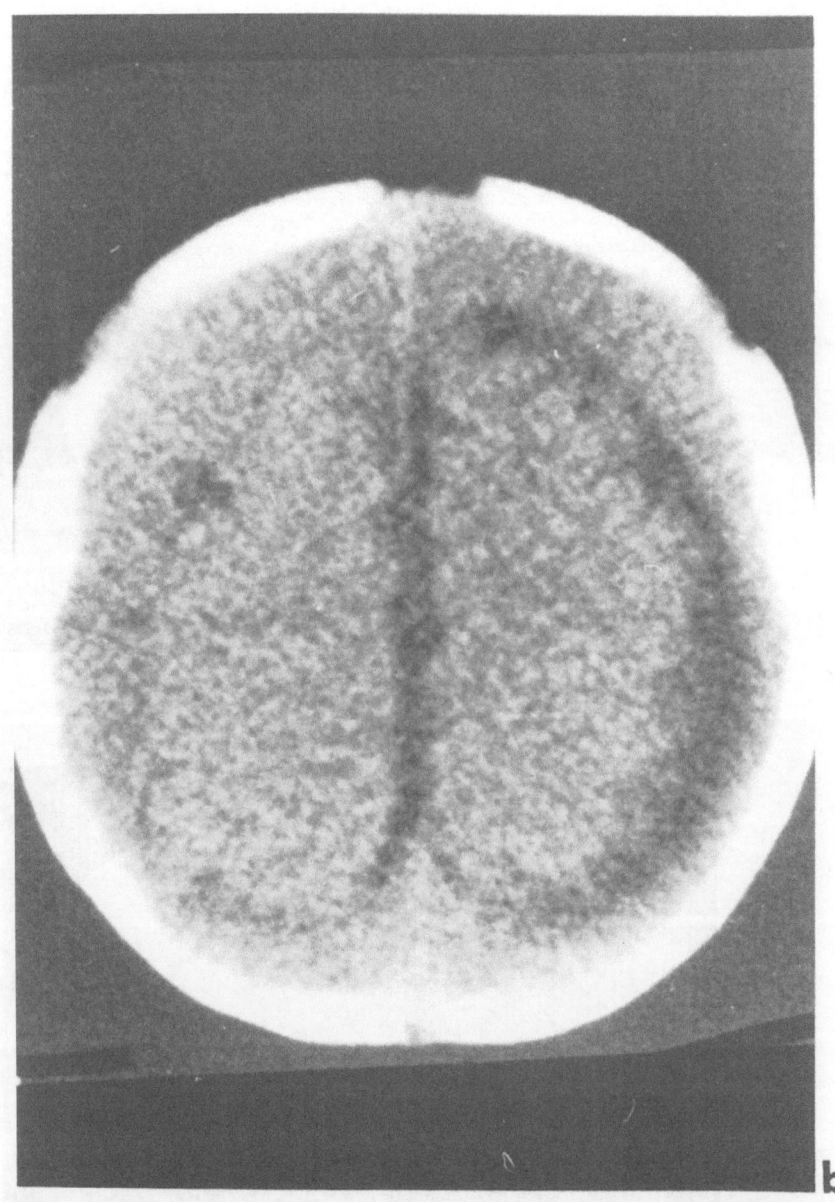

b

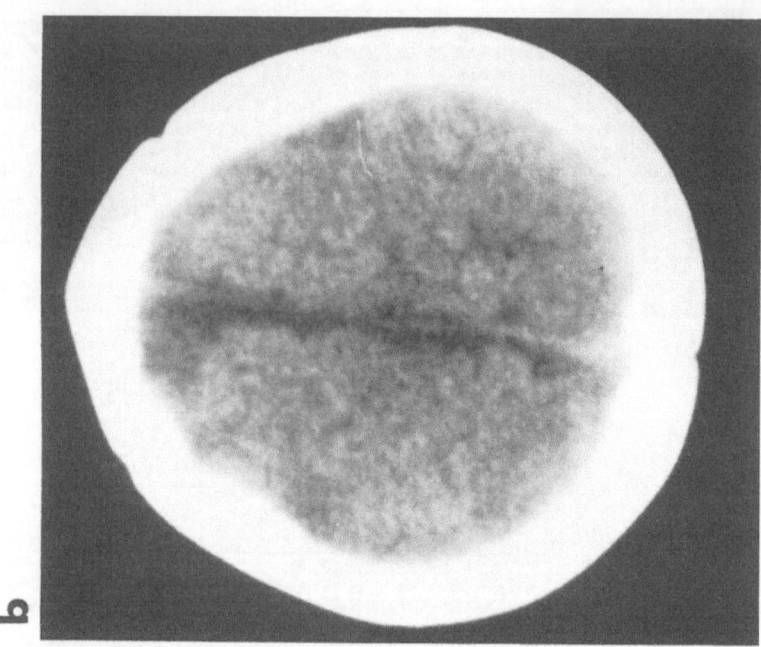

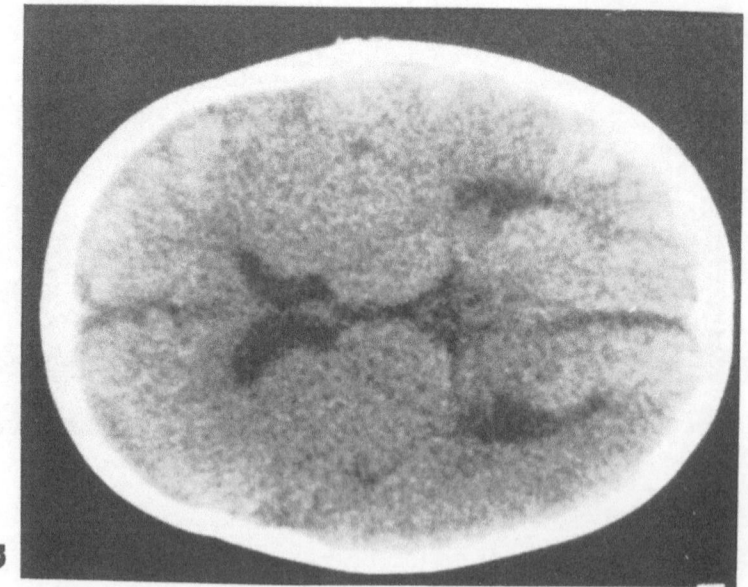

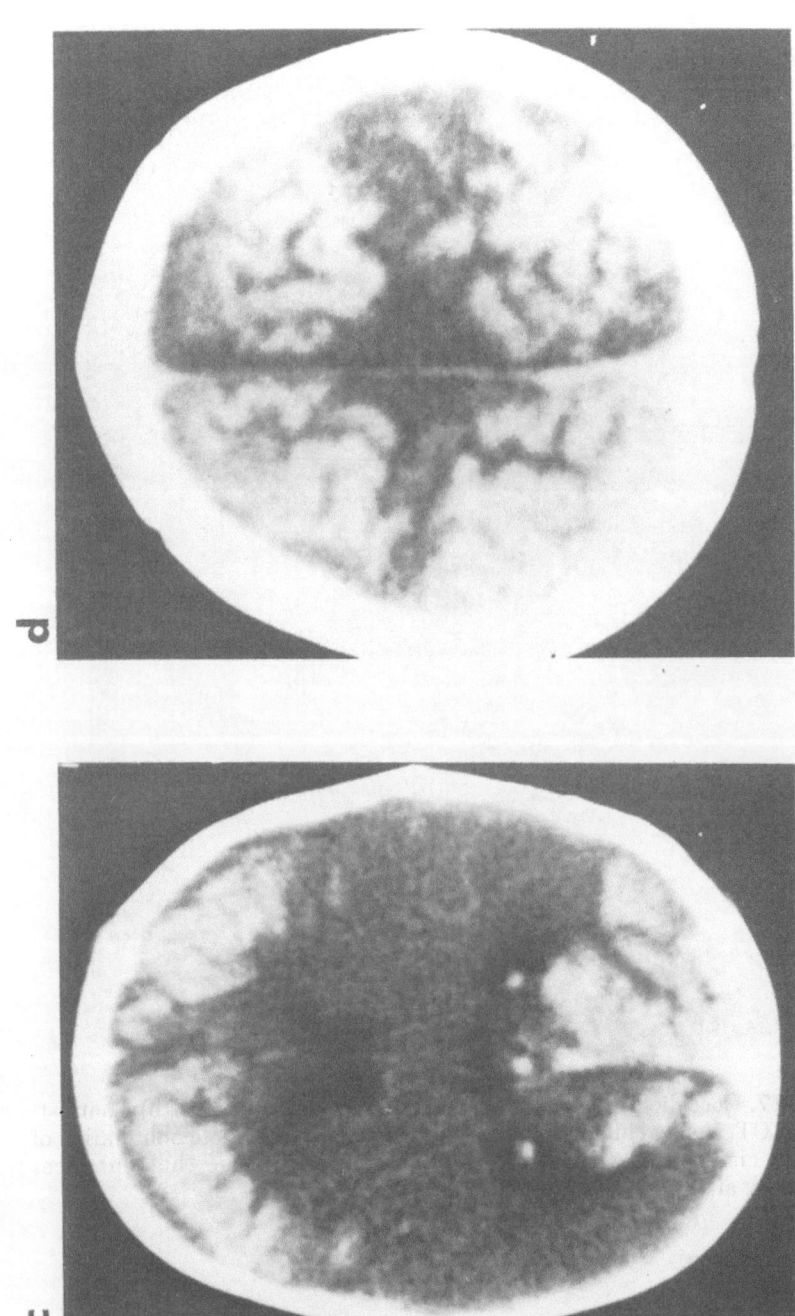

Figure 16. Hemophilus influenzae meningitis. (a, b) Unenhanced CT. (c, d) Contrast-enhanced CT. Striking contrast enhancement of the cortex is seen due to breakdown of the blood–brain barrier and possibly cortical congestion.

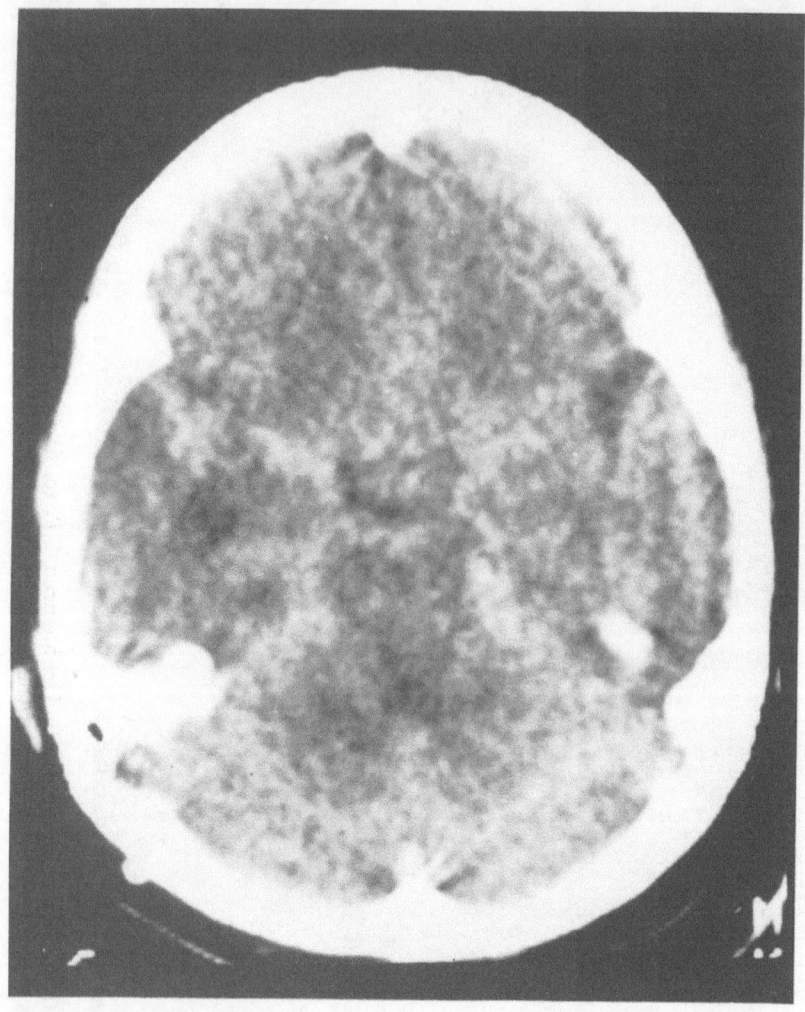

Figure 17. Coccidioidomycosis meningitis. (a) Unenhanced CT. (b) Contrast-enhanced CT. Young child with recent onset of meningitis. Note obliteration of the basal cisterns by slightly dense inflammatory tissue that enhances dramatically after contrast infusion.

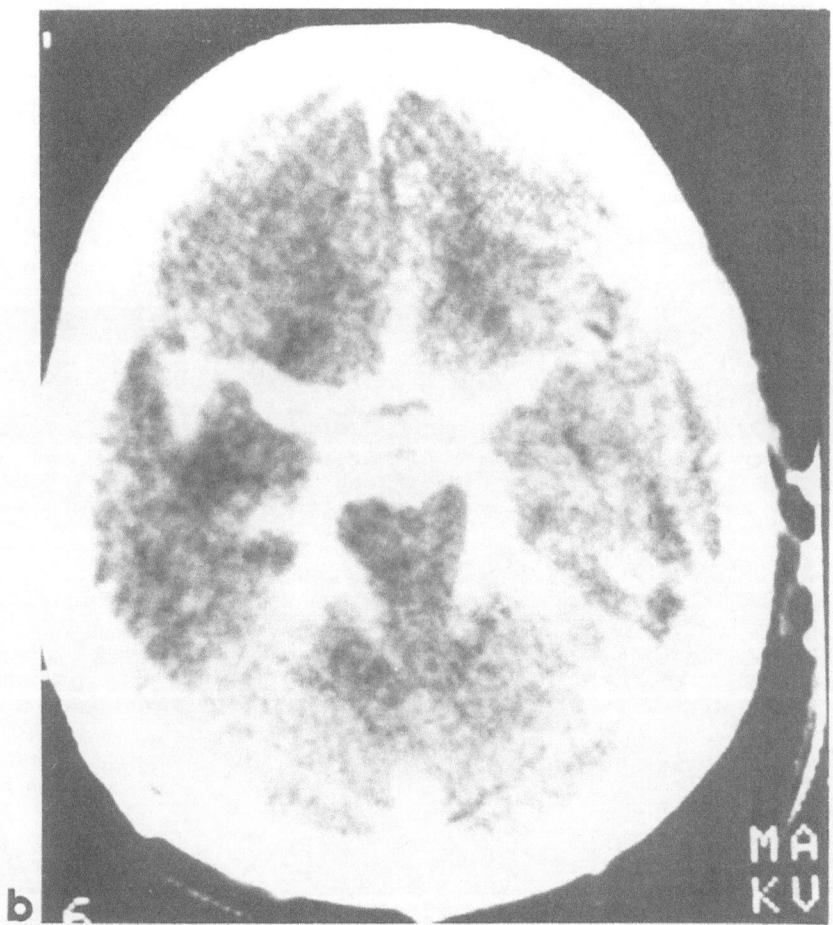

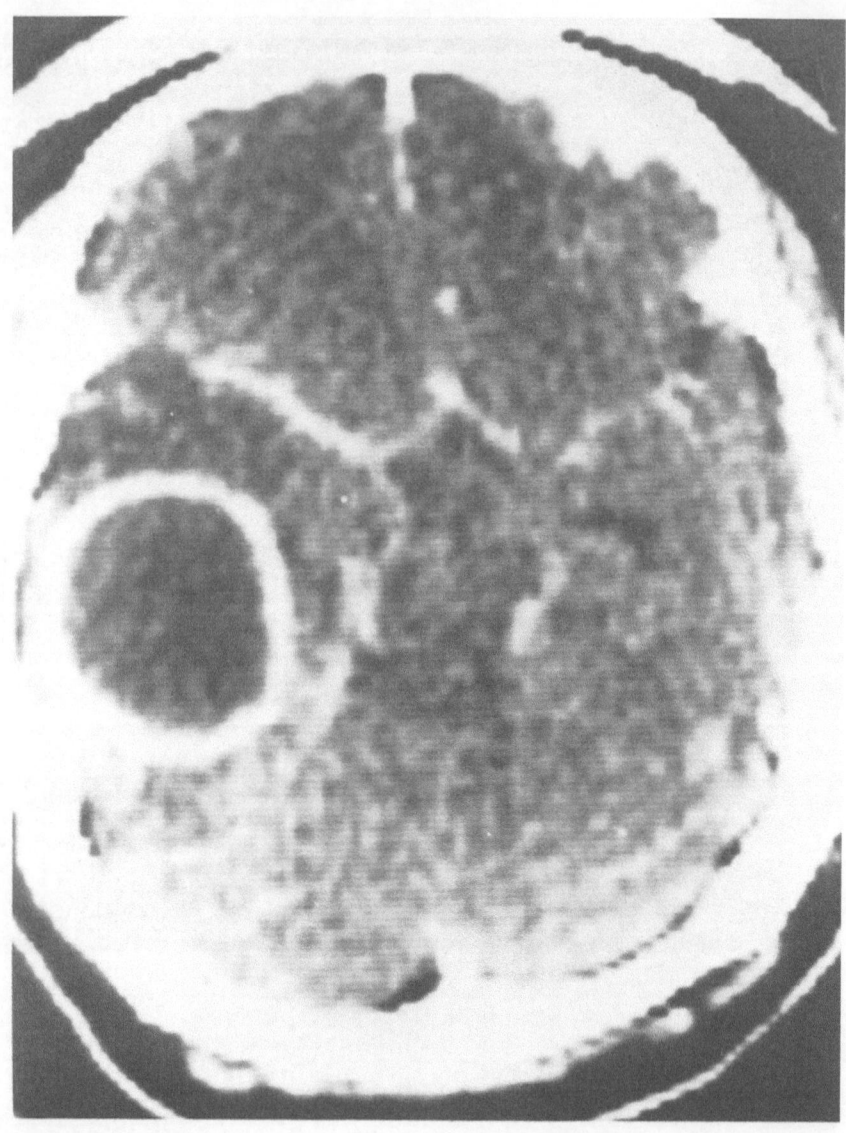

Figure 18. Brain abscess. Young male with history of chronic mastoiditis. Contrast-enhanced CT demonstrates ring enhancement and central lucency. Note stretching and displacement of the right middle cerebral artery by the mass effect.

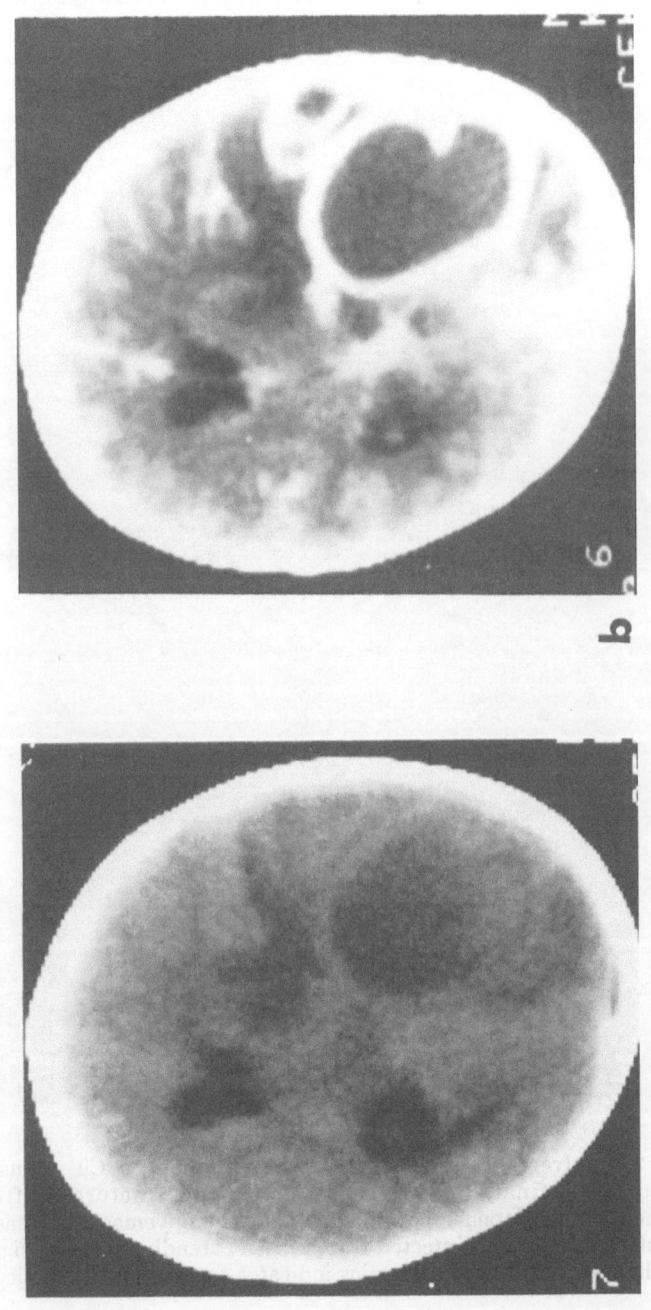

Figure 19. Brain abscess. (a) Unenhanced CT. (b) Contrast-enhanced CT. Infant clinically suspected to have meningitis. CT scan performed because of deteriorization after lumbar puncture shows a multiloculated abscess cavity with a medial nodular component consistent with a focal zone of cerebritis.

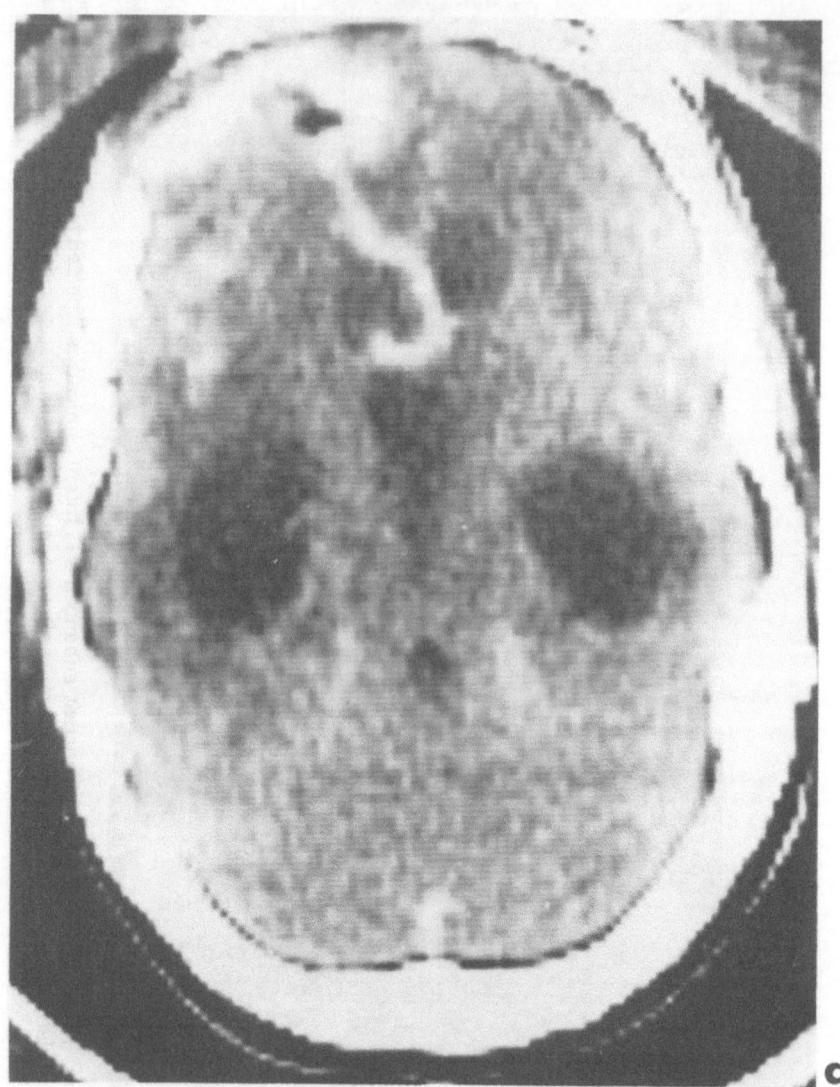

Figure 20. Intracranial abscesses. Contrast-enhanced CT scans. Patient sustained contaminated depressed frontal skull fractures. After initial debridement he developed subdural and epidural empyemas as well as multiple frontal lobe abscesses. An infected tract is seen extending into the right frontal horn. Enhancement of the ventricules indicates an associated ventriculitis.

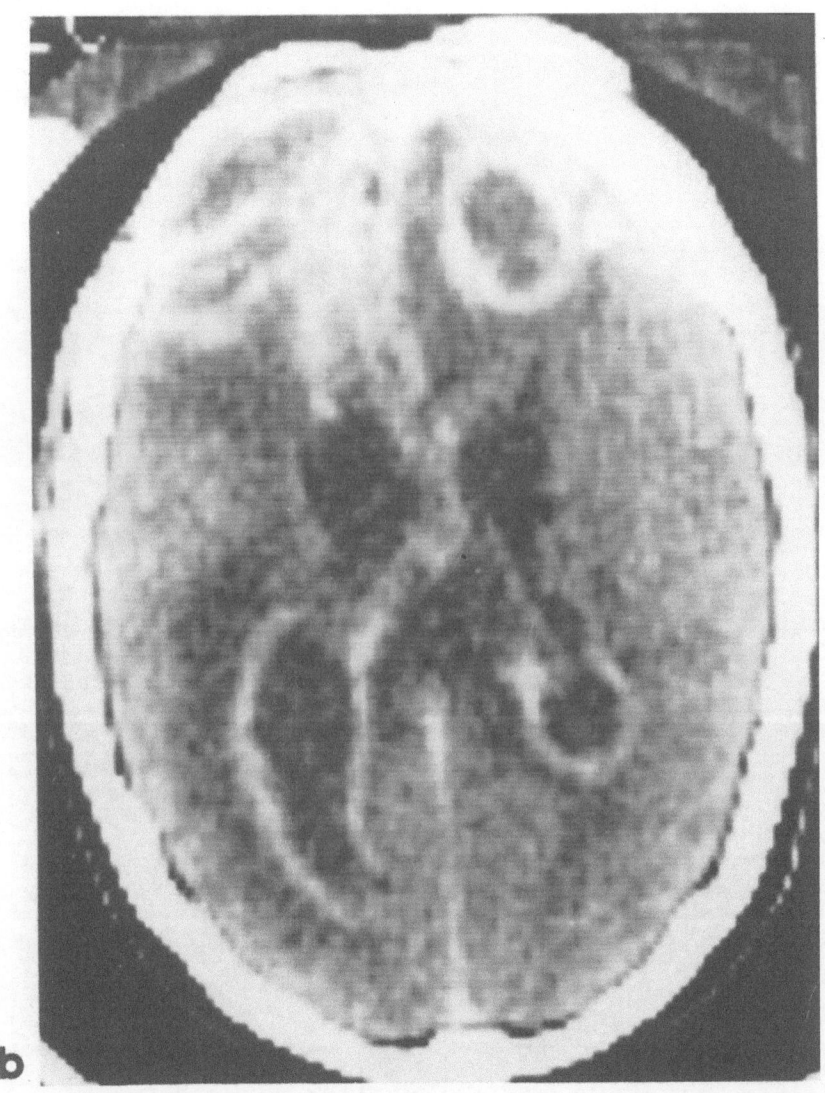

b

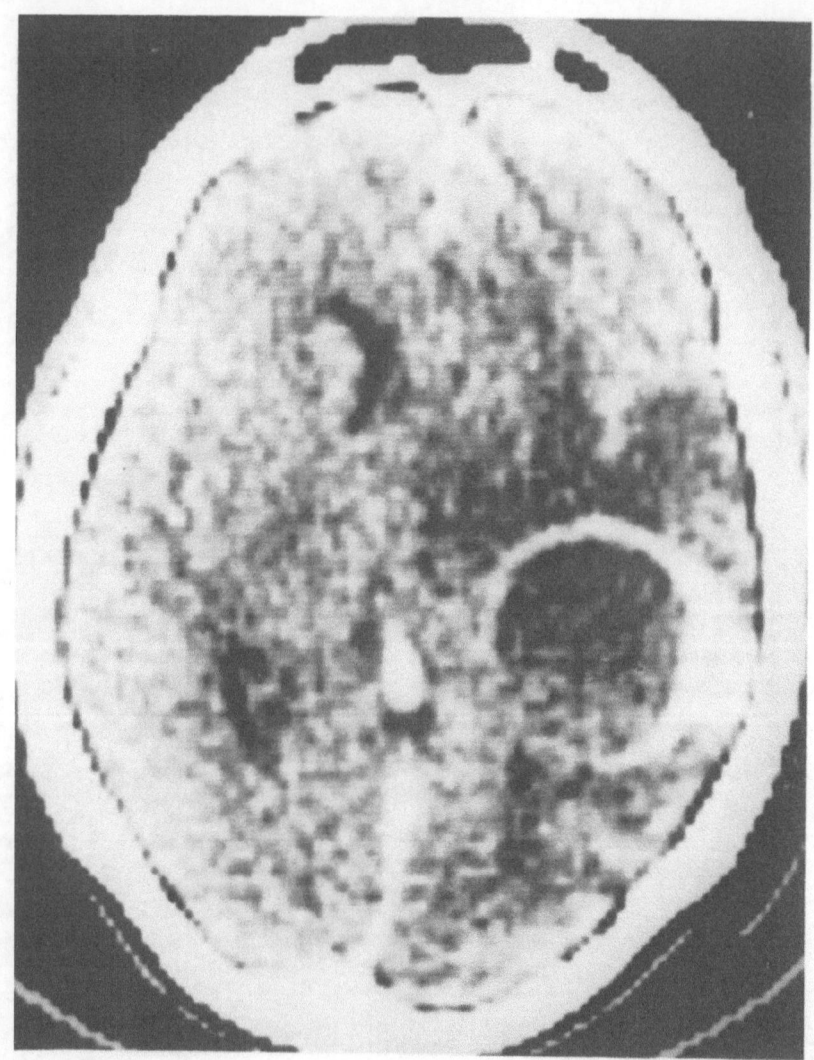

Figure 21. Nocardia brain abscess. (a) Contrast-enhanced computed tomography demonstrates a well-defined ring-enhancing lesion with a thick lateral rind. Central lucency, surrounding edema, and midline shift are associated findings. (b) Contrast-enhanced CT after catheter drainage shows reduction in the size of the abscess cavity.

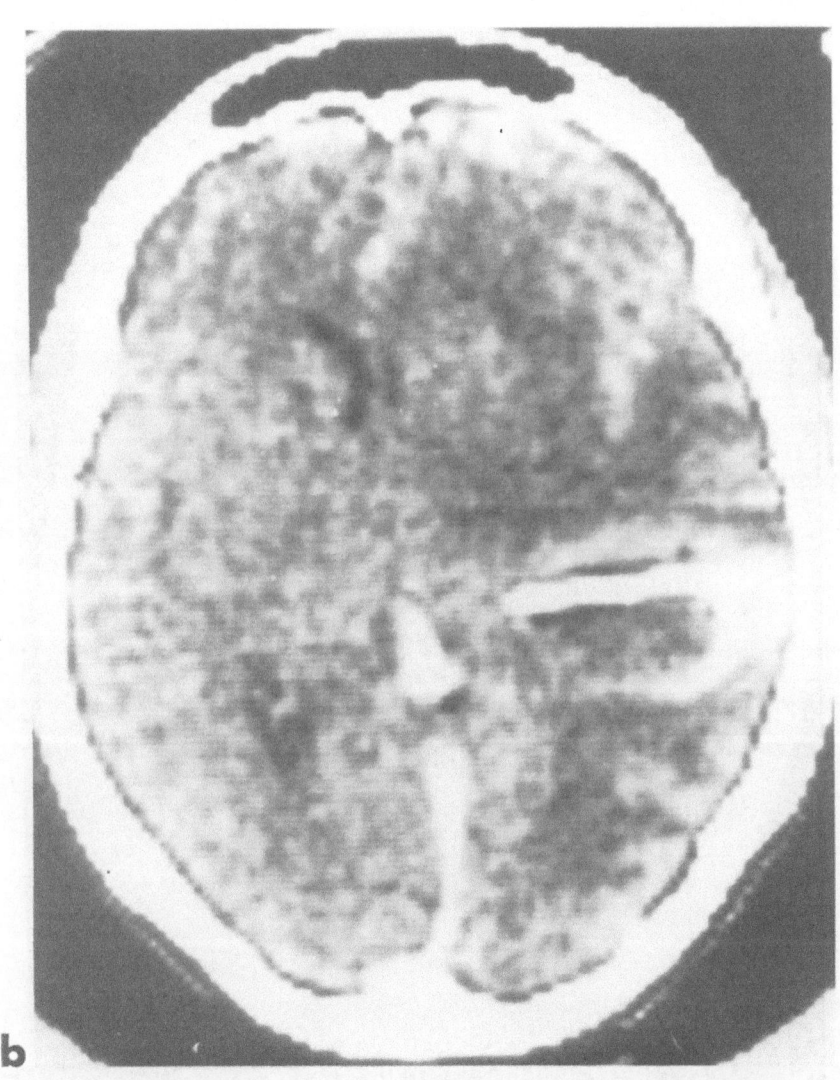

b

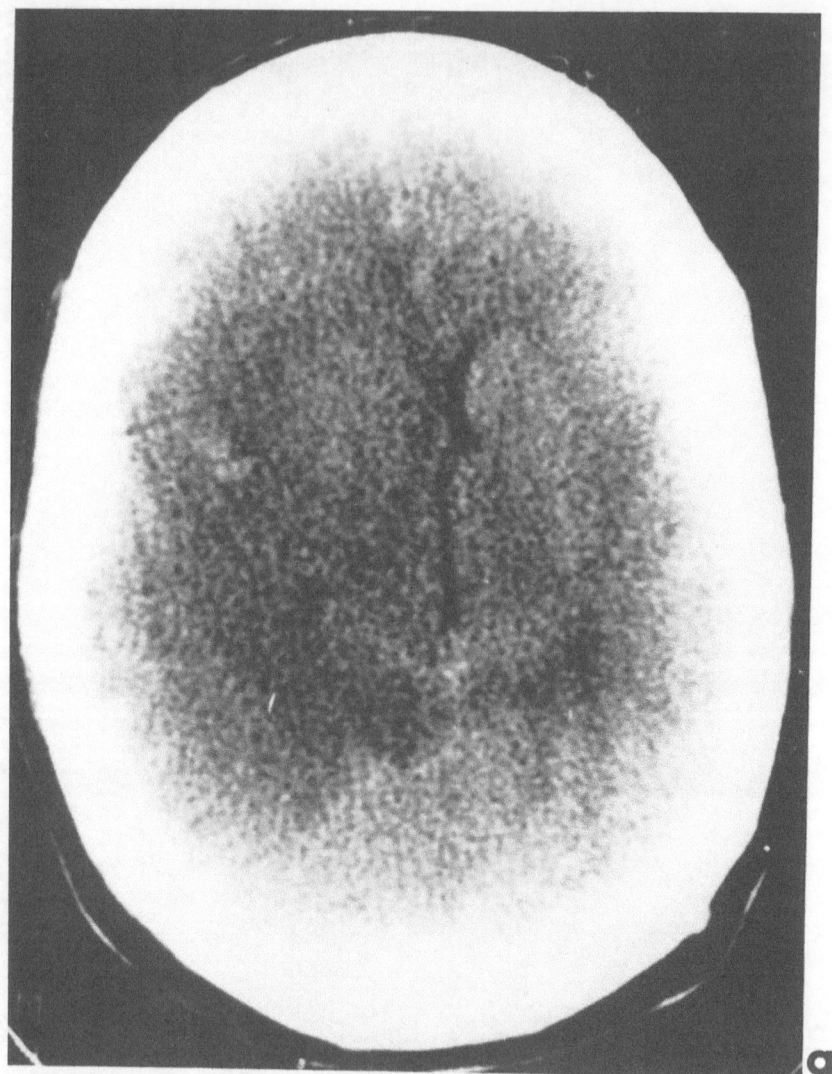

Figure 22. Herpes simplex encephalitis. (a) Unenhanced CT. (b) Contrast-
enhanced CT. Demonstrated are diffuse temporal and frontal lobe swelling on
the right with focal zone of hemorrhage. After contrast infusion, a diffuse area of
enhancement is seen in the anterior temporal lobe.

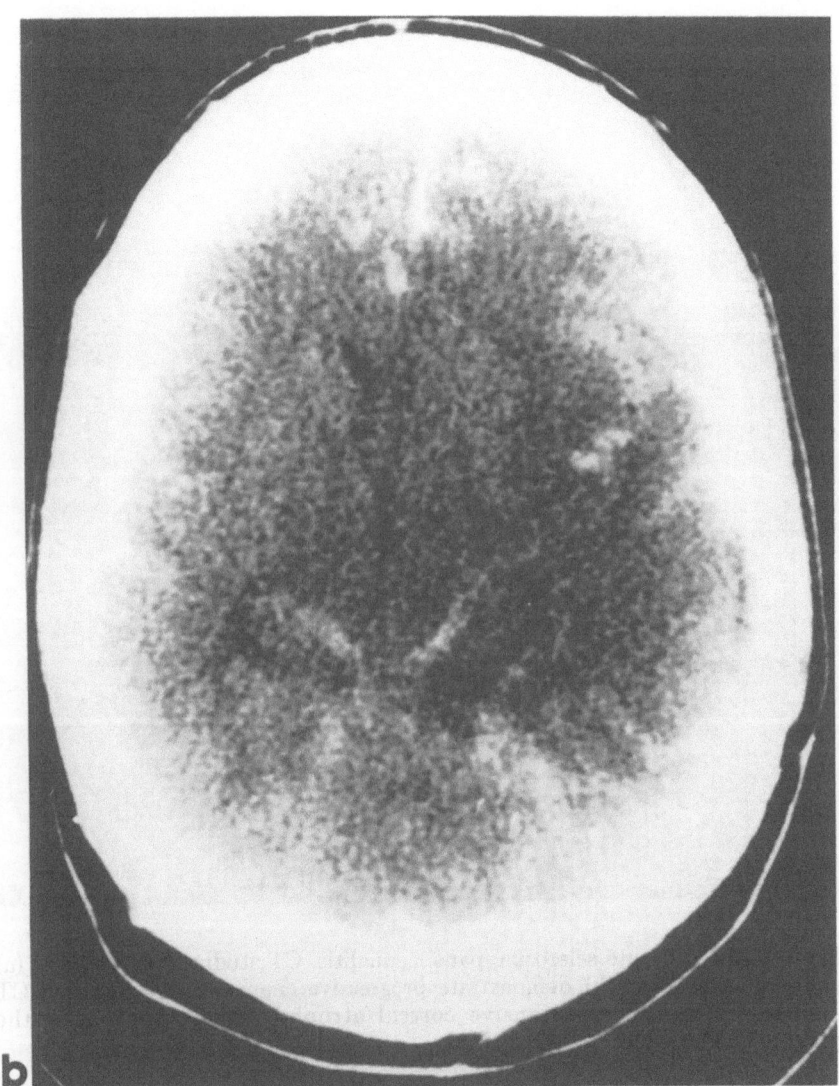

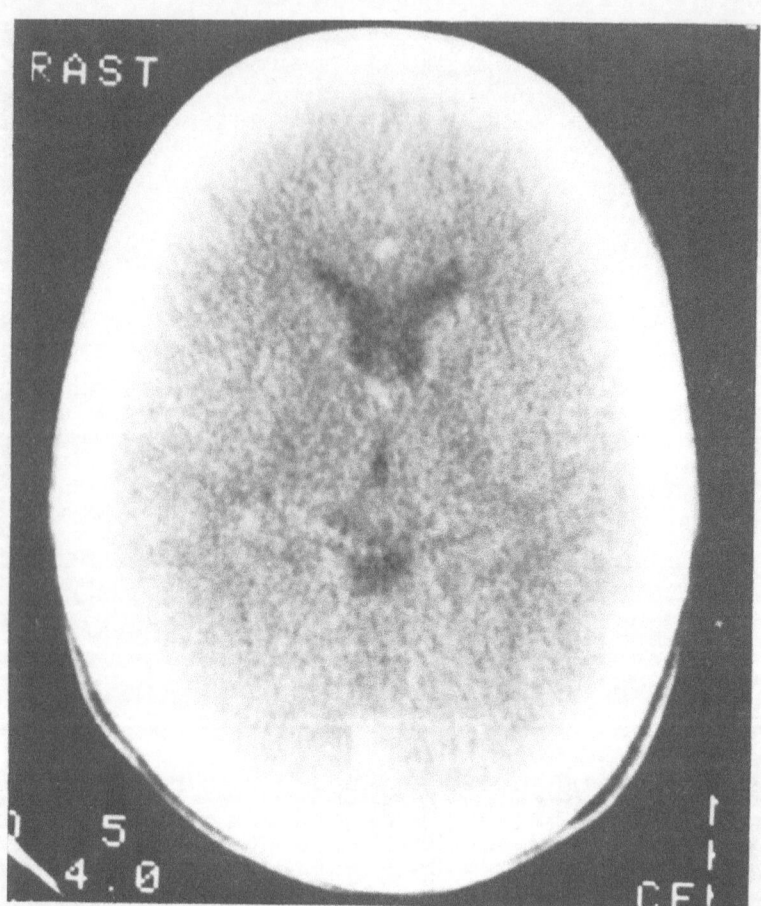

Figure 23. Subacute sclerosing panencephalitis. CT studies done initially (a) and 4 months later (b) demonstrate progressive changes from a normal CT appearance to one of extensive cortcal atrophy and diminution of the paraventricular white matter.

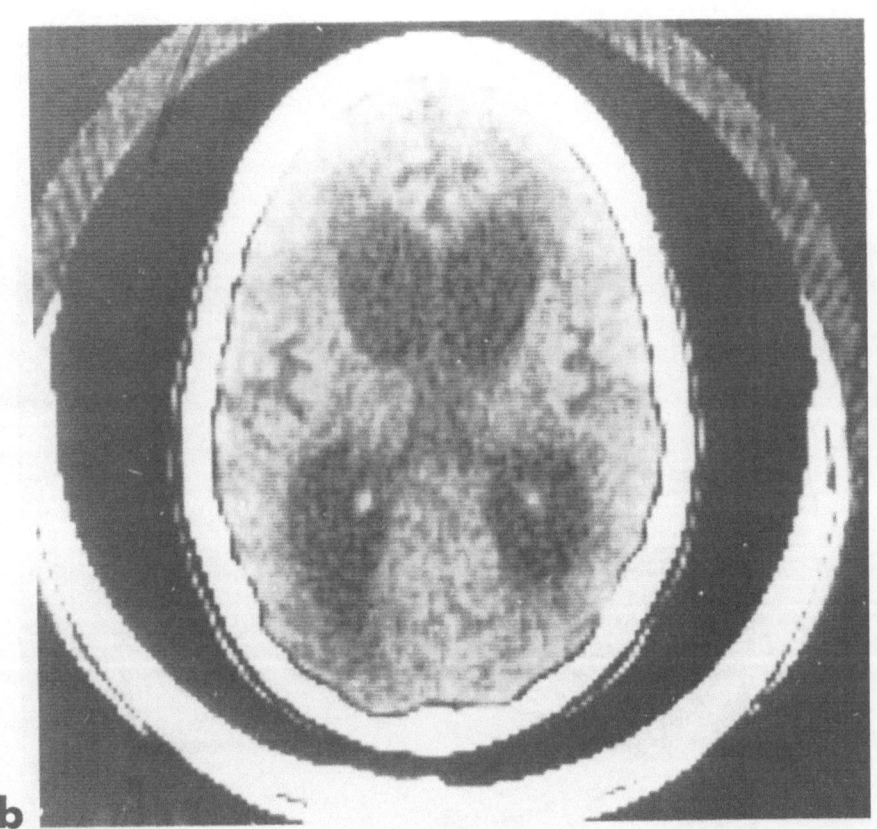

b

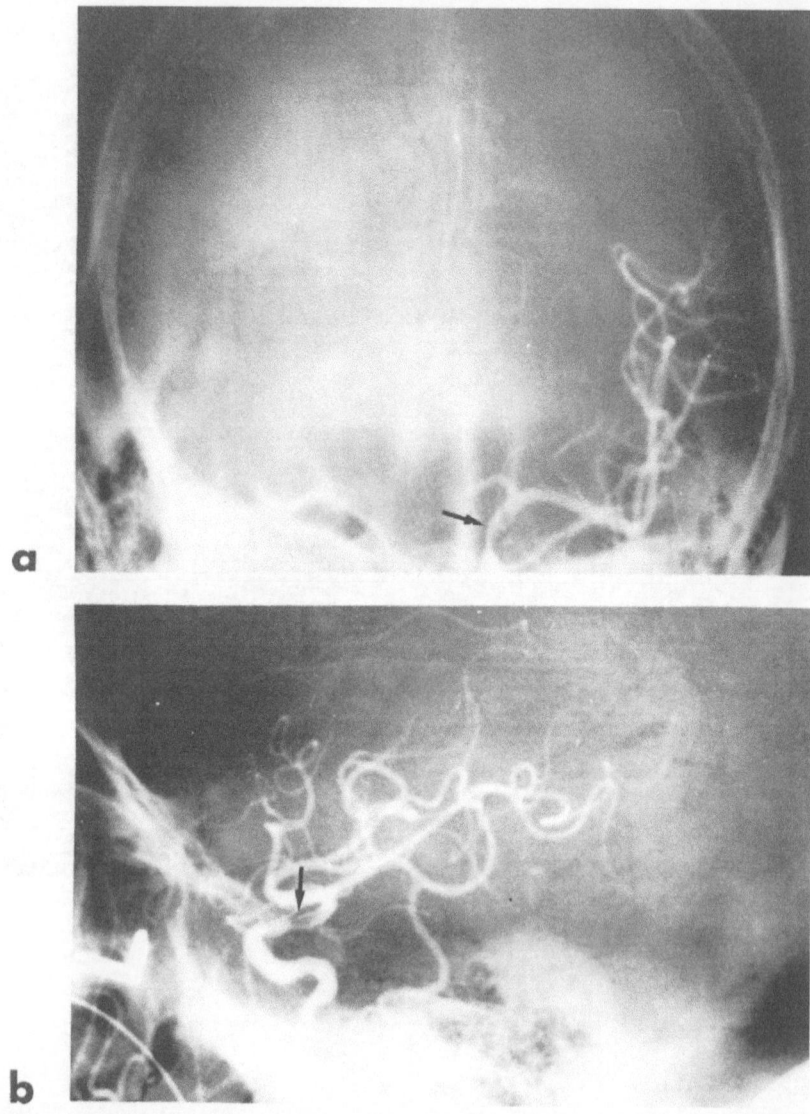

Figure 24. Mucormycosis. (a) Anteroposterior and (b) lateral cerebral angiograms. Filling defect (clot) is noted within the immediate supraclinoid internal carotid artery and there is occlusion of the ophthalmic artery. At autopsy, the microorganism was found within the clot. (c) Orbital venography demonstrates occlusion of the left superior ophthalmic vein. (d) CT clearly reveals proptosis of the left eye with a retrobulbar mass invading the ipsilateral ethmoid sinuses.

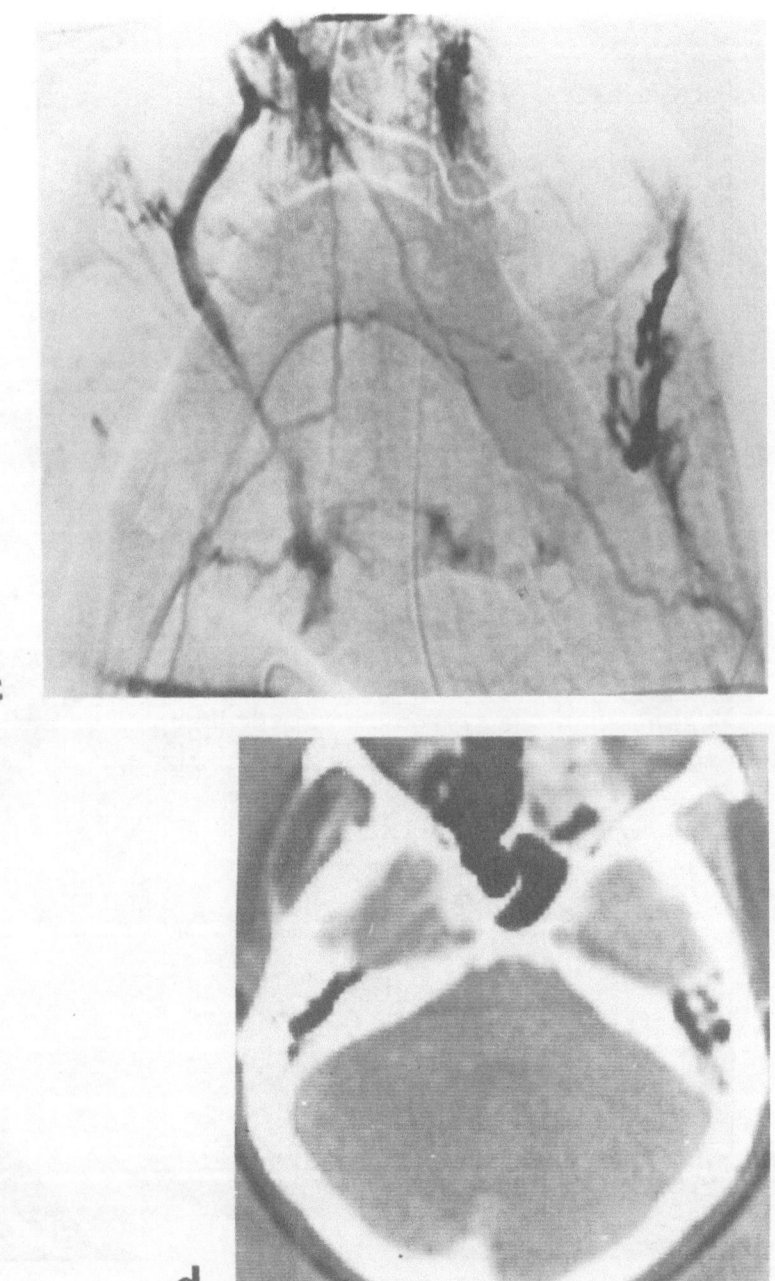

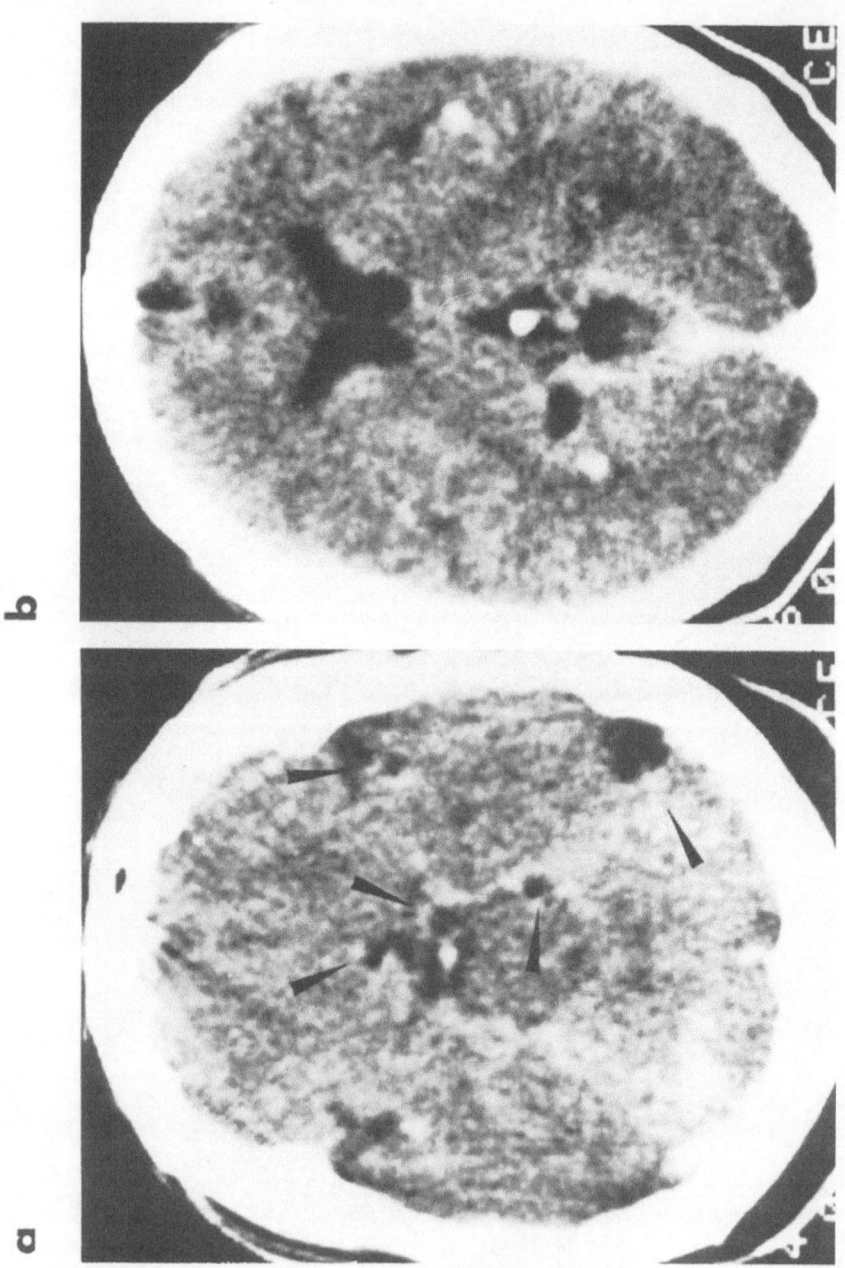

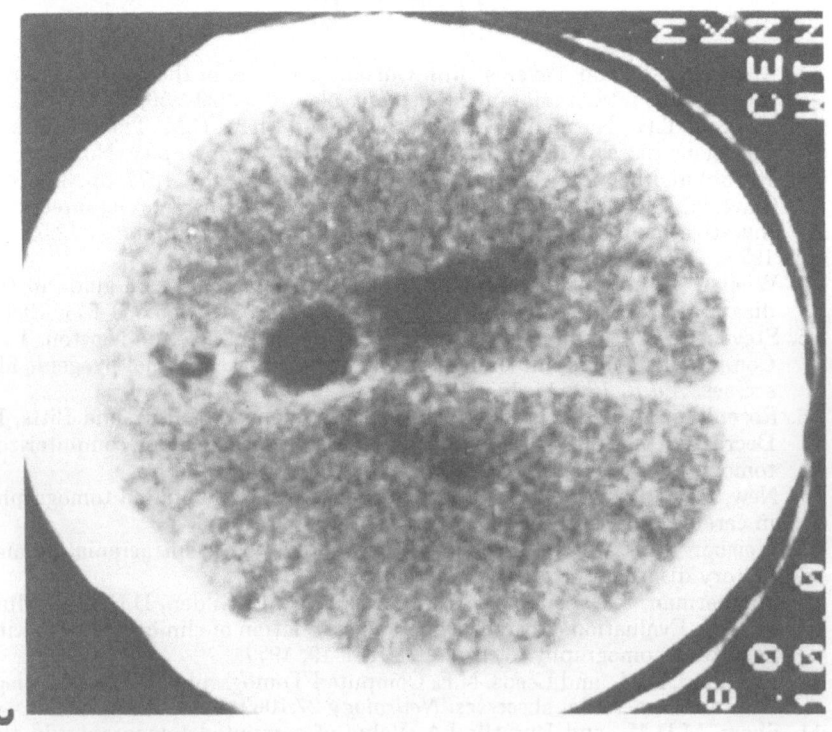

c

Figure 25. Cysticercosis. Contrast-enhanced CT scans. Leptomeningeal form of cysticercosis with sharply defined cysts in the basal cisterns, sylvian fissures, and the interhemispheral fissure. Note the small zone of contrast enhancement along the right sylvian fissure (b).

REFERENCES

1. Altemus, L.R. and Taveras, J.M. Current concepts in the neuroradiologic diagnosis of intracranial infection. *Adv. Neurol.* 6:229–256, 1974.
2. Newton, T.H., Norman, D., Alvord, E.C., and Shaw, C.M. The CT scan in infectious diseases of the CNS. In: *Computed Tomography.* Norman, D., Korobkin, M., and Newton, T.H., eds. St. Louis: Mosby, 1977, pp. 317–338.
3. Claveria, L.E., Du Boulay, G.H., and Moseley, I.F. Intracranial infections: investigation by computerized axial tomography. *Neuroradiology 12:*59–71, 1976.
4. Whelan, M.A., and Hilal, S.K. Computed Tomography as a guide in the diagnosis and follow-up of brain abscesses. *Radiology 135:*663–671, 1980.
5. Stevens, E.A., Norman, D., Kramer, R.A., Messina, A.B., and Newton, T.H. Computed tomographic brain scanning in intraparenchymal pyogenic abscesses. *A.J.R. 130:*111–114, 1978.
6. Rosenblum, M.L., Huff, J.T., Norman, D., Weinstein, P.R., and Pitts, L. Decreased mortality from brain abscesses since advent of computerized tomography. *J. Neurosurg.* 49:658–668, 1978.
7. New, P.F.J., Davis, K.R. and Ballantine, Jr., H.T. Computed tomography in cerebral abscess. *Radiology 121:*641–646, 1976.
8. Weisberg, L.A. Cerebral computerized tomography in intracranial inflammatory disorders. *Arch. Neurol.* 37:137–142, 1980.
9. Zimmerman, R.A., Bilaniuk, L.T., Shipkin, P.M., Gilden, D.H., and Murtagh, F. Evaluation of cerebral abscess: correlation of clinical features with computed tomography. *Neurology* 27:14–19, 1977.
10. Kaufman, D.M., and Leeds, N.E. Computed Tomography (CT) in the diagnosis of intracranial abscesses. *Neurology* 27:1069–1073, 1977.
11. Shaw, M.D.M., and Russell, J.A. Value of computed tomography in the diagnosis of intracranial abscess. *J. Neurol. Neurosurg. Psychiatry 40:*214–220, 1977.
12. Joubert, M.J., and Stephanov, S. Computerized tomography and surgical treatment in intracranial suppuration. *J. Neurosurg.* 47:73–78, 1977.
13. Rotherman, Jr., E.B., and Kessler, L.A. Use of computerized tomography in nonsurgical management of brain abscess. *Arch Neurol.* 36:25–26, 1979.
14. Berg, B., Franklin, G., Caneo, R., Boldrey, E., and Strimling, B. Nonsurgical cure of brain abscess: early diagnosis and followup with computerized tomography. *Ann. Neurol.* 3:474–478, 1978.
15. Lott, T., El Gammal, T., Dasiliva, R., Hanks, D., and Reynolds, J. Evaluation of brain and epidural abscesses by computed tomography. *Radiology 122:*371–376, 1977.
16. Dunker, R.O., and Khakoo, R.A. Failure of computed tomographic scanning to demonstrate subdural empyema. *J.A.M.A.* 246:1116–1118, 1981.
17. Sadha, V.K., Handel, S.F., Pinto, R.S., and Glass, T.F. Neuroradiologic diagnosis of subdural empyema and ct limitations. *Am. J. Neuroradiol. 1:*39–44, 1980.
18. Baker, A.S., Ojemann, R.G., Swartz, M.N., and Richardson, Jr., E.P. Spinal epidural abscess. *N. Engl. J. Med.* 293:463–468, 1975.
19. Chambers, A.A., Lukin, R.R., and Tomsick, T.A. Cranial and intracranial tuberculosis. *Sem. Roentgenol.* Vol. 14, No. 4, 1979.
20. Enzmann, D.R., Norman, D., Mani, J., and Newton, T.H. Computed tomography of granulomatous basal arachnoiditis. *Radiology 120:*341–344, 1976.

21. Burger, P.C., and Vogel, F.S. *Surgical Pathology of the Nervous System and Its Coverings.* New York: John Wiley and Sons, 1976.
22. Enzmann, D.R., Britt, R.H., and Yeager, A.S. Experimental brain abscess evaluation: computed tomographic and neuropathologic correlation. *Radiology 133*:113–122, 1979.
23. Enzmann, D.R., Britt, R.H., Lyons, B., Carroll, B., Wilson, D.A., and Buxton, J. High-resolution ultrasound evaluation of experimental abscess evolution: comparison with computed tomography and neuropathology. *Radiology 142*:95–102, 1982.
24. Whitley, R.J., Soong, S., Linneman, Jr., C., Liu, C., Pazin, G., Alford, C.A., and National Inst. of Allergy and Infectious Diseases Collaborative Antiviral Study Group. Herpes Simplex encephalitis. *J.A.M.A. 247*:317–320, 1982.
25. Whitley, R.J., Soong, S., Hirsch, M.S., Karchmer, A. W., Dolin, R., Galasso, G., Dunnick, J. K., Alford, C.A., and NIAID Collaborative Antiviral Study Group. Herpes simplex encephalitis—vidarabine therapy and diagnostic problems. *N. Engl. J. Med. 304*:313–318, 1981.
26. Landry, M.L., Booss, J., and Hsiung, G.D. Duration of vidarabine therapy in biopsy-negative herpes simplex encephalitis. *J.A.M.A. 247*:332–334, 1982.
27. Duda, E.E., Huttenlocher, P.R., and Patronas, N.J. CT of subacute sclerosing panencephalitis. *Am. J. Neuroradiol. 1*:35–38, 1980.
28. Hammock, M.K., and Milhorat, T.H., *Computed Tomography in Infancy and Childhood.* Baltimore/London: Williams and Wilkins, pp. 299–341, 1981.
29. Lazo, A., Wilner, H.I., and Metes, J.J. Craniofacial mucormycosis: computed tomographic and angiographic findings in two cases. *Radiology 139*:623–626, 1981.
30. Addlestone, R.B., and Baylin, G.J. Rhinocerebral mucormycosis. *Radiology 115*:113–117, 1975.
31. Centeno, R.S., Bentson, J.R., and Mancuso, A.A. CT scanning in rhinocerebral mucormycosis and aspergillosis. *Radiology 140*:383–389, 1981.
32. Whelan, M.A., Ster, J., and De Napoli, R.A. The computed tomographic spectrum of intracranial mycosis: correlation with histopathology. *Radiology 141*:703–-707, 1981.
33. Carbajal, J.R., Palacios, E., Azar-Kia, B., and Churchill, R. Radiology of cysticercosis of the central nervous system including computed tomography. *Radiology 125*:127–131, 1977.

9

Treatment and Prevention of Shunt Infection

Robert L. McLaurin and Peter T. Frame

Infection continues to be one of the most common complications of shunting for hydrocephalus, second only in frequency to mechanical shunt malfunction. In contrast to malfunction, however, the proper management of infection remains a matter of differing opinions. The following discussion, therefore, must be considered to present a point of view, but not necessarily the definitive consensus at this time.

INCIDENCE

The incidence of shunt infection as judged from the literature has varied considerably from one investigator to another. One reason for this variation is that some workers have calculated incidence on the basis of the ratio of infection into operations performed for shunt placement or revision while others have calculated on the basis of infection per patient. In 1973, Robertson[1] reviewed all major series of ventriculoatrial shunts and reported a variation of incidence from 7 to 31 per cent. The incidence in ventriculoperitoneal shunts was approximately 14 percent. The majority of reports, however, have indicated that the present incidence is from five to ten percent in peritoneal shunts. It has also been noted that the incidence of infection in the peritoneal shunts is considerably less than that with vascular shunts and it is also noteworthy that the consequences of shunt infection are less devastating with peritoneal shunts.[2]

145

TYPES OF INFECTION

Basically there are two principal forms of shunt infection. The first is an acute infection which occurs shortly after the insertion or revision of a shunt system. This is characterized by systemic signs of acute infection, including fever and leukocytosis, and frequently by evidence of infection along the tract of the shunt. This may be detectable either as reddened swollen inflammation along the course of the shunt or purulent drainage from one or more of the incisions. This type of presentation of infection is most likely to be due to staphyloccus aureus or Gram-negative organisms. This type of occurrence has in our experience been more frequent in neonates whose scalps are extremely thin and susceptible to decubitus ulceration over the hardware. It also may occur if the incision is directly overlying part of the shunt apparatus so that incisional dehiscence and infection may occur. It may be considered that the acute type of infection is primarily an infection on the outside of the shunt system. Although there is probably no absolute barrier between infections on the inside and those on the outside of shunt systems, the clinical presentations differ depending on the primary sight of infection.

The second type of infection is primarily within the shunt system and the cerebrospinal fluid compartment. Clinically, this is likely to present in a more subtle and less fulminating manner although it may occur in the early postoperative period. It can also be seen months after the last operative procedure although this type of presentation appears to be decreasing in incidence. The infection is usually not associated with evidence of acute inflammation but rather is accompanied by intermittent low grade fever, anemia, moderate leukocytosis, and if prolonged, the presence of hepatosplenomegaly. The cerebrospinal fluid infection is usually not a fulminating ventriculitis or meningitis and therefore signs of meningeal inflammation or neurologic dysfunction as a result of infection are generally not present. The organisms responsible for this type of infection are quite variable, although the most common organism has in the past been *Staphylococcus epidermidis*. During the past two years the experience in this clinic has been that the incidence of *S. epidermidis* infection has diminished while the occurrence of other organisms has increased in frequency.

While many types of organisms, including obscure varieties, have been responsible for shunt infections, one may conveniently consider that there are basically two sources of infection. The first of these includes contaminants from the skin; the principal organisms from this source are *S. aureus, S. epidermidis, Streptococcus viridans*, and diphtheroids. The second major source of contamination is from the enteric organisms. This includes *E. coli, Klebsiella, Enterobacteriaciae,* and enterococcus. This list of organisms includes the majority of those which have been treated in this clinic.

METHODS OF TREATMENT

There are three basic types of treatment used at the present time: (1) complete removal of the shunt apparatus followed by antibiotic therapy; (2) removal of an infected shunt with immediate replacement of a new system followed by antibiotic therapy; (3) antibiotic therapy alone without surgical removal of the shunt.

Ideally, the last method is the optimum type of treatment since it does not subject the patient to any surgical procedures or to risks of intracranial hypertension due to the absence of a shunt system. On the other hand, the use of antibiotics alone without surgical removal is not always successful and, therefore, has not been widely accepted as a means of treatment. It is believed, however, by this author that the incidence of cure of infection without surgical intervention is sufficiently high that it should in most instances be the first method of treatment. The following discussion will be concerned mainly with this form of management.

PRINCIPLES OF TREATMENT

Antibiotics

Several principles regarding the use of antibiotics are important to effective therapy. The first such principle is that very few of the antibiotics presently being used cross the blood-CSF barrier and, therefore, achieve very inadequate spinal fluid concentration. It must be recalled that in most shunt infections the meninges are not significantly inflamed and, therefore, those antibiotics which achieve access to the CSF only in the presence of inflammation do not approach therapeutic levels when administered parenterally. For example, penicillins and cephalosporins achieve very poor penetration to the CSF with uninflamed meninges and the cephalosporins do not penetrate adequately even in the presence of inflammation. The penetration of aminoglycosides into spinal fluid is

generally poor except during the neonatal period. Chloramphenicol has
been determined to penetrate into spinal fluid and also into brain tissue.
Vancomycin, however, achieves no significant penetration into spinal
fluid. It may be noted, however, that rifampin and trimethoprim have
been shown to penetrate the spinal fluid barrier quite adequately and
both of these preparations are administered orally. From the above brief
review of the pharmacodynamics of the antibiotics it becomes apparent
that only rarely can adequate CSF concentration be achieved by parental
therapy and therefore direct administration of antibiotic into the ventricular fluid is essential. In most instances, the principal site of infection
is inside the shunt system. This site is well protected from antibiotic
concentration in the tissues surrounding the shunt. It is an essential
principle of treatment, therefore, that a high concentration of antibiotic
be administered to the inside of the shunt. This principle has somehow
been ignored by many previous observers. Schoenbaum et al.,[3] in a review
of 91 patients with infected shunts, condemned the use of antibiotics
alone to control such infection although no patient received antibiotics
by direct installation into the CSF.

There are several principles of antibiotic therapy which have been
learned from the treatment of endocarditis. One such principle is that
sterilization of the inside of a shunt system is mainly a function of the
fluid bathing that surface since the patient's phagocytic system has no
access to it. Therefore, the antibiotic regimen must provide a bactericidal
titer to the CSF to compensate for the absence of the patient's natural
phagocytic defense system. In addition, it is necessary that a sufficient
time of exposure to bactericidal concentrations be allowed. Although this
latter principle is recognized it has not been determined at present what
the optimal period of treatment may be.

Another principle of treatment involves the use of the CSF inhibitory or bactericidal titer rather than relying on antibiotic concentration in
relation to *in vitro* mean inhibitory concentration in monitoring the
effectiveness of treatment. This principle also derived from early work
with endocarditis and resulted from the rationale that the bacterial killing must be achieved by the effectiveness of the antibiotic within the
patient's body fluids, in this case the CSF. The inhibitory or bactericidal
titer is obtained by testing the effectiveness of the spinal fluid, obtained
at a trough level, against the offending organism. It is presently accepted
that bacterial killing should be achieved at a concentration of 1:8 or
less.

The required frequency for intraventricular antibiotic administration, in order to achieve adequate trough levels, has been determined in

a series of observations reported by Wald and McLaurin[4] These observations were made in 20 patients with documented shunt infections and daily intraventricular injections of either methicillin, cephalothin, or gentamycin were performed. Trough levels were obtained in all patients at 24 hours and in many instances at 48 and 72 hours after the last injection. In all cases the antibiotic level within the ventricular system was well above the Minimum Inhibitory Concentration (MIC) of that organism 24 hours after intraventricular injection. At 48 hours the ventricular levels were usually above the MIC but in a few instances inadequate concentrations were found. The goal of therapy at the time of that study was to establish an antibiotic level at least five times the MIC and inhibitory and bactericidal titers were not being used. The conclusion reached on the basis of those observations was that there is essentially never any need for intraventricular injection more frequently than every 24 hours in the presence of a well-functioning shunt. Only rarely does administration need to be more often than every 48 hours although it has been our practice to continue 24 hourly injections.

Finally, appropriate antibiotic therapy may involve the use of multiple synergistic agents; this is amplified below.

Surgical

There are two main surgical principles to be kept in mind for effective antibiotic treatment of shunt infection if the shunt apparatus is to be left *in situ*. Both of these principles are dependent on the concept that a bactericidal concentration of antibiotic must be delivered to the inside of the apparatus. The first of these is the need to insure that the shunt is functioning satisfactorily. If malfunction of a shunt is present it is very unlikely that the shunt can be sterilized effectively. This applies not only to malfunction due to proximal shunt failure but also to distal malfunction which may occur as a result of the infection itself causing a peritoneal cyst around the distal end of the catheter. The corollary to this principle therefore, is that it is essential to determine that there is no peritoneal cyst around the distal catheter tip. This can best be achieved by the use of ultrasound which should be a routine procedure before antibiotic therapy.

The second surgical principle involves the presence of retained shunt components within or adjacent to the ventricular system. Any such retained components which are not functioning cannot be sterilized since there will be no access of the antibiotics to their internal surfaces. Therefore, if such retained components exist, it is necessary that they be removed before therapy.

Specific Recommendations for Antibiotics

Table 1 summarizes our present recommendations for therapy. It is noted that chloramphenicol, despite its access to CSF, is not recommended because it is basically not bactericidal, a function which was noted earlier to be essential in sterilizing a foreign body. It is also to be noted that methicillin is not included in the recommendations. Although methicillin is a very effective antistaphyloccal antibiotic it is considered less desirable than nafcillin for three reasons: (1) here is a higher incidence of interstitial nephritis with methicillin than with nafcillin; (2) nafcillin is five to ten times more active against staphylococci on a weight basis; and (3) nafcillin is more efffective against streptococci than methicillin.

The recommended antibiotic regimen includes the use of multiple antibiotics. Antibiotic synergism (bacterial inhibition or killing which is greater than the effect of either antibiotic alone) is an important part of our present therapy of shunt infections. In general, synergism occurs between a betalactam antibiotic (a penicillin or cephlosporin) and an aminoglycoside. Synergistic activity is usually present when the organism is sensitive to both the beta-lactam and the aminoglycoside. It must be kept in mind that antibiotic antagonism can occur but is generally seen when one antibiotic of the combination is a bacteriostatic agent such as chloramphenicol or tetracycline. For this reason, these agents are not recommended in the management of shunt infections. As noted above, the synergistic combined effectiveness of the antibiotics can be determined only by the use of the inhibitory or bactericidal titer of the "trough" spinal fluid specimen. Our most recent experience with shunt infections has included treatment with antibiotic regimens consisting of orally

TABLE 1. Selection of Antibiotics in Shunt Infections

1. *Staphylococcus aureus* and *Staphylococcus epidermidis*:
   a. If sensitive (MIC < 1.0 mg/ml) nafcillin, cephalothin, or cepharpirin intravenous (IV), intraventricular (IVT), plus gentamicin IVT.
   b. If resistant to nafcillin, cephalothin, and cephapirin: rifampin, po, plus TMP/sulfa, po, plus vancomycin, IV and IVT (Trimethoprim alone may be given in place of TMP/sulfa).
2. *Enterococcus:* ampicillin IV, IVT, plus gentamicin IVT. If intravascular shunt, gentamicin IV also.
3. Other streptococci: either a staphylococcal or enterococcal regimen.
4. Aerobic Gram-negative rods: according to susceptibilities, should use both a beta-lactam and aminoglycoside IV and IVT.
5. *Corynebacterium* sp. and *Propionibacterium* sp. (diptheroids)
   a. Penicillin sensitive: use enterococcal regimen.
   b. Penicillin resistant: vancomycin IV, plus IVT.

administered antibiotics supplemented by daily intrashunt injections.
Nine patients have been treated in this manner and they all received
trimethoprim-sulfamethoxasole in doses designed to achieve serum concentration of 75 to 150 µg of sulfamethoxasole. Seven patients also received oral rifampin in doses ranging from 10 to 20 mg/kg/24 hours.
Seven of the patients received vancomycin in the ventricular system
while the other two received cephapirin and kanamycin, respectively.
Inhibitory titers of the spinal fluid remained well above 1:8 in all instances.

The results of therapy in this group of patients are shown in Table
2. It is noted that seven of the nine patients were treated with the shunt
remaining *in situ* while two patients required complete removal of the
shunt. There was one therapeutic failure in the group. The duration of
"cures" so far seems to indicate that this method of treatment may be
effective in a significant percentage of patients. The advantages of the
use of oral rather than parenteral therapy of antibiotics in, of course,
obvious.

As stated previously, the duration of antibiotic treatment necessary
to achieve cure of the shunt infection is not known. From experience with
endocarditis it is appreciated that rather prolonged therapy may be
desirable. In this clinic an arbitrary treatment time of 14 days has been
used and the results seem to indicate that this has been effective in most
cases.

TABLE 2. Patients Treated with Oral and Intraventricular Antibiotics

| Patient | Organism | Surgery | | | | Duration of "cure" (months) |
		None	Externalized	Revised	Removed	
A'de M	*Pseudomonas*				x	30
	S. epidermidis					
BW	*S. aureus*			x		15 (died, other cause)
SJ	*Micrococcus*				x	22
CW	*S. epidermidis*			x		1 (died, other cause)
GS	*S. aureus*		x			8
	Enterococcus					
TA	*S. epidermidis*	x				5
EW	*Corynebacterium*		x			4
JU	*S. epidermidis*	x				Failed
MB	*S. epidermidis*	x				3

PROPHYLACTIC USE OF ANTIBIOTICS

Prophylactic antibiotic therapy to patients undergoing surgery has been advocated for many surgical procedures but has proved to be of benefit in relatively few. In genral terms, antibiotic prophylaxis has been shown to be useful in procedures which have a high postoperative infection rate. As noted previously, the incidence of infection after shunting procedures has varied considerably but most frequently has been reported to be in the 5 to 15% range. It would be anticipated, therefore, that antibiotic therapy would be of benefit in this type of surgery. Although numerous reports have advocated varying prophylactic antibiotic regimens, there is little or no conclusive evidence of its effectiveness. Indeed, in a review of 840 CSF shunting procedures it was found that the surgeon performing the shunt was the largest single factor in determining the incidence of shunt infection.[5] In this particular report, the uncontrolled use of prophylactic antibiotics had no effect.

In a consideration of prophylactic antibiotics two principles should be kept in mind. The first of these is that tissues must contain adequate concentration of antibiotics before the onset of surgery and this tissue concentration should be maintained during surgery. This indicates, therefore, that the antibiotic must be given before the surgical procedure and must be given in dosages which achieve adequate tissue concentration of the drug during the entire surgical procedure. This may require repeated administration during the surgical procedure if it is prolonged.

The second principle of antibiotic prophylaxis demonstrated by many studies is that prolonged administration of antibiotic after surgical procedure is not required. Indeed, patients who receive extended courses of antibiotics are likely to be colonized by antibiotic-resistant hospital associated organisms.

Utilization of these two principles indicates that if prophylaxis is to be attempted, the drugs should be administered before surgery, should be given in adequate dosages to insure high concentration during the entire surgical procedure, and should be stopped within 24 hours after surgery. The regimen that is being followed in this clinic is noted in Table 3.

TABLE 3. Antiobiotic Prophylaxis in Shunt Operations

1. Intravenous: Cefazolin
   Dosage, Adults: 2 g
     Children: 25 mg/kg
     Newborns: 12 mg/kg (second dose 6 mg/kg)
   Timing: First dose started 1 hour before surgery; administration time:
   approximately ½ hour; second dose 6 hours after first dose
2. Intraventricular:
   Gentamycin: 4 mg during surgery
3. Alternative to be used in case of allergy to cephalosporins:
   Vancomycin, 1 g IV, 2 hours before surgery, no second dose.
   Gentamycin, 4 mg, IVT.

RESULTS OF TREATMENT

Although emphasis has been placed on antibiotic management of shunt infections in this clinic for approximately 15 years, numerous changes have occurred during this time in the availability and modes of administration of antibiotics and also in the surgical procedures utilized. For this reason it seems appropriate to summarize the results during the past three years only, since other variable factors have been at a minimum during this interval. Seventeen patients have been treated for shunt infection. In three of these patients it was not possible to obtain bacteriologic cure without shunt removal. In eight of the 17 patients it was necessary to perform a shunt revision to achieve a functioning shunt during treatment, but in these patients the shunt was never removed. In one patient, shunt removal was done for mechanical reasons because of erosion of the skin overlying the pumping device. In summary, therefore, bacteriologic cure was apparently achieved in 13 of the 17 patients without the assistance of shunt removal. It is concluded, therefore, that a trial of intensive antibiotic therapy, systemic and intraventricular, associated with frequent monitoring of CSF inhibitory titer is justifiable and to be recommended before surgical removal of the shunt apparatus.

REFERENCES

1. Robertson, J.S., Maraqua, M.I., and Jennett B Ventriculoperitoneal shunting for hydrocephalus. *Br. Med J. 1*:289–291, 1973.
2. George, R., Leibrock, L., and Epstein, M. Long-term analysis of cerebrospinal fluid shunt infections. *J. Neurosurg. 51*:804–811, 1979.

3. Little, J.R., Rhoton, A.L., Jr., and Mellinger, J.F Comparison of
   ventriculoperitoneal shunts for hydrocephalus in children. *Mayo Clin. Proc.*
   47: 396–401, 1972.
4. Schoenbaum, S.C., Gardner, P., and Shillito, J. Infections of cerebrospinal
   fluid shunts: epidemiology, clinical manifestations, and therapy. *J. Infect.
   Dis. 131*:543–552, 1975.
5. Wald, S.L., and McLaurin, R.L Cerebrospinal fluid antibiotic levels during
   treatment of shunt infections. *J. Neurosurg. 52*:41–46, 1980.

10

Incidence and Prevention of Infection After Neurosurgical Operations

T. Forcht Dagi, Robert G. Ojemann, and Nicholas T. Zervas

INTRODUCTION

At about the time of the Boston Tea Party, King George III of England was troubled by a sebaceous cyst of the scalp. He summoned the renowned surgeon Sir Astley Cooper to attend to him and remove the wen. Sir Astley did so successfully, but with reluctance. "Wounds of the scalp," he is quoted to have said, "are not so trifling as they first might appear. Inflammation very often follows, erisipelas etc, and many die in consequence of the injury done to the scalp ... I was called upon to remove a tumor from the scalp of a lady; it was unfortunately attached to the tendon of the occipito-frontalis muscle and I necessarily had to remove a part of this tendon. The operation was done on a Wednesday, she seemed quite well after its removal, but on Sunday she was seized with rigor, succeeded by heat—she became feverish and on the Tuesday she died. Therefore, you will, I trust, be upon your guard and never make an unnecessary cut on any part of the scalp for such a practice is dangerous and you will not know what may follow such a wound."[1]

Many illustrious physicians and surgeons have contributed to the control of infection. Ambrose Pare recognized that wounds healed better when they were treated gently than when they were bathed in caustic substances. Semmelweiss established the importance of handwashing in the prevention of puerperal sepsis. Angostino Bassi ascribed the cause of infection to a living organism. Louis Pasteur studied bacterial pathogenesis and was the first to note that some organisms impeded the growth of others. Robert Koch established the role of bacteria in disease and formulated guidelines for proving that a given organism was responsible for a specific infection.

Joseph Lister was the first surgeon to use antiseptics to reduce the incidence of surgical infection. In the late 1850s, he was troubled by the high mortality rate from sepsis following amputation despite meticulous cleanliness, drainage of the wound, and frequent dressing changes. He became aware of Pasteur's experiments and hypothesized that chemical agents might be used to prevent the growth of micro-organisms. On August 12, 1865, he first treated a compound fracture of the tibia with carbolic acid. The wound healed perfectly with no infection. In 1867, he first published the results of "Antiseptic Surgery," and applied the principles to surgery of the spine and joints.[2]

Other surgeons adopted and modified Lister's methods. Some denied that bacteria caused infection, but nevertheless they insisted on surgical cleanliness and washed their hands and the operative site with soap and scrub brushes. Von Bergmann, a general surgeon who operated on the brain, insisted that his instruments and surgical linens be boiled. In 1877, Horsley recommended that the scalp be prepared as follows: "the day before the operation, the patient's head is shaved and washed with a soft soap and then ether; next the position of the lesion is ascertained by measurement and marked on the scalp. The head is covered with lint, soaked in 1 in 20 solution of carbolic acid, oiled silk and cotton wool, being thus thoroughly carbolised for at least twelve hours before operation."[3]

Mikulezc, one of Billroth's assistants, was the first to use cotton gloves for surgery. Halsted first ordered rubber gloves to control irritation produced by the mercuric chloride solution he used as an antiseptic. "In the winter of 1889 and 1890—I cannot recall the month—the nurse in charge of my operating room complained that the solutions of mercuric chloride produced a dermatitis of her arms and hands. As she was an unusually efficient woman, I gave the matter my consideration, and one day in New York requested the Goodyear Rubber Company to make as an experiment, two pair of thin rubber gloves with gauntlets."[4] In a picture taken at the opening of the new surgical amphitheater at Hopkins in 1904, Halsted is seen gowned, gloved, and caped, but leaning unmasked over the patient.

REPORTED INFECTION RATES IN NEUROSURGICAL PROCEDURES

Wright[5] reviewed the early reports of neurosurgical infection in cranial operations. Von Eiselberg and Ranzi, in 1913, reported 20 deaths from meningitis or sepsis in 168 cases[5] Cushing,[6] in 1915, mentioned only one case of postoperative sepsis in 249 operations for brain tumors. In 1916 he claimed, "There has never been an infection, even of a stitch in the scalp, in something over 300 cranial operations in the writer's series."[7] In his monograph on acoustic neuromas in 1917, infection as a postoperative complication is not even discussed.[8] In 1931, he related two fatalities to meningitis in 113 operations on 74 cerebellar astrocytomas.[9] In the treatise on meningiomas, Cushing records that in 522 operations on 281 patients, there were three cases of draining sinus after retained cottonoids, and three cases of meningitis, one of which followed a transsphenoidal operation.[10]

Hugh Cairns[11] was the first to report the effect of antibiotics on infection rates in neurosurgery. Between May 1938 and November 1944, there were 51 infections in 1,169 operations (4.4 percent). Six of these infections were fatal. After November 1944, he instilled a mixture of penicillin and sulphamethazine at the time of operation. In 670 cases, only six infections (0.9 percent) were noted and none were fatal.

In his monographs Wright reviewed the reports of postoperative infections in craniotomies up to 1966 and in spinal operations up to 1970.[5,12,13] Infection rates ranged from less than 1.0 percent to over 6 percent. Wright and Burke reported the infection rate in clean cases at the Massachusetts General Hospital for the period 1952 to 1966 to be 5.3 percent in craniotomies (ranging from 2.0 to 9.4 percent per year) and 4.1 percent in laminectomies (ranging from 0.9 to 7.8 percent per year).[5] Between 1952 and 1957, almost every patient undergoing intracranial operation received intramuscular injections of penicillin and streptomycin for periods of four to seven days postoperatively. After 1958, bacitracin solution was used to irrigate the wound after closure of the dura in most procedures. No difference was found in the infection rate when antibiotics were given but it was emphasized that in almost all cases the antibiotic had been started in the immediate postoperative period.

In 1967, Balch[14] reported an overall infection rate of 3.06 percent in 1,767 neurosurgical procedures. This report points out the importance of analyzing the incidence relative to the type of operation and the frequency of each procedure. The incidence differed depending on the type of operation: craniotomy 5.0 percent, laminectomy for tumor 7.6 percent, disc excisions 1.4 percent, thalamotomy 1.2 percent, sterotactic hypophysectomy 9.8 percent, shunts 1.5 percent, and miscellaneous 1.0 percent. The miscellaneous group and thalamotomy were the most common procedures, accounting for almost half of the total number of cases. No local or systemic antibiotics were used in clean cases.

INCIDENCE OF INFECTION IN NEUROSURGICAL PROCEDURES AT THE MASSACHUSETTS GENERAL HOSPITAL, 1970 to 1979

Patient Population and Data Retrieval

All patients who were admitted to the neurosurgical services of the Massachusetts General Hospital and who were operated between January 1, 1970 and December 31, 1979 were included in this study. A total of 11,910 neurosurgical procedures were performed. William Sweet's series of patients with intractable facial pain treated by injection of lidocaine or by a radiofrequency procedure was considered separately. A personal series (RGO) of 181 consecutive posterior fossa operations (including 132 for acoustic neuroma) with long-term follow-up was also analyzed.

The incidence of postoperative infection was determined by reviewing the weekly departmental reports of death and complications filed by the resident staff. A random sample of 1,000 patients who underwent neurosurgical operations during this period was reviewed. It is possible that delayed infections that did not manifest themselves during the hospitalization were missed by this review. The charts of every patient who was recorded to have had postoperative infection was reviewed. The anesthesia notes, bacteriologic reports, and postoperative orders were examined to ascertain whether and how antibiotics were utilized, the details of the infection, and what complicating factors might have been present.

From 1970 to 1977, almost all scheduled cases were operated in neurosurgical operating rooms with ultraviolet (UV) lights on 24 hours a day. Emergency operations were often performed in other rooms. After July, 1977, the regular use of UV irradiation was stopped. The total number of cases operated without UV was estimated from the total of emergency cases performed between 1970 and July 1977 and all cases performed between July 1, 1977 and December 31, 1979 where ultraviolet lights were known to have been off.

The criteria for infection included the presence of one or more of the following:

1. Demonstration of serous or purulent collection or drainage in or from a wound with positive cultures of Gram stain.

2. Unexplained fever, leukocytosis, and/or abnormally elevated erythrocyte sedimentation rate in a patient with a red, warm, swollen, and tender wound.

3. Meningismus, leukocytosis in the cerebrospinal fluid (CSF) and spinal fluid glucose 50 percent or less of blood glucose or, in the absence of simultaneous blood glucose, below an absolute level of 45 mg/100 ml.

4. Positive CSF Gram stain or culture.

During the period of the study, prophylactic antibiotics were used at the discretion of the surgeon. Most patients received the antibiotic just before the incision and the drug was continued for a variable period of time after surgery, usually one to five days. Nearly all patients having shunt procedures, cranioplasty, or operations with contaminated wounds received antibiotics. In transphenoidal operations, prophylactic antibiotics were routinely continued for 48 hours postoperatively by intravenous injection and for three to five days orally therafter. No infection occurred without CSF leak.

It has been the practice to irrigate the extradural space with a solution of bacitracin over the entire course of this study. Bacitracin is active against many Gram-positive organisms but not against most Gram-negative organisms. Its action is not affected by blood, pus, or the products of tissue necrosis and it has a low incidence of local hypersensitivity reactions.

Results

The overall infection rate in neurosurgical procedures performed between 1970 and 1979 at Massachusetts General is shown in Table 1. The mean yearly infection rate was 1.22 percent, with a standard deviation of 0.32 percent. The mean yearly infection rate was constant over the past decade. This incidence represents a substantial drop when compared with the rate reported by Wright for the 1952 to 1965 period.[5] It is higher than the rate in the first three years (1966 to 1968) when UV lights were used even when the operations with shunts and foreign bodies are excluded.[15] The use of UV lights is discussed in the next section.

There was no change in the focus of infection over the course of the study. Table 2 shows that 57.8 percent of the infections occurred in the wound; 18.4 percent were meningitis, 10.2 percent involved CSF and the wound, and 9.5 percent involved a ventriculostomy or a shunt.

The total number of cases performed each year has not changed substantially. There has been a steady slight decrease in the proportion

TABLE 1. Overall Infection Rate in Neurosurgical Procedures at MGH (1970–1979)

Year	Cases	Infections	Rate (%)
1970	1,111	7	0.63
1971	936	10	1.06
1972	1,147	16	1.39
1973	1,268	19	1.50
1974	1,367	20	1.46
1975	1,268	12	0.95
1976	1,291	12	0.92
1977	1,054	12	1.14
1978	1,211	17	1.40
1979	1,257	22	1.75
Total	11,910	147	$\bar{x}$ = 1.22
	$\bar{x}$ = 1,191	$\bar{x}$ = 14.7	sd = 0.32%

TABLE 2. Focus of Infection (1970–1979)

Year	N	Wound (%)	CSF (%)	Ventricular catheter or shunt (%)	Combined infections (%)	Other subdural empyema sellar abscess
1970	7	4 (57.1)	1 (14.3)	1 (14.3)	1 (14.3)	0
1971	10	6 (60.0)	1 (10.0)	0	3 (30.0)	0
1972	16	11 (68.8)	3 (18.8)	1 (6.3)	1 (6.3)	0
1973	19	13 (68.4)	3 (15.8)	1 (5.3)	1 (5.3)	1 (5.3)
1974	20	12 (60.0)	7 (35.0)	1 (5.0)	0	0
1975	12	7 (58.3)	2 (16.7)	1 (8.3)	0	2 (16.6)
1976	12	5 (41.7)	3 (25.0)	3 (25.0)	1 (8.3)	0
1977	12	5 (41.7)	1 (8.3)	1 (8.3)	3 (25.0)	2 (16.6)
1978	17	8 (47.1)	2 (23.5)	4 (23.5)	3 (17.6)	0
1979	22	14 (63.6)	4 (18.2)	1 (4.5)	2 (9.1)	1 (4.5)
Totals	147	85 (57.8)	27 (18.4)	14 (9.5)	15 (10.2)	6 (4.1)

of spinal procedures performed and an increase in the proportion of shunts and carotid procedures. Whereas in the first two years of the decade many of the procedures on the carotid artery were litigation or application of carotid clamps for a gradual carotid obliteration in the treatment of internal carotid artery aneurysms, carotid interruptions have become fairly rare and most of the neck cases from 1974 on represent carotid endarterectomies. With the advent of the CT scan, fewer exploratory burr holes for trauma have been performed. The number of trauma and emergency cases has remained about the same.

Signs of wound infection were usually noted between the fifth and eleventh postoperative days. A review of the case histories may suggest a reason why that patient developed the infection. Of 98 infections expressed at the wound site, 53 could be explained at least partially by such specific predisposing factors as insertion of a foreign material, an open traumatic wound, immunosuppression, systemic infection, severe diabetes, a recognized source of external contamination during the operation, prolonged external drainage, and CSF leak. The use of epidural drainage for 24 hours or less did not affect the incidence of wound infection. If those cases with specific predisposing factors were excluded, the incidence of infection would be 0.38 percent.

The onset of meningitis was most frequent from the fifth to seventh day after operation. In 27 of 34 cases with CSF infection, there was clinical evidence of miningitis. In 23 patients a predisposing factor such as brain abscess, wound infection, presumed intraoral or intranasal contamination during a stereotactic procedure, external ventricular drains, and CSF leaks was noted. No infection of the CSF occurred without opening the dura or CSF leak.

In the 147 infections, 47 percent grew out flora that frequently reside on the skin or in the upper respiratory tract (e.g., streptococcus and staphylococcus species), 18 percent were Gram-negative or anaerobe organisms, 5 percent were mixed, and 31 percent produced no bacterial growth (Table 3). When the proportion of infections with Gram-positive skin and upper respiratory flora is examined year by year, it will be seen that yearly variation is minimal. However, in 1979 four staphyloccocus infections in a fairly short period of time led to an intensive investigation and the discovery that a resident involved in all operations was carrying staphylococcus in his nose. The resident was treated and the epidemic ceased.

TABLE 3. 147 Infections in Ten Years.
Distribution of Organism by Year and Type

Year	Infections (%)	Skin flora (%)	GN or anaerobes (%)	Mixed (%)	None isolated (%)
1970	7 (0.63)	4 (57.1)	2 (28.6)	1 (14.2)	0
1971	10 (1.06)	5 (50.0)	2 (20.0)	0	3 (30.0)
1972	16 (1.39)	7 (43.8)	1 (6.3)	1 (6.3)	7 (43.8)
1973	19 (1.50)	8 (42.1)	3 (15.8)	0	8 (42.1)
1974	20 (1.46)	8 (40.0)	5 (25.0)	0	7 (35.0)
1975	12 (0.95)	7 (58.4)	3 (25.0)	2 (16.7)	1 (8.4)
1976	12 (0.92)	5 (41.7)	2 (16.7)	1 (8.4)	4 (33.4)
1977	12 (1.14)	6 (50.0)	1 (8.4)	0	5 (41.7)
1978	17 (1.40)	7 (41.2)	4 (23.5)	1 (5.9)	5 (29.4)
1979	22 (1.75)	10 (45.5)	3 (13.6)	0	9 (40.9)
Mean	14.7 (1.22)	6.7 (47.0)	2.6 (18.3)	0.6 (5.2)	4.9 (30.6)

GN=gram-negative.

We are unable to estimate how many uninfected patients received prophylactic antibiotics. In the infected cases, 36.7 percent had received prophylactic antibiotics. The proportion of infections due to Gram-positive, Gram-negative, or anerobic organisms were the same irrespective of whether prophylactic antibiotics had been given. A special study of the use of antibiotics in posterior fossa operations is discussed in the next section.

Through the courtesy of Dr. Sweet, we were able to review and report his experience with 931 procedures for the injection of lidocaine or glycerine, or for radiofrequency retrogasserian differential thermal rhizotomy in Meckel's cave percutaneously, via Hartel's route performed from January 1, 1970 to July 30, 1980 (Table 4). The overall infection rate was 0.54 percent. One case of meningitis after a lidocaine injection was probably aseptic. The microbiology of the temporal lobe abscess is unknown.

PROPHYLACTIC ANTIBIOTICS

Use of Prophylactic Antibiotics in Nonneurosurgical Operations

Much of the recent literature on surgical antibiotic prophylaxis is difficult to evaluate.[16–21] From these studies prophylactic antibiotics seem to be effective in reducing infection in hysterectomy and cesarian section, emergency appendectomy, total hip arthroplasty, and extensive operations for cancer of the pharynx and larynx.[17,22,23] In the study on prophylaxis of postoperative infection of the hip, two widely separated hospitals did a double-blind study of 171 major hip operations.[22] One group of

TABLE 4. Infection Rates for Percutaneous Puncture
of Meckel's Cave. All Attempted
and Completed Procedures Are Included

804 Radiofrequency differential thermal rhizotomies	
127 Lidocaine injections	
(in 5 cases, followed by injection of glycerine)	
931 Procedures via Haertel's route (1/1/70–7/30/80)	
RFL	1 temporal lobe abscess
RFL	1 meningitis (Neisseria)
Injection	2 meningitides (streptococci)
Injection	1 meningitis (aseptic)
Overall Infection Rate 0.54%	

RFL=radiofrequency lesion.

patients received prophylactic cloxacillin; the other received a placebo. The first group had no postoperative infections, while the second had 12 in 88 patients. Ten of the 12 infections were staphylococcal.

The role of antibiotics in general surgery is not established. Some studies suggest a benefit, especially in biliary and bowel surgery, but others do not.[16–20,24,25] Chodak and Plaut[17] concluded that there is a suggestion that prophylactic antibiotics are useful in clean contaminated general surgical procedures. In cardiac surgery, prophylaxis is almost universally used but no controlled studies document this need.[20,23]

Use of Prophylactic Antibiotics in Neurosurgical Operations

In a review of the literature to 1979, Haines[24] stated that there are no unequivical indications for antibiotics prophylaxis in neurosurgery. Using the designations proposed by the National Academy of Science—National Research Council, he divided neurosurgical procedures into (1) clean neurosurgical procedures; (2) clean neurosurgical procedures with implanted foreign body; (3) clean contaminated procedures (including those where a paranasal or mastoid sinus was entered and external ventriculostomies); (4) contaminated neurosurgical procedures. He could find only a few reports on the use of prophylactic antibiotics for clean neurosurgical procedures without implanted foreign bodies. A few retrospective analyses suggested that prophylactic antibiotics might be of benefit. The largest of these was the report of Horwitz and Curtin[26] on 530 laminectomies. In 402 patients given prophylactic antibiotic, the infection rate was 1.0 percent compared with 9.3 percent in 128 patients not given antibiotics.

In a personal series (RGO) of 181 consecutive posterior fossa operations between 1974 and 1979, there were six infections (Table 5). During the later part of the series, a planned program of prophylactic antibiotics was used because of the suggestion that infection could be virtually eliminated by their use. Oxacillin (or Cephalothin where allergy to

**TABLE 5.   Infection Rate in 181 Posterior
Fossa Operations (1974–1979)**

No Antibiotics (141)	
Infections	5 (3.5%)
Shunt	1
Delayed around suture	2
Wound	2
Prophylactic antibiotics (40)	
Infections	1 (2.5%)
Meningitis	1

penicillin was suspected) was administered shortly before making the skin incision, during the operation, and for 24 hours thereafter. All 181 patients had bacitracin irrigation at the time of surgery. The incidence of infection without systemic antibiotics was 3.5 percent (5 in 141 operations) and with prophylactic antibiotics 2.5 percent (1 in 40 operations). Analysis of the five patients who did not receive antibiotics revealed that one had a shunt infection with meningitis, two developed delayed small infections around sutures three months and three years after operation which healed with removal of the suture, and only two (1.4 percent) had the typical type of wound infection. The single patient who developed infection despite the use of prophylactic antibiotics developed meningococcal meningitis on the fifth postoperative day. He completely recovered. No statistical advantage to the use of prophylactic antibiotics was demonstrated.

The report by Malis in 1979[25] presented a strong case for the use of prophylactic antibiotics routinely in neurosurgical operations. After analyzing the wound infections recorded over a five-year period, he chose a combination of bactericidal antibiotics known to be sensitive to the Gram-positive and Gram-negative organisms cultured in the institution. Gentamycin, 80 mg IM, and vancomycin, 1 g IV, were given at the induction of anesthesia. Streptomycin, 50 mg, was added to each liter of irrigating saline solution. Subsequently, tobramycin, 80 mg IM, was substituted for gentamycin. The vancomycin was given over about one hour to avoid the risk of hypotension. No postoperative antibiotics were used. In a series of 1,732 cases, there was no postoperative infection and no evidence of toxicity. This series included patients with cranioplasty, shunts, and those in whom the mastoid and paranasal sinus were opened.

Quartey and Polyzoidis[27] also followed a program similar to that outlined by Malis. After reviewing cultures of previous infections, they used the combination of 80 mg of gentamycin IM and 1 g of vancomycin IV as soon as the patient was anesthetized. They decided that the effectiveness of topical antibiotics had not been established so omitted the streptomycin irrigating solution. The average infection rate before this antibiotic program was 2.62 percent and after was 0.8 percent. Haines and Goodman[23] used the same antibiotic program as Malis and found an infection rate of 0.9 percent in 878 consecutive neurosurgical operations. It is not clear how this antibiotic program related to the sensitivity of organism cultures from wound infections in the 12 months just before the use of the prophylactic program when the infection rate was 2.7 percent. There were no toxicity problems related to the medication program. Although Haines and Goodman concluded that antibiotics were effective in reducing the postoperative infection rate, the fact that this rate is similar to the lowest rate previously reported without the use of antibiotics, known fluctuations in infection rates, and other variables made them suggest that interpretation was difficult.

In a report by Savitz and Katz,[28] analysis of wound infections in neurosurgical procedures led to a program of antistaphylococcal prophylaxis. In the five years before starting routine prophylaxis, the infection rate was about 4 percent and the predominant organism was staphylococcus. Cephalothin, 2 g IV, was administered as the incision was made. In clean contaminated cases, where a paranasal sinus or mastoid sinus was entered, the same drug was used. Before closure the wound was irrigated with bacitracin (50,000 units in 50 ml of saline solution). In contaminated cases cephalothin was started in the emergency room and given every six hours until the sutures were removed five to seven days later. Bacitracin was also used. When foreign bodies were to be implanted, 1 g of methicillin was given IV and every six hours until the patient could take oral medication; then, dicloxacillin, 500 mg, was given orally four times a day until sutures were removed. If the patient had a known allergy to either penicillin or cephalothin, erythromycin was given instead. There were no primary wound infections in 1,000 cases (817 clean, 20 clean contaminated, 62 contaminated, and 101 with implantation of a foreign body). There were two delayed infections, one in a patient with a shunt and another who had a reexploration for a subdural hematoma, who later developed *Pseudomomas pneumonia* and a wound infection with the same organism while receiving antibiotics. There were no problems from toxicity to the antibiotic drugs.

Haines[24] also examined the evidence favoring the use of antibiotics in cranioplasty operations. Convincing evidence for the use of prophylactic antibiotics, when a foreign material is implanted surgically, has been demonstrated only for total hip arthroplasty.[22] The use of antibiotics in cranioplasty and operations where acrylic is used for bone fusion has not been studied systematically. However, most neurosurgeons use antibiotics under these circumstances.

Choice of Antibiotics for Prophylaxis

It is preferable to use bactericidal antibiotics whenever possible. The antibiotics should be as specific as possible for the organisms which statistically are known to cause postoperative infection in each institution. It may be necessary to change the prophylactic antibiotic regimen from time to time as the causative organisms and sensitivities change.

The antibiotic must be capable of achieving bactericidal levels in the tissue which is most likely to be infected. Much attention has been given to the need in neurosurgical operations for an antibiotic to penetrate the blood-brain barrier. In point of fact, most neurosurgical infections arise in the wound, and meningitis or brain abscess are less common. Thus, it is most reasonable to select an antibiotic which achieves rapid, bactericidal levels in skin and soft tissue regardless of its ability to pass the blood-brain barrier. Fourth generation cephalosporins such as cefoxitin, cefataxine, and moxalactam pass the blood-brain barrier very well and have a very wide spectrum of effectiveness. These drugs are recognized for their particular advantages in meningitis caused by enteric Gram-negative bacilli, but, except in extremely unusual circumstances, they should not be used for routine prophylaxis since they offer no advantage and should be reserved for infections due to resistant organisms.[29]

Savitz and Katz[28] chose cephalothin for prophylaxis because cultures of prior wound infections showed sensitive staphylococcus. These cephalosporin-type antibiotics tend to reach substantial wound levels one to two hours after administration.

Malis[25] used vancomycin because it is bactericidal and no other antibiotic was as consistently sensitive to Gram-positive organisms isolated in his institution. The half life of vancomycin in the circulation is six hours. The drug does not cross the normal blood-brain barrier but rapidly enters areas that are traumatized, inflamed, or infected. A 1 g dose should be given over 60 to 90 minutes. More rapid administration may result in hypotension. Tobramycin is bactericidal and is effective against Gram-negative organisms. It does not cross the uninjured blood-brain barrier efficiently. No evidence of renal toxcity or ototoxicity has been noted from the single administration of these drugs. Streptomycin was used for topical irrigation because it is bactericidal to a wide range of organisms. At the dosage used it is not injurious to nervous tissue and it is reported to have a broader range of sensitivity than bacitracin.

Timing of Admi.iistration of Antibiotics

Burke[30] showed that there is a definite "decisive period" lasting about three hours from the time of bacterial contamination of a wound during which infection may be suppressed by antibiotics. Antibiotics were maximally effective when they were present in the tissues before the bacteria were implanted. He also demonstrated that there is a "critical mass" of bacteria required to cause infection. The volume of this mass differs depending on whether foreign material is present. In one study, 10^6 organisms injected subcutaneously around a buried nylon suture sufficed to cause a staphlococcal infection; although in the absence of foreign material, no infection occurred.[31] Other studies confirm that a concentration of 10^6 to 10^7 bacteria/ml or greater is required to cause staphylococcal infection.[32,33] The "critical mass" for the other organisms or for the immunosuppressed or otherwise debilitated patient may also differ.

The clinical situation may differ from the experimental setting in that a series of subcritical innocula may accumulate in a wound over a period of time and excede the critical level. In that case, the "decisive period" may be prolonged, but no experiments along these lines have been performed. Measures which reduce the absolute number of proliferating bacteria in a wound may lower the incidence of infection. For example, irrigation of the wound with saline solution to remove debris or with topical antibiotics to kill bacteria may prove as important or more important than systemic prophylaxis in some case.

It is known that some antibiotics equilibrate in tissues more quickly or differently than others. The studies from the literature cited indicate that if the correct antibiotic is chosen, adequate prophylaxis will be obtained from one preoperative loading dose, intraoperative coverage, and one dose postoperatively. In any event, treatment for more than 24 hours appears to be unnecessary unless there is an ongoing portal of potential bacterial contamination.

Risks of Administering Antibiotics

Although antibiotics are on the whole relatively benign drugs, the surgeon should be aware of adverse reactions which accompany their use. Caldwell and Cluff[34] reported on 21,877 courses of antibiotics administered to 7,775 patients over a three-year period. Adverse reactions were reported in 5.4 percent. In 45 percent of these reactions, hospitalization was increased by one or more days, and in 14 percent by four days or longer. Fifty-eight percent of the reactions were severe enough to require treatment, extend the duration of hospital stay, or be life-threatening.

The risks of giving prophylactic antibiotics can be broken down into the following categories:

1. Alteration of normal flora resulting in the overgrowth of pathogens which replace the organisms eliminated by the antibiotics.

2. Prothrombin deficiency caused by the elmination of certain enteric organisms

3. Allergic and hypersensitivity responses ranging from insignificant skin eruptions to idiosyncrotic marrow depression after a single dose.

4. Toxicity, usually dose-and-time-related, affecting the ear, liver, and kidney. These are of particular concern with the use of streptomycin, gentamycin, kanamycin, and cephaloridine.

5. The development of resistant organisms.

6. Unpleasant adverse effects such as nausea, vomiting, and diarrhea.

The patients reported by Caldwell and Cluff can be presumed to have received a full course of antibiotics, and for this reason they would be more subject to dose-related toxicity. It is very unlikely that the adverse reactions to antibiotics used in the short course of prophylactic treatment would occur as often, or be as severe. Since the infection rate in neurosurgical procedures is already low, it is necessary to consider any complications and morbidity antibiotic administration may cause.

OTHER FACTORS AFFECTING POSTOPERATIVE WOUND INFECTIONS

The main source of random bacterial contamination continues to be airborne staphylococcus species from skin folds and from the upper respiratory tract of the operating room team.[28] Sudden increase in the incidence of wound infection can often be traced to a staphylococcal carrier. Excellent reviews of the effects of operating room environmental factors on postoperative infection rates have been written.[15,35]

The use of ultraviolet lights has been reported to be of benefit. Woodall et al.[36] found that before the use of UV lights, the overall evidence of neurosurgical infection in clean cases was 9 percent. With the use of UV lights, the infection rate was 1.05 percent in 1,228 craniotomies and 1.9 percent in 1,334 laminectomies. Later, Odom reported that over a 15-year period (1941 to 1955) during which UV lights were used, there was 0.4 percent infection in 1,342 craniotomies and 0.6 percent in 3,774 laminectomies.[36] Wright and Burke reported that before the use of UV lights at the MGH, the average infection rate over 13 years was 5.3 percent in craniotomies and 4.1 percent in laminectomies.[36] During the three years after UV lights were placed, the infection rate dropped to 0.7 percent in 669 craniotomies and 0.3 percent in 579 laminectomies. However, other changes in technique were made at the same time which included more extensive masking and gowning required for protection from UV lights and fewer personnel entering the operating room. Ultraviolet lights were used at the MGH until July 1977. Between 1974 and 1979, approximately 4,490 operations were performed under the UV lights and 2,957 operations were performed without them. There was no significant difference in the incidence of postoperative infection in these two groups (See Table 2). The need for special eye and skin protection, required when UV lights are used, has prevented more widespread use of intraoperative UV irradiation. Many surgeons cannot use the operation microscope when wearing protective glasses. Theoretically, the lights must be in constant use to confer any advantage over routine antiseptic precautions.[37]

For several years we have used a pHisoHex® wash or shampoo on the patient the evening before surgery. It has recently been reported that the practice of washings of the scalp twice with hexachlorophene before operation reduced the infection rate from 2 to 0.5 percent.[38]

Various programs have been used for preparation of the skin. Draping must be done carefully with the use of plastic drapes that adhere to the skin and provide waterproof barriers. The details of our technique are outlined in the next section.

Wright reported that the incidence of infection was related to the duration of the operation.[5] However, this has not been the finding in recent reports and we did not find this correlation in analysis of the recent MGH experience.[25] The use of high-dose steroids does not appear to influence the risk of infection.[5,39] It has been shown that simple irrigation of a wound washes out bacteria and reduces the inoculum from the skin. We know of no study comparing irrigation with bacitracin to irrigation with similar amounts of saline solution or other substance.

The use of drains at the time of craniotomy was also considered by Wright but this factor did not by itself significantly increase the rate of infection.[5] In most of those cases, the drains were removed within one to two days. We found no increase in infection rate when drains were left up to 24 hours. In Malis'[25] series of no infections in 1,732 cases, closed suction drainage was used for the first 24 hours after operation. On the other hand, Wyler and Kelly,[40] in reviewing 70 patients with 102 ventriculostomies that were in place a mean of five days, found 7 of 26 (27 percent) not receiving antibiotics became infected while 4 of 44 (9 percent) who had prophylaxis, usually with ampicillin, became infected.

PREVENTION OF POSTOPERATIVE WOUND INFECTION

Measures designed to reduce the rate of postoperative infection can only be assessed in comparison to a baseline incidence. This incidence is likely to vary from hospital to hospital and from year to year. Factors seemingly remote from the operating theater may affect this figure, and determine which organisms are responsible. As the types of operation vary, both the incidence and the character of postoperative infections may change.

We have found the following plan to be associated with a low incidence of infection.

1. If a systemic infection is present, it should be treated and surgery delayed if possible. Systemic factors which must be considered in assessing preoperative risks include immunosuppression and severe diabetes.
2. The evening before surgery, the appropriate area is washed with pHisoHex or a pHisoHex shampoo is used.
3. The skin at the operative site is not shaved until immediately after the induction of anesthesia. We believe it very important to avoid injuring the skin in the hours before surgery.
4. The skin is scrubbed with a soap solution followed by application of a 70% solution of isopropanol which is allowed to dry. The incision is then marked with a sterile marking pen.
5. In addition to the usual fabric drapes, the operative area and adjacent part of the field is covered by a sterile adhesive plastic drape.
6. Careful technique must be practiced by the operating room team.

Prophylactic antibiotics are considered. If prophylactic antibiotics are to be used the following principles are followed:

1. Prophylaxis with antibiotics is indicated when after controlling technical and environmental factors, there is an unacceptable rate of infectious complication which antibiotics can be shown to lower. Rates of infection vary from hospital to hospital as does the microbiology. The organisms and their sensitivities must be known, and the infection rate strictly monitored. The culture results of organism sensitivities from wound infections in the preceding months should be reviewed at frequent intervals.
2. Antibiotics should be bactericidal whenever possible. Bacteriostatic antibiotics are generally ineffective, especially when foreign material is implanted. The antibiotic chosen must cover a significant number of the organisms implicated in the infections to be prevented. In most hospitals this will usually mean some antistaphylococcal drug.
3. The antibiotic that is chosen must attain adequate levels in tissue before the time the incision is made. Our plan is to give the antibiotic just before or after induction of anesthesia, during the procedure, and for 24 hours thereafter.
4. Antibiotic prophylaxis is not a substitute for meticulous adherence to surgical techniques which are known to decrease the risk of infection, for surveillance of the operating room environment to eliminate contributory factors, and for scrupulous attention to aseptic techniques.

From information available, it would appear that prophylactic antibiotics are indicated in the following circumstances:

1. Whenever paranasal sinus or mastoid air cells are to be entered.
2. When a foreign material is being implanted.
3. When an external ventricular drain is planned.
4. When there has been a recent systemic infection.
5. In contaminated wounds.
6. In the patient with rheumatic heart disease, prosthetic heart valve, severe diabetes, immunosuppresion, or other debilitating illness.

Based on the recent literature, a case can be made for using antibiotics as outlined in all patients who are having neurosurgical operations. Toxicity is apparently not a problem. It remains to be proven that this treatment is really necessary.

REFERENCES

1. Cope, Z. *Sidelights on the History of Medicine*, pp. 157–158. London: Butterworth, 1957.
2. Lister, J. On the antiseptic principle in the practice of surgery. *Lancet* 2:353–356, 1867.
3. Saugous, E. (ed.). Annual of the Universal Medical Sciences, p. 15. Philadelphia: Davis, 1885. (Quoted from *Weekly Medical News*, 1877.)
4. MacCallum, W. G. *William Stewart Halsted*, p. 81. Baltimore: Johns Hopkins, 1920.
5. Wright, R. L. *Postoperative Craniotomy Infections*. Springfield, IL: Charles C Thomas, 1966.
6. Cushing, H. Concerning the results of operation for brain tumor. *JAMA* 64:189–195, 1915.
7. Cushing, H. Surgery of the head. In: *Surgery, Its Principles and Practice*, vol. 3, W. W. Keen (ed.), pp. 17–276. Philadelphia: W. B. Saunders, 1912.
8. Cushing, H. *Tumors of the Nervus acusticus and the Syndrome of the Cerebellopontine Angle*. Philadelphia: W. B. Saunders, 1917.
9. Cushing, H. Experiences with the cerebellar astrocytomas: A critical review of seventy-six cases. *Surg. Gynecol. Obstet.* 52:129–204, 1931.
10. Cushing, H., and Eisenhardt, L. *Meningiomas, Their Classification, Regional Behaviour, Life History and Surgical End Results*. Springfield, IL: Charles C Thomas, 1938.
11. Cairns, H. Bacterial infection during intracranial operations. *Lancet* 1:1193–1198, 1939.
12. Wright, R. L. A survey of possible etiologic agents in postoperative craniotomy infections. *J. Neurosurg.* 25:125–132, 1966.
13. Wright, R. L. *Septic Complications of Neurosurgical Spinal Procedures*. Springfield, IL: Charles C Thomas, 1970.
14. Balch, R. E. Wound infections complicating neurosurgical procedures. *J. Neurosurg.* 26:41–45, 1967.
15. Ritter, M.A., Eitzer, H. E., French, M. L. V., and Hart, J. B. The effect that time, touch, and environment have upon bacterial contamination of instruments during surgery. *Ann. Surg.* 184:642–644, 1976.

16. Berger, S. A., Nagar, H., and Weitzman, S. Prophylactic antibot antibiotics in surgical procedures. *Surg. Gynecol. Obstet. 146*:469–475, 1978.

17. Chodak, G. W., and Plaud, M. E. Use of systemic antibiotics for prophylaxis in surgery. *Arch. Surg. 112*:326–334, 1977.

18. Jacoby, J., Mandell, L. A., and Weinstein, L. The chemoprophylaxis of infection. *Med. Clin. North Am. 62*:1083–1098, 1978.

19. Lewis, R. T. Antibiotic prophylaxis in surgery. *Can. J. Surg. 24*:561–566, 1981.

20. Antimicrobiologic prophylaxis for surgery. *Med. Lett. 23*:77–80, 1981.

21. Moellering, R. C., Kuntz, L. J., Poitras, J. W., et al. Microbiologic basis for the rational use of prophylactic antibiotics. *South. Med. J.* 70 (suppl. 1):8–14, 1977.

22. Ericson, C., Lidgren, L., and Lindberg, L. Cloxacillin in the prophylaxis of postoperative infection of the hip. *J. Bone Joint Surg. (Am.) 55*:808–813, 1973.

23. Haines, S. J., and Goodman, M. L. Antibiotic prophylaxis of postoperative neurological wound infection. *J. Neurosurg. 56*:103–105, 1982.

24. Haines, S. J. Systemic antibiotic prophylaxis in neurological surgery. *Neurosurgery 6*:355–361, 1980.

25. Malis, L. I. Prevention of neurological infection by intraoperative antibiotics. *Neurosurgery 5*:339–343, 1979.

26. Horwitz, N.G., and Curtin, J. A. Prophylactic antibiotics and wound infections following laminectomy for lumbar disc herniation. *J. Neurosurg. 43*:727–737, 1975.

27. Quartey, G. R. C., and Polyzoidis, K. Intraoperative antibiotic prophylaxis in neurosurgery: A clinical study. *Neurosurgery 8*:669–671, 1981.

28. Savitz, M. H., and Katz, S. K. Rationale for prophylactic antibiotics in neurosurgery. *Neurosurgery 9*:142–144, 1981.

29. Landesman, S. H., Corrado, M. L., Shah, P. M., et al. Past and current roles for cephalosporin antibiotics in the treatment of meningitis. *Am. J. Med. 71*:693–703, 1981.

30. Burke, J. F. The effective period of preventive antibiotic action in experimental incisions and dermal lesions. *Surgery 50*:161–168, 1961.

31. Rodeheaver, G., Edgerton, M. T., Smith, S., King, H., Kurtz, I., and Edlick, R. F. Antimicrobial prophylaxis of contaminated tissues containing suture implants. *Am. J. Surg.* 133:609–611, 1977.

32. Halasz, N. A. Wound infection and topical antibiotics. *Arch. Surg. 112*:1240–1244, 1977.

33. Krizek, T. J., and Robson, M. C. Biology of surgical infection. *Surg. Clin. North Am. 55*:1261–1267, 1975.

34. Caldwell, J. R., and Cluff, L. E. Adverse reactions to antimicrobial agents. *JAMA 230*:77–80, 1974.

35. Schonholtz, G. J. Maintenance of aseptic barriers in the conventional operating room. *J. Bone Joint Surg. 58A*:439–445, 1976.

36. Wright, R. L., and Burke, J. F. Effect of ultraviolet radiation on postoperative neurosurgical sepsis. *J. Neurosurg. 31*:533–537, 1969.

37. Woodhall, B., Neill, R. G., and Dratz, H. M. Ultraviolet radiation as an adjunct in the control of post-operative neurosurgical infection. II. Clinical experience, 1938–1948. *Ann. Surg. 129*:820–825, 1949.

38. Kourtopoulos, H., and Burman, L. G. Prophylaxis of neurosurgical infec-

tions by improverd preoperative disinfection of the scalp. *Scand. J. Infect. Dis. 11*:175–176, 1979.

39. Quadery, L. A., Medlery, A. V., and Miles, J. Factors affecting the incidence of wound infection in neurosurgery. *Acta Neurochir. (Wein) 39*:133–141, 1977.
40. Wyler, A. R., and Kelly, W. A. Use of antibiotics with external ventriculostomies. *J. Neurosurg.* 37:185–187, 1972.

11

Medical and Surgical Considerations
of Coccidioidomycosis Infection

Harvey W. Buchsbaum

Coccidioidomycosis is probably one of the best understood of the systemic fungal infections. A number of excellent reports have reviewed the aspects of coccidioidal meningitis,[1-7] but this remains a disease where diagnosis and problems in management may be complicated.

The purpose of this presentation is to briefly review the history of diagnosis and treatment of coccidioidal meningitis and to review our personal experience in forty cases.

Ophuls in 1905[11] described the first case of central nervous system involvement by *C. immitis*. Smith clearly delineated the epidemiology of coccidioidal meningitis and contributed greatly with his coccidioidin skin test, serum precipitin, and complement fixation studies. Much of this work was continued later by Pappagianis.[9,12-18] Winn and Einsten also made significant contributions to treatment with amphotericin B.[5,7,19-22]

C. immitis is a fungus restricted to certain western hemisphere deserts. In the United States and Mexico, the lower Sonoran life zone, made up mainly of California, Arizona, and Northern Sonora and to a lesser degree Texas, Nevada, New Mexico, and Utah, are the areas where *C. immitis* resides in the soil. Guatemala, Honduras, Venezuela, Argentina, and Paraguay are also endemic areas.

Almost all cases are acquired via inhalation and initial pulmonary involvement. Ideal conditions to acquire coccidioidomycosis require a dry desert soil after a rainy season near active construction sites.

Approximately 90 percent of patients with coccidioidal meningitis die in the first year of illness if untreated. There are a few well-documented survivals of 10 and 25 years, respectively, of untreated coccidioidal meningitis.[10] Even with treatment, approximately 50 percent will eventually die from coccidioidal meningitis. From 25 to 50 percent of survivors are left with neurological deficit.[1]

Coccidioidal meningitis may occur with acute coccidioidal pulmonary or disseminated disease, years after known acquisition of coccidioidal disease, or with no antecedent history of infection.

Patients may rarely have a fulminating course simulating bacterial meningitis (Case IV, this chapter), but indolent courses over months with long periods of headache, mental changes, symptoms, and findings of increased intracranial pressure or focal neurologic abnormalities are more common.

In our experience with 40 cases of coccidioidal meningitis we have never had an acellular CSF. Ninety percent of our patients initially had 25 to 500 WBC/mm^3 in the CSF. Usually a majority of the cells are lymphocytes, with a high incidence of CSF eosinophilia. Two thirds of our patients had CSF sugars less than 50 mg/100ml and three fourths had CSF proteins greater than 50 mg/100ml. Forty percent had a CSF protein greater than 100 mg/100 ml initially. Over 80 percent of our patients have had a positive coccidioidal complement fixation test in the CSF. The diagnosis of *C. immitis* meningitis was made in the rest of our patients (with one exception) by positive culture for *C. immitis* in the CSF.

The diagnosis is usually made by a reactive CSF coccidioidal serology (complement fixation) with the exception of immunologically suppressed or very early patients; in these two groups the serology may be nonreactive. When this nonreactivity occurs, the organism can usually be cultured. Humans can tolerate, and actually clinically need, larger doses of intracisternal amphotericin B than are usually recommended. *C. immitis* meningitis needs to be treated for long periods with intracisternal amphotericin B in hope for "cure" which might be defined as the development of negative CSF findings and the development of a positive coccidiodal skin test. Some patients have to be treated with intracisternal amphotericin B for a lifetime, and may not be amenable to cure.

Twelve of our 40 cases will be discussed to emphasize specific problems with diagnosis and, particularly, management.

CASE I

A 40-year-old man in June 1967 had a pneumonic process presumed to be coccidioidomycosis, although his skin test at that time was negative. In December 1967, he had a three-week history of headache. Spinal fluid contained 850 white cells/mm^3 with 91% lymphocytes, protein of 320 mg/100 ml, and a spinal fluid complement fixation test that was positive at 1:16 dilution. Cisternal amphotericin B therapy was begun with 0.5 mg given on alternate days, in addition to intravenous amphotericin B. In June, when the spinal fluid titer had dropped to 1:2, the interval between treatments was increased to once every week and sometimes once every other week. He was treated continuously until June 1971 when an intracisternal injection of amphotericin B was followed by loss of hearing in the left ear, numbness of the left face, and tingling of the legs. At that time, therapy was discontinued. The following month the spinal fluid serology was nonreactive and the patient was lost to follow-up until October 1972. When seen then, he was totally asymptomatic except for the left hearing loss. Spinal fluid examination, including cocci serology, in November 1972 was entirely normal. He had a positive skin test at 1:100 with an erythema of 70 X 40 mm present at 48 hours. In 1980, he continued to be asymptomatic.

This case remains the longest of our recorded cases of apparent cure. We still insist that "cure" implies a negative or trace positive CSF coccidioidal complement fixation test and essentially a normal CSF sugar and cell count with the concomitant development of a positive skin test result. We continue to treat many patients every two to four weeks until these criteria are met. We have treated patients with this regimen for as long as four years.

We have now recorded five patients with normal CSF and negative skin test results who have exacerbated nine, 12, 14, 17, and 62 months later.

In our cured group, we have 13 patients and no exacerbations of disease.

CASE II

A 21-year-old Mexican-Japanese man entered the hospital after two months of headaches and low-grade fever; the highest temperature was 102°. He had had several episodes of transient left hemiparesis and was referred to the United States for evaluation. He had an unremarkable neurologic examination except for meningismus and fever. Lumbar puncture produced spinal fluid with a sugar of 40 mg/100 ml and a white cell count of 124/mm^3 with 61% lymphocytes. All studies of the spinal fluid had negative findings for infective organisms except a 1:4 positive complement fixation test for cocci. His blood titer was 1:8. Chest x-ray and sputum and urine cultures were consistently negative. Antecedent history revealed no past respiratory illnesses.

Amphotericin B treatment was begun with intracisternal injections. Because of no evidence of lung, urine, or other systemic involvement, we elected to treat the patient only with intrathecal injection every other day. The patient, after his initial two months' hospitalization, maintained a constant 1:4 titer in the spinal fluid. In January 1973 he was readmitted to the hospital after an untoward incident described as follows.

Preparation of the amphotericin B solution was shifted from the emergency room to the pharmacy. At the pharmacy, the final dilution of amphotericin B was not made, so the 2 ml/sent for injection contained 10 mg of amphotericin B instead of 0.5 mg. After cisternal installation of this concentrated solution, the patient became violently ill with high fever, meningismus, nausea, vomiting, and myalgia. He was treated symptomatically for three days and discharged. When he returned from Mexico the following month, his spinal fluid serology was totally negative for the first time. Subsequent cisternal taps were done for installation of amphotericin B. His spinal fluid serology remains nonreactive and his skin test one year later converted to a positive result.

We have given, on at least four other occasions, 5 mg of amphotericin B intrathecally, but never with the dramatic results of our first case. Two of the four treatments did produce marked improvement in the CSF abnormalities. The other two treatments did not produce any substantial change. With 5 mg intracisternally, patients were sicker than with the 1 mg injection, but they never became as ill as our first patient.

Three other cases, all men in their twenties, with evidence of *C. immitis* meningitis without other documentable organ system involvement, were treated only with intracisternal amphotericin B; all had apparent cures. All had initial serum complement fixation to *C. immitis* of greater than 1:8. The longest a patient has survived subsequently without treatment is seven years.

CASE III

A 47-seven-year-old woman had a long history of Hodgkin's disease, documented as stage III in 1968, and had received chemotherapy. She was admitted in both October and December of 1971 with problems related to her Hodgkin's disease. One admission was for a pneumonitis which improved with antibiotics. In December 1971, she was thought to have disseminated coccidioidomycosis on the basis of culture and blood serologic findings. She had negative spinal fluid studies at that time. She returned to the east where in July 1972 she developed headache. In August she was admitted to a hospital in New Jersey and remained there until September. Spinal punctures were reported to show elevated spinal fluid protein with cell counts of 200. She was treated with systemic antibiotics, but her condition deteriorated. She was transferred to Arizona, at which time repeat spinal fluid examination revealed 191 white cells/mm^3 a majority of which were lymphocytes, glucose of 35 mg/100 ml, and protein of 48 mg/100 ml. Serum complement fixation tests for *C. immitis* were positive at 1:2, but spinal fluid serologies on repeated occasions were nonreactive. However, *C. immitis* was cultured from the spinal fluid. She was treated with intrathecal and systemic amphotericin B, but died in October 1972.

CASE IV

J.G. was a 46-year-old man with a long history of Stage 4-B Hodgkin's disease, who developed diffuse pulmonary coccidioidomycosis in August 1981, before his final admission on October 28, 1981. He was placed on ketoconazole with regression of his pulmonary symptoms. A lumbar puncture on August 4, 1981 was within normal limits. One day before admission he developed fever, headache, and confusion. He then developed a left hemiplegia, gaze palsy, and had a lumbar puncture which revealed 1100 WBC/mm^3—92% Segs, a sugar of 22 mg/100 ml, and a protein of 147 mg/100 ml. A cocci CSF serology was negative, but *C. immitis* was cultured. The patient died November 1, 1981, five days after CNS symptoms.

These two cases are representative of four patients with lymphoma who never developed positive CSF coccidioidin complement fixation titers, but from whom *C. immitis* was cultured from their CSF. Another patient with lymphoma, who was also receiving immunosuppressive therapy, had less than a 1:16 CSF complement fixation for *C. immitis* with the initial lumbar puncture. We have one patient who, after extensive treatment with amphotericin B intracisternally, developed a positive complement fixation for *C. immitis* with negative CSF cultures at all times, but had a complication and died from later pulmonary problems; only at autopsy was the diagnosis of Hodgkin's made.

Our experience with six cases of *C. immitis* meningitis in patients with lymphoma reveals that the longest survival is less than six months. J.G. presented clinically as an acute bacterial meningitis with CSF consistent with acute bacterial meningitis and died in a matter of days with *C. immitis* as the organism being cultured within 48 hours.

J.G. is of interest also because of the normal CSF followed by the development of meningitis while receiving treatment with ketoconazole.

CASE V

A 32-two-year-old woman was first hospitalized in June 1971 with cutaneous coccidioidomycosis of the jaw. She had no pulmonary symptoms, but later had a positive chest x-ray. She had a negative coccidioidomycosis skin test, but *C. immitis* was cultured from the wound and the blood titer was reactive at 1:256. Spinal fluid examination produced a nonreactive serology. She was treated with intravenous amphotericin B for a total dose of two grams. In February 1972 the patient gave a history of headaches over a matter of a month and had a spinal fluid examination showing 290 white cells/mm^3, 80% lymphs, a sugar of 25 mg/100 ml, and protein of 33 mg/100 ml. Initial spinal fluid titers were 1:8 and 1:16. The patient was treated in the hospital over a three-week period with a course of 0.5 mg of cisternal intrathecal amphotericin B injection daily, and then every other day. She continued to have outpatient cisternal injections once a week, gradually tapering to once a month. In August 1972, at the time of an attempted cisternal puncture, arterial blood was returned and the needle was promptly withdrawn. Three hours later the patient complained bitterly of headache and became somnolent. She developed retinal hemorrhages and began intermittent decerebrate posturing. She was rushed to the operating room where a posterior fossa hematoma was removed. The site of the bleeding was unknown. The patient did well initially. Because of increasing somnolence, however, she had a ventricular tap which revealed the ventricles to be under pressure. A day later, she underwent ventriculoperitoneal shunting, following which she became hemiplegic. After a stormy six-week course, she left the hospital with no significant deficit except mild hyperreflexia on the left. At the time of discharge her spinal fluid complement fixation titer was 1:4. Within the next two months her titer rose to 1:64. Because of the multiple problems in the past and because the patient was asymptomatic, it was elected not to continue treatment. She was followed until July 1973 at which time she had been totally asymptomatic over a nine-month period despite a rising spinal fluid titer and presumed increasing coccidioidal activity in the spinal fluid.

The patient then began to deteriorate mentally and was readmitted to the hospital with the shunt still functioning. Her CSF examination yielded a positive coccidioidal complement fixation titer of greater than 1:64, over 500 cells/mm^3, and sugar under 20 mg/100ml. Because of shunt tubing in both ventricles, an Ommaya reservoir was placed with the tubular end in the cisterna magna and the reservoir under the scalp at the occipitocervical junction. She was again treated with amphotericin B twice a week for six weeks and then weekly. She subsequently recovered and was intermittently treated until the middle 1970s. She is alive and well and still has her Ommaya reservoir.

This case is an example of a complication of cisternal amphotericin B injection with the development of a posterior fossa hematoma. It was also the first case in which a cisternal Ommaya reservoir was used. The rest of our complications are: unilateral deafness with transient paraparesis (one case), unilateral deafness with transient hemiparesis (one case), transient brainstem stroke (two cases), transient third nerve palsy (two cases), paraplegia (one case). Table 1 summarizes our experience with 15 such cases. When looking at our data seven months ago, there was a striking lack of change in spinal fluid formulas.

However, during the last six months we have been using increased dosages of intra-Ommaya-reservoir amphotericin B (minimum of 1.5 mg per injection) and have seen markedly improved results. In the cases of R.E. and P.P., we gave a few 5 mg injections and found both reservoirs

TABLE 1. Cisternal Ommaya Reservoirs

Patient	Reservoir complications	Comment and course
SM-1	None	1-year treatment, CSF almost negative
SM-2	None	Less than one-year treatment, CSF almost negative
JB[a]	Plugged cisternal reservoir	New reservoir in lumbar area — treated nine months — untreated six months — doing well
HO	None	Less than one year of treatment — lost to follow-up with markedly improved CSF
SC	None	18 months of treatment with markedly improved CSF — lost to follow-up
P-1[a]	Plugged less than one year	Cisternal arachnoiditis
P-2[a]	Plugged less than six months	Cisternal arachnoiditis
RK	None	5 mg injection, did well and discharged — lost to follow up
RG	CSF leak — taken out	Receiving chronic steroids for prior ten years — died
HE[a]	Taken out	Ventricular CSF negative, cisternal equivalent not under treatment
PP	Plugged and replaced	Occurred after 5 mg injection — doing well, still under treatment two years
CA[a]	None	Ventricular and cisternal CSF negative after eight months
MM[a]	None	Not under treatment for five years — reservoir still in
EI[a]	Plugged after 5 mg injection	Replaced — died of shunt complications but CSF improved
JK[a]	Replaced once	Alive after stormy course

[a] Patients with hydrocephalus and ventriculoperitoneal shunts.

required replacement because they were plugged with amphotericin B crystals. However, we have had no bacterial infections with the cisternal reservoirs, in contrast to the frequency of this complication with intraventricular reservoirs.[1,8] Six of the patients' Ommaya reservoirs plugged, and one patient receiving chronic high-dose corticosteroids had an Ommaya reservoir removed because of lack of wound healing with CSF leak. We do not know whether the lack of superimposed infections is fortuitous or whether it is due to other factors, including a larger area for the dispersement of injections.

CASE VI

J.F. was a 44-year-old man who had the onset of cough, chest pain, and fever and days later of headache in November 1980. He developed a positive 1:4 complement fixation to cocci after having a negative one two weeks before admission. His peripheral eosinophile count was 2,224 and chest x-rays revealed a right middle lobe pneumonia. An initial lumbar puncture revealed 800 WBC/mm^3 with eosinophilia with a normal protein, sugar, and negative complement fixation and precipitin test for *C. immitis*. CSF cultures were negative. Sputum cultures subsequently grew out *C. immitis*, but CSF cultures and complement fixation tests for *C. immitis* were constantly negative. With intrathecal amphotericin B, he normalized his CSF in one year, developed a positive skin test for *C. immitis*, and has now been followed to the present with no further therapy. He was never treated with IV amphotericin B.

This case represents our only case where neither CSF culture nor serology was ever positive for *C. immitis*, but clinically there was no doubt that the patient had coccidioidal meningitis. Perhaps the extremely early treatment had much to do with the lack of later development of a positive coccidiodal complement fixation test in the CSF in this patient. He was another of the men who received no systemic therapy for *C. immitis*.

CASE VII

G.S. at age twenty-five, after eight years in Arizona and one year with steroids for systemic lupus erythematosus (SLE), developed fulminating disseminated coccidioidomycosis. He had pulmonary, bone, urinary, and bone marrow involvement with five blood cultures positive for *C. immitis*. He had four months of systemic treatment with IV amphotericin B and eight months later developed *C. immitis* meningitis. He was treated with cisternal amphotericin B for 20 months. Less than a year later he recurred. After six months of further treatment with intracisternal amphotericin B, his spinal fluid became totally normal. He has, over the last year, been treated monthly with intracisternal injections of amphotericin B. He had two bouts in his clinical course of unexplained hypercalcemia.

This is the only patient with any underlying immunologic problem (SLE + steroids) who has done very well. He has now received a year of monthly intracisternal treatments. We have treated two other patients with monthly intracisternal amphotericin B between two and three years who finally converted their coccidioidin skin tests and have not had recurrences. We are trying to accumulate enough cases of treated patients whose CSF became normal, but remain skin test negative and who are then treated intracisternally infrequently for long periods, to see if recurrences are prevented.

CASE VIII

This is a 38-year-old woman whose significant medical history begins in 1979 at which time she had a febrile illness with eosinophilia and a pneumonic process treated with dexamethasone. She subsequently developed skin lesions, followed one month later by meningitis; coccidioidal dissemination was diagnosed. She then was transferred to our care and was found to have hydrocephalus. In February 1980, a ventriculoperitoneal shunt was placed. She then had a Ommaya reservoir placed and was treated with intrathecal amphotericin B in the shunt tubing and into the Ommaya reservoir. She was treated with ketoconazole and amphotericin B IV for six months.

The complications off and on through the hospitalization, which had stretched intermittently to June 1981, were progressive osteomyelitis of her lower lumbar spine, hypercalcemia that caused intermittent obtundation, and coma, and a plugged reservoir that was replaced. The serum calciums had been in excess of 15 mg/100 ml with low serum proteins. For these episodes she had been treated with mithramycin with some success. Lumbar punctures could not be done because even with fluoroscopy she had what seemed to be a dry space in the lumbar area. Because of abnormal cisternal fluid, she had continuous intracisternal treatment. She had been treated intraventricularly and her last spinal fluids from her ventricular space were all normal.

She was discharged with a functioning shunt, negative intracisternal CSF, positive complement fixation tests from the cisternal space but complicated by protein values that were in excess of 3 g. We felt that the spinal fluid values were uninterpretable because of the protein. She was discharged on ketoconazole and periodic IV amphotericin B. She has improved mentally, but remains in a nursing home. She has no evidence of active coccidioidal meningitis, but by x-ray she still has active bone disease.

This patient is the second of our patients who had significant neurologic problems with hypercalcemia that had to be treated.

Studies done did not suggest the hypercalcemia as being due to an absorptive mechanism. Vitamin D levels were low. She had multiple parathormone levels measuring both C terminal and intact hormones which were all somewhat low. She had an elevated nephrogenic cyclic AMP. Tumor work-up was negative, and tumor probably could be excluded clinically because of the 1.5 year's duration of the elevated calciums. Our conclusion was that somehow this patient's disease state with *C. immitis* caused the elaboration of a material that acts in a way similar to parathormone.

This patient and three others who were initially receiving high dose steroids have either died or have been left with substantial neurological deficit. Steroids were started because one of the patients was thought to have pseudotumor, one to have a vasculitis because of lung and kidney involvement, and one to have increasing asthmatic problems. When they

received very high-dose steroids, all developed obvious meningeal involvement and neurologic signs, and coccidioidal meningitis was finally
diagnosed. All had stormy courses.

We have had three patients with known cocci who were given in
excess of 12 mg of Decadron a day for other reasons with chest x-rays
before and after demonstrating widespread pulmonary dissemination
within days. Two of these patients were given the steroids for presumed
strokes and one for a severe hypotensive episode. Figures 1 and 2 show
the x-rays taken before dexamethasone. Figures 3 and 4 show the x-rays
taken after dexamethasone. These x-rays were three to seven days apart.
Sputum samples were positive for *C. immitis*.

We think the use of steroids, either short or long-term, in patients
with *C. immitis* infections (active or as in the case of one of our patients
previously treated and thought to have stable disease) is fraught with a
real danger of dissemination. We also think that the use of steroids in
pneumonia without proven origin in areas endemic for *C. immitis* can be
disastrous.

CASE IX

J.B. in June 1979 was traveling over dirt roads for miles and within a week
developed chest pain and cough. The second week he had a continuous headache
and had a lumbar puncture and CSF with 466 cells/mm^3 (50% lymphs), a glucose
of 35 mg/100 ml, protein of 62 mg/100 ml, and negative CSF *C. immitis* serologies.
Cultures were positive for *C. immitis*. After six weeks of intracisternal amphotericin B, the patient developed hydrocephalus and had to have a ventriculoperitoneal shunt. Cisternal taps were discontinued after we could not return fluid even
with fluroscopically assisted taps. An Ommaya cisternal reservoir was put in
place even though there was evidence of arachnoiditis and a very small CSF
cisternal space. This became blocked within five weeks. A lumbar puncture was
performed and the CSF fluid clotted with proteins in excess of 2 g. A cauda
equina reservoir was put in place. Treatment was instituted both through the
on-off ventricular shunt and through the reservoir. Within four weeks, the intraventricular fluid was perfectly normal and therapy through the shunt was
discontinued. Therapy through the caudal Ommaya reservoir was discontinued
a year later with the development of hoarseness and upper cervical findings. The
patient is now off treatment for six months and doing well. His CSF has been
normal continuously from the ventricles and uninterpretable from the lumbar sac
with CSF proteins measured in grams.

This patient's condition reflects the problem of two space infections
when hydrocephalus complicates cocci meningitis. In this situation, both

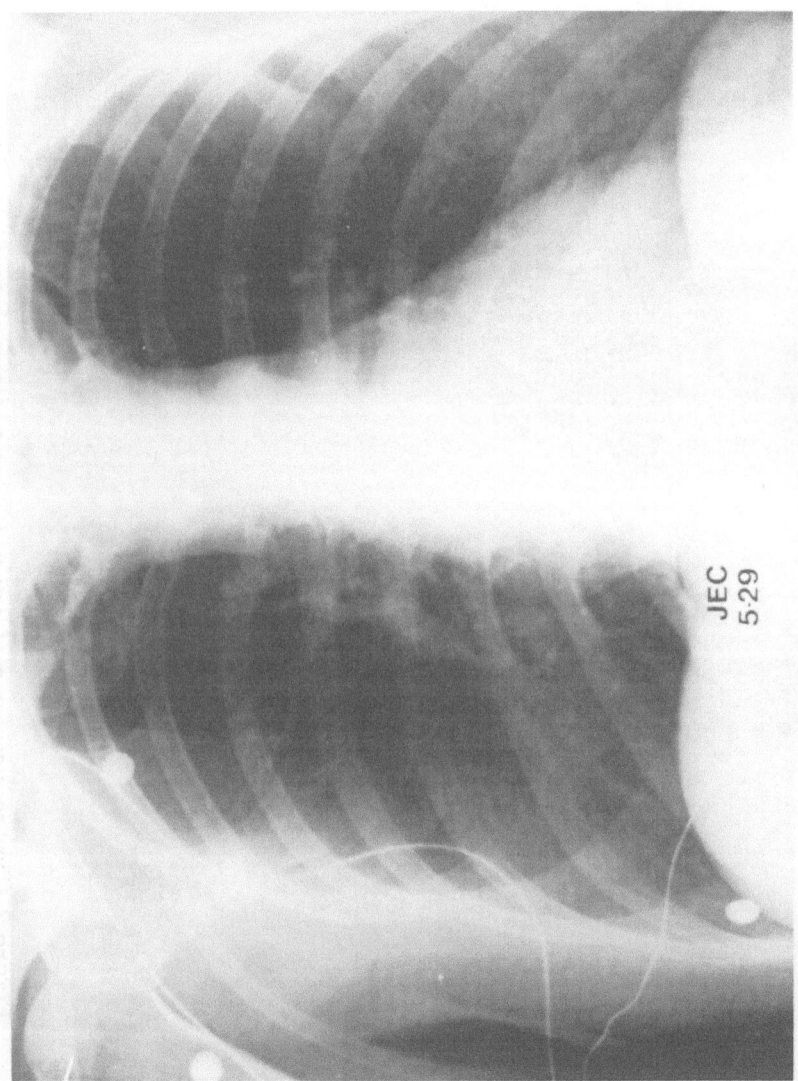

Figure 1. Chest roentgenogram of Patient JEC before dexamethasone administration.

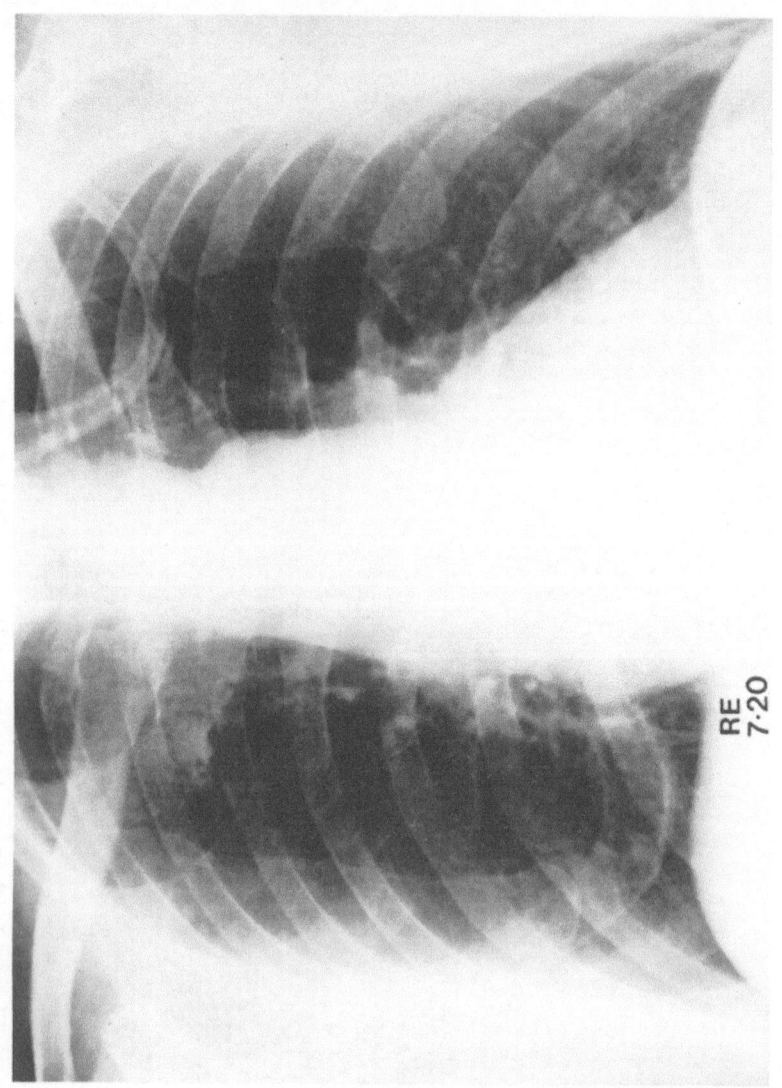

Figure 2. Chest roentgenogram of Patient RE before dexamethasone administration.

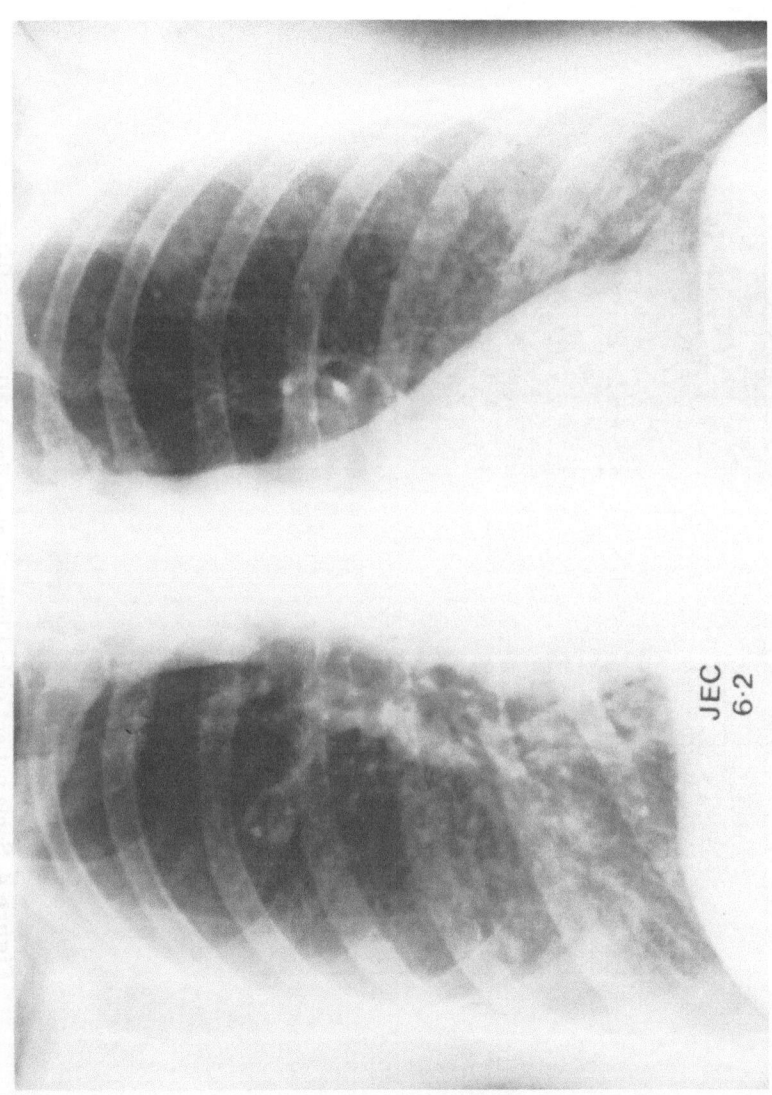

Figure 3. Same patient as in Figure 1, after dexamethasone administration.

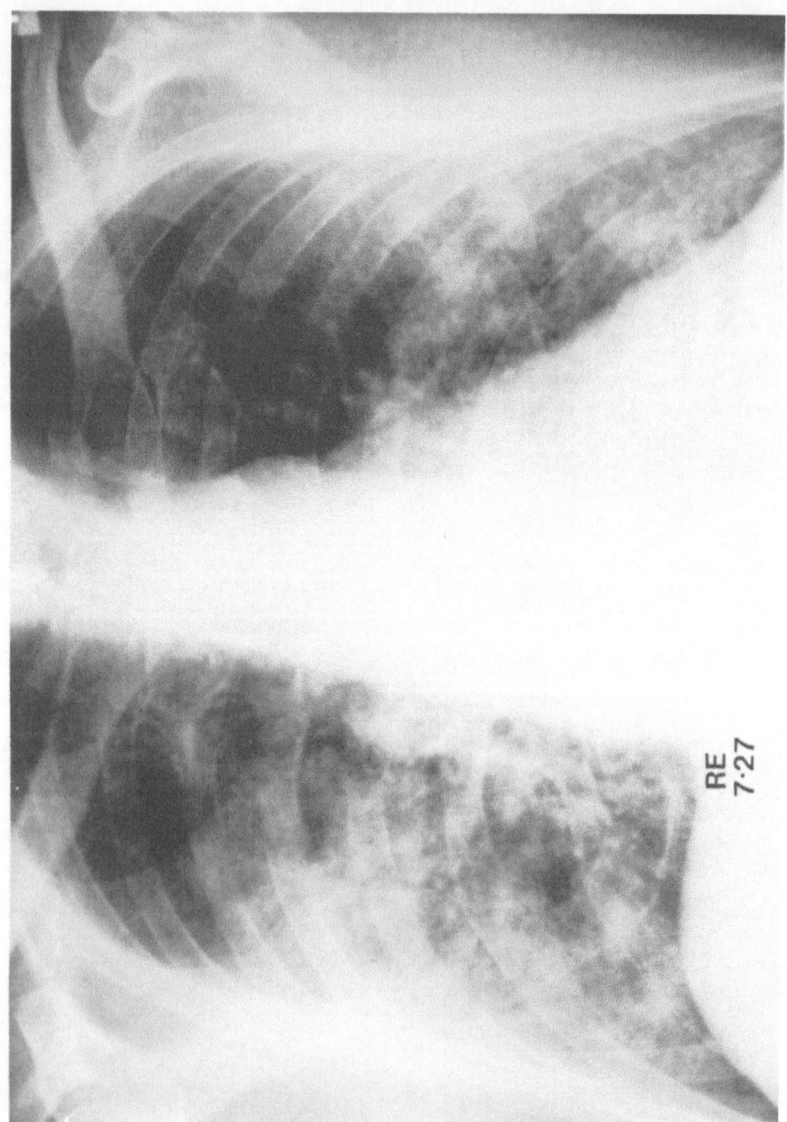

Figure 4. Same patient as in Figure 2, after dexamethasone administration.

spaces have to be treated. It is, in our experience, easy to normalize the ventricular CSF even in the very sick or immunosuppressed patient. We have elected to continue treatment in the cistern if possible even in the face of enormously high CSF proteins until the patient develops a positive skin test, or to discontinue treatment if it is technically impossible to continue, or if signs compatible with arachnoiditis start to develop. When CSF protein exceeds 2 g, cell counts, sugars, and serologies are so variable as to be meaningless.

We inserted the lumbar Ommaya reservoir reluctantly because all of our patients from the late 1960s with lumbar intrathectal injections of amphotericin B developed arachnoiditis. It worked out well, but we think we perpetuated the brain stem and cervical arachnoiditis.

This is one of three patients who had negative CSF serologies when CSF studies were done after less than six weeks of initial symptoms. All, however, had positive cultures.

CASE X

J.Y., a 27-year-old woman, in the third trimester of her pregnancy in September 1980 developed cough and had a chest x-ray which showed diffuse infiltrates. She had a serum complement fixation test for *C. immitis* that was positive at 1:512 with sputum samples that were culture positive for *C. immitis*. Spinal fluid exam revealed the CSF to contain 43 WBC/mm^3, a glucose of 49 mg/100 ml, and a protein of 17 mg/100 ml. She was then given one 0.2 mg dose of amphotericin B but the CSF drawn at the time of injection was normal. She had no further intracisternal treatment and no headache. She had another lumbar puncture on January 28 with 6 WBC/mm^3, normal protein and sugar, negative CSF complement fixation for *C. immitis,* and negative culture. In February, she had another lumbar puncture with one WBC/mm^3, normal protein and sugar. At this time she was receiving IV amphotericin B because of her pulmonary picture. In June 1981 she complained of headache again and had a lumbar puncture with CSF having 150 WBC/mm^3, a sugar of 18 mg/100 ml, and a protein of 76 mg/100 ml. Her *C. immitis* complement fixation test was positive at 1:8. She is still undergoing intrathecal amphotericin B treatment at present with her latest CSF complement fixation down to 1:2.

We are at a total loss to explain the headache, transient meningeal involvement, apparent spontaneous clearing of the CSF, and then the subsequent development of coccidioidal meningitis. One wonders about the possibility of transient meningeal involvement with spontaneous clearing in other cases and the possibility that infection can take place in the ependyma and that it can take a while for frank meningeal involvement to occur.

CASE XI

J.R., a 59-year old insulin-dependent diabetic, post four-vessel coronary bypass and a chronic gallbladder disease patient, developed headache and a pulmonary infiltrate. CSF exam revealed 150 to 200 WBC/mm^3, proteins of 80 mg/100 ml, to 112 and sugar of 40 to 82 mg/100 ml. Her CSF complement fixation test was greater than 1:16. With her first intracisternal injection of amphotericin B, she developed chest pain with electrocardiographic changes and CPK and LDH elevation, and was diagnosed as having a acute myocardial infarction. After two weeks, amphotericin B was reinstituted and she was treated at least three times a week for over four months. During the last year she has been treated about weekly and over the last months every other week because of other medical problems. Her CSF complement fixation test has remained at 1:4 with cell counts of 15 to 27/mm^3.

Because of her fifth episode of cholecystitis, she finally had her gallbladder removed and is recovering.

This patient represents the type that, we think, has little hope for cure. She has been functional between bouts of cholecystitis, with bi-weekly to every other week intracisternal injections and interestingly maintaining her CSF formula relatively constant at a low level of activity. We think that there are many such patients who, for technical or other medical reasons, might be treated in this manner.

CASE XII

C.A., a 25-year-old man, was diagnosed in late 1980 in another city of having coccidioidal meningitis and was treated for three months and discharged in January 1981. In July 1981, he developed headaches and in August had a lumbar puncture with CSF having 74 WBC/mm^3 (57% lymphs) with a protein of 30 mg/100 ml and a glucose of 40 mg/100 ml. CSF complement fixation test was positive at 1:2. During the hospitalization, the patient developed progressive hydrocephalus and was shunted with an on-off ventriculoperitoneal shunt. A cisternal Ommaya was also put in place because of difficulty with cisternal punctures and the history of two previous neurologic deficits with treatment intracisternally before our assuming care. Intraventricular amphotericin B normalized the ventricular CSF within six weeks. Four months later, the cisternal fluid was normal. Twice the patient was found somnolent with neurologic findings and was found to have the shunt off. Within hours, the patient neurologically cleared with the shunt being put on.

This represented the ideal case to present for efficacy of the use of cisternal Ommaya reservoir. The patient had complications with cisternal puncture because of arachnoiditis, developed hydrocephalus, and with vigorous treatment both CSF compartments' complement fixation tests and other studies returned to normal values with negative serologies.

However, the complication with the on-off shunt valve being off was not an isolated problem. We have had two other patients with coccidioidal meningitis and hydrocephaly develop significant problems; one died later, possibly as an indirect result of the valve being off. We have had one patient with cryptococcal meningitis who most certainly died from her valve being off.

DISCUSSION

In the course of treatment of our 40 patients, none developed erythema nodosum and only two developed erythema multiform. Three of our four black patients we consider cured. The fourth was transferred out of state to another institution and lost to follow-up. The alternative therapies of miconazole in two patients resulted in problems that led to one death and in one patient led to being restarted on smaller doses of amphotericin B. Oral ketoconazole up to doses of 800 mg/day has not been helpful in any way in the treatment of coccidioidal meningitis, but we have not had any significant complications from its use.

Table 2 summarizes the patients who have died. The data imply the patients with rheumatoid arthritis, chronic steroid use, lymphoma, SLE, immunosuppression and very young pediatric patients are likely to die from *C. immitis* meningitis despite vigorous treatment. It would seem from this and our other data,[1,2] the preferred route of amphotericin B administration in patient with CSF involvement with *C. immitis* should be the cisterna magna, whatever way amphotericin B can be delivered into it. Although there have been complications (listed earlier), these are

TABLE 2. Deaths

Three RA

One SLE

Six lymphoma

One unspecified immunologic problem

Two congenital abnormalities in early childhood

One shunt problem

One chronic lung disease patient receiving high doses of steroids for greater than ten years

RA=rheumatoid arthritis, SLE=systemic lupus erythematosus.

certainly acceptable as compared with the superimposed bacterial infections of the Ommaya reservoir used intraventricularly[8] or with direct lumbar instillation.[1] We would hope our data with cisternal Ommayas and amphotericin B therapy hold. However, we still only put reservoirs in patients with whom we have had complications or difficulty with percutaneous treatment, or who have refused percutaneous intracisternal punctures and would have stopped treatment.

SUMMARY

1. The diagnosis of *C. immitis* meningitis is usually made by a CSF positive complement fixation serology.
2. Eight of 40 patients had negative CSF *C. immitis* serologies. Four had lymphoma, three were early onset cases and had positive CSF cultures, and one had negative serology and negative cultures (CSF).
3. Our past experience with ventricular Ommayas was complicated by bacterial infection.
4. Our past experience with lumbar amphotericin B was complicated by arachnoiditis.
5. Our present experience with cisternal Ommayas is certainly better than ventricular Ommayas. In the future we think we will use it more often.
6. Chronic or acute steroid usage can precipitate pulmonary spread or disseminated cocci.
7. If there is no other indication to treat with IV amphotericin B other than the meningitis, we do not.
8. Oral ketoconazole has been a disappointment in conventional doses.
9. Miconazole has been a disappointment.
10. Hypercalcemia is an uncommon complication of coccidioidal meningitis and is difficult to treat.
11. We have continued to treat most of our patients until the spinal fluid has cleared and their skin test results have converted to positive.
12. Hydrocephalus should be treated promptly.
13. Patients with underlying immunosuppressive problems usually survive less than one year.
14. Cisternal puncture with amphotericin B injection still remains the most reliable form of therapy in our hands.
15. Like most other series, young men do very well with this disease.
16. One patient received 10 mg of amphotericin B intracisternally and his CSF promptly cleared of abnormality.

17. Through cisternal Ommaya reservoirs, we have started to give up to 5 mg of amphotericin B at a time.
18. Thirty-seven of 40 patients had negative coccidiodal skin test results initially.
19. There were no cases of meningitis with erythema nodosum.
20. Five patients in whom therapy with intracisternal amphotericin B was stopped because of consistantly normal CSF have had recurrences of meningitis. All five patients had negative skin tests for *C. immitis* at the time of discontinuance of therapy.

REFERENCES

1. Bouza, B., Dreyer, J.S., et al. Coccidioidal meningitis. *Medicine 60*: 3, 1981.
2. Buchsbaum, H.W. Clinical management of coccidioidal meningitis, in coccidioidomycosis. In: *Current Clinical and Diagnostic Status*. L. Ajello, ed. Miami, Fl: Symposia Specialists, pp. 191, 1972.
3. Caudill, R.G., Smith, C.E., and Reinarz, J.A. Coccidioidal meningitis. A diagnostic challenge. *Am. J. Med. 49*:360, 1970.
4. Drutz, D.J., and Catanzaro, A. Coccidioidomycosis. *Am. Rev. Respir. Dis. 117*:559, 727, 1978.
5. Einstein, H.E., Holeman, C.W., Sandidge, L.L., and Holden, D.H. Coccidioidal meningitis. The use of amphotericin B in treatment. *Calif. Med. 94*:339, 1961.
6. Einstein, H.E. Spinal fluid in coccidioidal meningitis. *Ann. Intern. Med. 78*:621, 1973.
7. Einstein, H.E. Coccidioidomycosis of the central nervous system. In: *Advances of Neurology*. Vol. 6. R. A. Thompson and J. R. Green, eds. New York: Raven Press, pp. 101, 1974.
8. Graybill, J.R., and Ellenbogen, C. Complications with the Ommaya reservoir in patients with granulomatous meningitis. *J. Neurosurg. 38*:477, 1973.
9. Loofbourow, J.C., Pappagianis, D., and Cooper, T.Y. Endemic coccidioidomycosis in Northern California. An outbreak in the Capay Valley of Yolo County. *Calif. Med. 111*:5, 1969.
10. Norman, D.D., and Miller, Z.R. Coccidioidomycosis of the central nervous system. A case of ten years duration. *Neurology 4*:173, 1954.
11. Ophuls, W. Coccidioidal granulomas. *J.A.M.A. 14*:1291, 1905.
12. Pappagianis, D. Coccidioides in the soil and the meninges. *Calif. Med. 119*:51, 1973.
13. Pappagianis, D., and Crane, R. Survival in coccidioidal meningitis since introduction of amphotericin B, in coccidioidomycosis. In: *Current Clinical and Diagnostic Status*, L. Ajello, ed. Miami, Fl: Symposia Specialists, pp. 223, 1977.
14. Pappagianis, D., Lindsay, S., Beall, S., and Williams, P. Ethnic background and the clinical course of coccidioidomycosis. *Am. Rev. Respir. Dis. 120*:959, 1979.
15. Smith, C.E., Beard, R.R., Whiting, E.G., and Rosenberger, H.G. Varieties of coccidioidal infection in relation to the epidemiology and control of the diseases. *Am. J. Public Health 36*:1394, 1946.

16. Smith, C.E., Beard, R.R., and Whiting, E.G. Effect of season and dust control on coccidioidomycosis. *J.A.M.A. 132*:833, 1946.
17. Smith, C.E., Saito, M.T., Beard, R.E., Kepp, R.M., Clark, R.W., and Eddie, B.U. Serological tests in the diagnosis and prognosis of coccidioidomycosis. *Am. J. Hyg. 52*:1, 1950.
18. Smith, C.E., Saito, M.T., and Simons, S.A. Pattern of 39,500 serologic tests in coccidioidomycosis. *J.A.M.A. 160*:546, 1956.
19. Winn, W.A. The use of amphotericin B in the treatment of coccidioidal disease. *Am. J. Med. 27*:617, 1959.
20. Winn, W.A. The diagnosis and treatment of coccidioidomycosis. *Ariz. Med. 19*:211, 1962.
21. Winn, W.A. Coccidiodomycosis and amphotericin B. *Med. Clin. North Am. 47*:1131, 1963.
22. Winn, W.A. The treatment of coccidioidal meningitis. The use of amphotericin B in a group of 25 patients. *Calif. Med. 101*:78, 1964.
23. Michell Parker, M.D. (personal communication).

12

Parasitic Infestation of the Central Nervous System

W. Eugene Stern

In a tabulation of parasitic infestations which may involve the central nervous system, the following (from the table of contents of Brown and Voge[1]) should be considered: (1) amoebiasis, (2) toxoplasmosis, (3) malaria, (4) trypanosomiasis, (5) schistosomiasis, (6) trematode infections, (7) cysticercosis, (8) hydatid disease and other tapeworm infections, (9) eosinophilic meningoencephalitis, (10) gnathostomiasis, (11) onchocerciasis and loiasis, (12) other filarial infections, (13) visceral larvae migrans, (14) other roundworm infections, (15) miyasis.

The focus in this chapter is primarily upon those conditions which have surgical implications.

AMOEBIASIS

The protozoon *Entamoeba histolytica* is transmitted by cyst stages which are passed by way of the stool of infected individuals and are accidentally ingested through contaminated materials. This organism is the amoeba which produces dysentery in man and may, through the bloodstream, invade other organs, notably the liver. In addition to *E. histolytica* there are free-living amoeba, notably *Naegleria* and *Acanthamoeba*, culpable in central nervous disease. The neural manifestations of these infections include a meningoencephalitis which can be associated with cerebral edema and a purulent encephaloleptomeningitis. The leptomeningeal manifestations are associated with a leukocytosis and mimic meningitides of other etiologies and, unless a "wet mount" of the cerebrospinal fluid is performed, the diagnosis may not be made.[2]

Brain abscess may be caused by the *Entamoeba histolytica*. Such lesions may be solitary or multiple and, though it is rare, brain abscess may occur in patients with neither liver abscesses nor other extraintestinal lesions. As is the case with brain abscesses of bacterial origin, the lesions may break into the subarachnoid space or into the ventricle with associated diffuse spread of purulent exudate. Solitary brain abscesses are amenable to excision, but in the absence of other evidence of the disease the diagnosis of the amoebic cause of such a lesion will be difficult. In suspected cases stool examination is warranted and serum serologic and immunofluorescent tests may be of value. Takaro and Bond[3] calculated a 3.7 percent incidence of brain abscess among patients infested with *E. histolytica*. A history of residence in tropical countries, especially if associated with swimming in bodies of warm, fresh water, may alert the physician to such a possibility. Lest one consider the amoebic threat very remote, I would note the recent recognition of infestations peculiar to local homosexual communities and cite the statistic that in the month of October 1981, there were reported 104 cases of amebiasis in the County of Los Angeles.[4]

Quite apart from any surgical implications, the drugs for therapy include miconazole, amphotericin B, metronidazole, emetine hydrochloride, and chloroquine phosphate. Control of leptomeningitis is likely to require intrathecal medication.[2]

TOXOPLASMOSIS

Infestation with *Toxoplasma gondii* (a tiny intracellular protozoon) recalls the frequent association of the organism with felines, whereby the tissues of the cat may be widely involved. The organisms are excreted by the animal and can remain active in contaminated soil for long periods of time, but the definitive points of contact with the infectious material may be difficult to discern. Congenital forms and acquired forms, particularly those associated with suppressed immunity, are well recognized. In the congenital forms severe involvement of the parenchyma of the brain may occur with necrosis, scarring, involvement of the periventricular tissues, aqueductal obstructions, hydrocephalus, and cyst-like formations. Although surgical management of hydrocephalic states resulting from this entity probably has been undertaken, I have found no comment nor have I any personal experience.

MALARIA

With respect to malaria, the neurosurgical armamentarium for the control of increased intracranial pressure (should it occur in association with the coma of cerebral malaria) will take second place to antimalarial therapy. Plasmodium falciparum is the malarial species responsible for the central nervous system syndromes, but, fortunately, the cerebral forms of the disease are infrequent. The report by Daroff et al. in 1967[5] may be consulted for more detailed descriptions, and the recent report by Warrell et al.[6] discrediting the use of dexamethasone for the condition is worthy of attention.

SCHISTOSOMIASIS

My first contact with this condition involved an American soldier released from Japanese incarceration where he had worked in the rice paddies in the Leyte Gulf area of the Philippines. (The alert physician will be suspicious of extended travel or of the residence of patients in areas of endemicity for this as well as most other parasitic processes.) He presented with signs of increased intracranial pressure and was found to have a parieto-occipital lobe granuloma which was excised surgically.

The infective larval stages of the schistosomes, the cercariae, emerge from the intermediate host, the snail, and penetrate the skin of people wading or swimming in infested water. The larvae migrate to the lungs and then enter the hepatic portal vascular system. The granulomatous reaction which is observed appears to be part of a sensitivity reaction to antigenic materials of either dead worms or eggs (ova). The greatest number of symptomatic cases are produced by Schistosoma japonicum, and this species involves primarily the brain and rarely the spinal cord. By contrast, S. mansoni predominantly involves the cord and, to far less extent, the brain. S. haematobium can involve the brain, but more particularly, the spinal cord. Ova of any of the species may be found in CNS tissue without any clinical signature; for example, in hepatosplenic disease the ova of S. mansoni were discovered in the brain in 12 of 46 autopsied cases without clinical neurologic findings.[7]

In a comprehensive review of central nervous system involvement by schistosomiasis, Marcial-Rojas and Fiol[8] identified 26 cases of brain involvement. Nineteen of these cases were surgical specimens, each of which had presented as a mass which was resected at the time of operation. It was the ova which appeared to accumulate and excite a granulomatous formation. The latter, in turn, developed as an expanding mass in the brain parenchyma. Of the 19 cases reported from surgical experience, there was, in general, improvement after the resection. Spinal cord involvement was identified in 24 cases, seven from surgical biopsies and 17 from autopsy examinations. Here, again, it was the ova which accumulated in the spinal cord and produced paralysis of function. Reyes et al.[9] believed that both hematogenous embolization with ova and adult worm involvement were the two mechanisms responsible for the production of the intracranial mass process. All the patients reviewed by Marcial-Rojas and Fiol[8] had either visited or were resident in endemic areas, usually in the Samar and Leyte regions of the Philippines.

In the report by Reyes et al.,[9] from the University of the Philippines, 25 cases were studied. Ten of the group were verified cases of cerebral involvement from surgical experience or from autopsy examinations (eight surgical, two autopsy). These ten patients presented with seizures but, in addition, other neurologic deficit was described as a result of the development of mass lesions. In the experience of these authors, there were no plain radiologic findings of diagnostic value, and cerebral angiography revealed only the signature of a mass lesion. Feces examinations were positive in the majority of cases, and a rectal mucosal biopsy was positive in nine of 11 cases in which it was done. (Examination of the urine for ova should not be neglected.) Skin testing with a somatic antigen was positive in 12 of 14 cases. The circumoval test, utilizing precipitins against ova with the patient's serum, was found to be highly sensitive and specific. When this test was applied to the cerebrospinal fluid it was positive in four of five cases. The masses removed at the time of operation were described as irregular granulomata, varying from pin-head tubercles to a 6 cm diameter mass in the gray and underlying white matter. The location was parietal in five examples and one each in the frontal and occipital lobes. There was firm adherence to the dura mater in some cases. The lesions were fairly easily dissected, albeit they produced an "iceberg" presentation, with a small surface signature of a much larger, submerged mass. They lent themselves to excision with a satisfactory outcome.

Jackson[10] noted two cases of spinal cord involvement in which a CSF pleocytosis with an increased eosinophile count were observed. Spinal granulomata, although at times diffuse, may be circumscribed and amenable to resection. Thus, it is clear that indications may exist for surgical therapy in this disease even though the preoperative diagnosis will require prescient medical sleuthing. The pharmacologic therapeutic armamentarium is far from standardized. Oxamniquine has been used against S. mansoni, praziquantel against both S. mansoni and S. japonicum; Amoscanate is on trial in China.

PARAGONIMIASIS

The organism responsible, the lung fluke, is contracted by ingesting encysted metacercariae in fresh water crabs, crayfish, or their raw products. The metacercariae leave the cysts and invade the wall of the intestine; they become free in the abdomen, penetrate the diaphragm and lungs, and mature into adult worms. Proliferative, inflammatory, and cystic lesions may be encountered anywhere in the brain. In 1971, Higashi et al.[11] reported ten cases of cerebral infestation with Paragonimiasis westermani over a 14-year period in Japan. Seven of the ten patients developed seizures as the primary presenting complaint; the other three had headache and clinical evidence of increased intracranial pressure, with or without seizures. Calcification, visible in plain skull x-rays, was observed in seven out of the ten cases occurring as fleck-like or congregated round and oval calcifications most frequently in the temporal and occipital regions. Skin testing in all five patients in which it was used was positive. Chest roentgenograms may reveal pulmonary paragonimiasis, and ova should be looked for in sputum and stool specimens. Nine of the patients reported upon by these authors were treated by craniotomy. At the time of operation the lesions consisted of congregated granulomatous and/or cystoid masses connected by fibrous gliosis. Ova were found, and, in one case, an adult fluke body. Multiple masses may be encountered above or below the tentorium. Bithionol vermifuge therapy is indicated in addition to any indications or neurosurgical intervention.

HYDATID DISEASE

This is a condition which I first associated with Basque sheepherders who ran flocks of sheep in the Sierra Nevada. The central nervous manifestations are produced by the larval stage of the tapeworm *Echinococcus granulosus,* and the epidemiologic foundation is frequently based upon contact by man with sheep and dogs. Dogs (definitive hosts) acquire the infection by eating the meat of sheep or wild herbivores (intermediate hosts) that contain hydatid cysts. These domestic animals harbor the adult tapeworm, the eggs of which are passed by feces to contaminate food-stuffs that are, in turn, ingested by herbivores. The embryo hatches in the intestine, penetrates the walls of the capillary and is carried through the portal circulation to various parts of the body. People who own infected dogs are at risk and may accidentally ingest eggs which follow the same cycle. The dog–sheep–man cycle is relatively simple, but if multiple carnivores are involved as definitive hosts and multiple herbivores as intermediate hosts the epidemiologic complexities mount.[12] The growth of the larval stage is slow, and cyst size may take several years to evolvé. It is the larval stage that causes most of the difficulty in man, although it is possible to acquire an infestation with an adult worm by ingesting meat harboring the larval form. It is, however, the ingestion of the eggs that is the dangerous maneuver. The larval cyst develóps in the tissues and is filled with a clear fluid. The germinative layer of a fertile cyst proliferates scoleces, and it is these that provide the cyst with a gritty consistency yielding the name "hydatid sand." Secondary cysts may proliferate within the primary cyst and disseminate in the event of rupture. Some of these secondary cysts may be sterile (acephalocysts), and some may be fertile and contain scoleces of their own. In the general distribution of the disease in man the liver is the most common site, followed next by the lung with the brain far less frequently involved. The reported frequency of encountering hydatid cysts in the brain varies from clinic to clinic. Seventeen of 500 brain tumor cases were reported by Kaya et al.[13] from Turkey, whereas five of 1500 cases were reported by Abbassioun et al.[14] from Iran. In Kaya's series, 335 patients with hydatid disease were reviewed. Liver was the focus in 63 percent, lung 24 percent, intracranial disease 4.8 percent, and intraspinal disease 1.5 percent. It is to be noted that the osseous system (including the skull and the orbit) may be involved, but particularly the vertebral column. When bone is involved it is the spinal column that is most frequently the target, and severe vertebral body destruction from disease in the cancellous bone can result in distortion and neural compression. Involvement of the skull produces severe and grotesque distortion but is rarely associated with neurologic problems. An unusual example of a hydatid cyst involving the calvarial wall with thinning of the inner table and dura mater and spreading of the Sylvian fissure was reported by Geiger in 1965.[15] In the orbit, the most common manifestation is a unilateral proptosis. The review by Saidi[16] noted that the skull is the rarest site of the areas of concern to us. It is reported that only two percent of all hydatid cysts involve the skeletal system, but in clinics with a neurologic orientation the frequency of skull, orbital, and vertebral column involvement will appear greater. As an example: in the experience of Arana-Íñigues and Lopez-Fernandez[17] who studied 117 cases from the Institute of Neurology in Montevideo, 76.9 percent were of the brain, 8.5 percent involved the cranium, and 17.9 percent involved the vertebral column. When the larval stages reach the brain, the conditions can be favorable to them. Initially, there is a focal inflammation response which gradually subsides. Slow development and encapsulation then proceeds into solitary, spherical, thin-walled cysts. Cysts may therefore be "primary" hydatid cysts, ie, those which develop from an embryo that are initially deposited from the bloodstream. "Secondary" hydatid cysts are those which are released from a primary cyst elsewhere and lodge, secondarily, in the brain. The lesions may be found in many parts of the brain, and may attain great size. The neural tissue is not infiltrated or invaded but is distorted with associated pressure atrophy. Toxic reactions and cerebral edema are not observed in the presence of an undisturbed cyst. The brain cyst was solitary in 15 of the 17 cases reported by Kaya et al.[13] in patients 17 years or older. When multiple cysts occur, the question arises as to the possible role of trauma or the possibility of cyst rupture into a vascular compartment (heart) with release of multiple secondary cysts. That the single (primary) cyst may contain multiple daughter cysts is well illustrated in the paper by Boles[18] in which, by accident, the lesions were demonstrated by positive contrast cystography at the time of attempted ventriculography. In Carrea, Dowling, and Guevera's[12] experience in the pediatric age group the brain cysts were also mainly solitary (27 of 29). The locations in decreasing frequency of involvement were parietal, frontal, temporal, and occipital lobes, but the posteria fossa may also be the site of disease.

Clues which may lead to the development of a clinical suspicion in diagnosis include the following: (1) the origin of the patient (particularly if from rural areas in an endemic region), (2) the youth of the patient, (3) the availability of contact with other hosts which could harbor the parasite, (4) the relatively slow evolution of the syndrome, and (5) the late appearance of progressive neural deficit (often preceded or overshadowed by the presenting symptomatology and findings of raised intracranial pressure). In the report by Carrea et al.[12] of 29 central cases 14 years of age or younger the clinical picture was documented. Presenting symptoms included convulsions (ten), progressive hemiparesis (nine), and headache with vomiting (eight). At the time of admission (average symptom duration, 11 months), 28 had severe papilledema, 25 were hemiparetic, and 15 were having seizures. Intradermal tests are of value if sterile hydatid fluid is available (no commercial source exists for this antigen at present). Serologic tests such as complement fixation, indirect hemagglutination, and indirect fluorescent antibody testing are more reliable. Peripheral blood eosinophilia as a nonspecific clue of possible parasitic infestation is well appreciated but occurs in a minority of reported cerebral cases.

In plain radiograms of the skull, a curved, fine calcific line, although rare, may be of diagnostic value and the skull may be quite asymmetrical. Before the days of CT scanning, angiography was the primary diagnostic tool and defined an avascular mass. With the advent of CT scanning (as noted by Abbassioun et al.[14]) the features of an echinococcus cyst became recognized as characteristic: a cystic lesion, spherical in shape, with sharply defined borders and absorption values similar to that of CSF. There is usually no perifocal edema. The cysts can be differentiated from brain abscesses by their lack of significant rim "enhancement" or perifocal edema and from cystic tumors by the absence of a solid portion to the mass as well as absent perifocal edema. Arachnoidal cysts are not completely spherical in shape, ie, the presence of one or more "straight" borders is of significance in excluding a hydatid cyst. Phonoencephalography, although described, has not received wide comment.

Surgical excision is the treatment of choice for hydatid cysts of the brain. Such treatment must accommodate the need to remove the cyst intact, without spillage of its contents. Anaphylactic shock and spread of the scolex-bearing fluid (sand) can be sequelae to cyst rupture; both may be fatal although the latter is not invariably so. It is, therefore, unwise to aspirate or open the cyst unless removal cannot otherwise be accomplished. Dowling and Orlando[19] in 1929 described a method of coping with the treacherously thin-walled cysts to deliver them without rupture. They employed hydraulic dissection and the lowering of the patient's head to "spill" the cyst out of the brain. Arana-Íñiguez (with San Julien and Rodriguez-Barrios)[20] pursued these methods to assist in cyst delivery without spillage. They also made use of air, injected into the lateral ventricle on the side opposite to the cyst, to encourage its delivery, but subsequently favored the dissection method via the means of injecting saline solution around the deep surface of the cyst to loosen the latter from its tenuous attachments and ease it from the brain. Arana-Íñiguez and Lopez-Fernandez[17] in their studies observed that the hydatid cyst is tolerated better by the brain than in the case of other cestode cysts which evoke a more violent reaction. Of 17 intracranial lesions reported as operated on by Kaya et al.[13] from Turkey, there were four postoperative deaths (one presumably due to anaphylactic shock secondary to rupture). Eight of the 17 left the hospital well with one known recurrence. In a second series, also from Turkey, Arasil and Erdogan[21] operated upon 20 intracranial cysts, including one in the cerebellum for which total extirpation was accomplished. Carrea et al.[12] utilized the senior Dowling's technique successfully to deliver intact cysts in 20 patients (one involved the spinal cord) with no mortality. Eleven patients were treated in whom cysts were broken either during diagnostic or excision maneuvers, but in only four of these patients did death occur (no anaphylactic shock) and these deaths were delayed four to 21 months postoperatively. In 1963, Samiy and Zadeh[22] reported 16 patients with spinal hydatid cysts. Two of these patients were paraplegic from extensive involvement of the vertebral column; in the others the lesions were limited to the laminae, spinous, and transverse processes. Arana-Ísñiguez and Lopez-Fernandez[17] note that for bony involvement only total extirpation is curative, but for vertebral body disease the challenge is obvious. The very rare occurrence of a primary intradural cyst involving the spinal cord and its suitability for surgical resection are noted by Sharma et al.[23] Orbital echinococcosus with exophthalmus presents its special challenges and the difficult task of removing the cyst without its rupture. Mebendazole appears to be the antihelminthic compound of some therapeutic promise.

COENUROSIS

The features of infestation with *Taenia multiceps multiceps* (cerebral coenurosis) have been reviewed in 1977 by Michal et al.,[24] who identified 27 reported examples of intracranial manifestations and added a patient of their own with intraparenchymatous cysts. They documented four cases of involvement of the eye and one case of spinal cord involvement. Recognized by them were examples of basilar-arachnoidal involvement with basal meningitis and chronic inflammation as well as several of the other manifestations encountered with cysticercosis (vide infra). It would appear that the epidemiologic, diagnostic, and therapeutic principles that pertain to cysticercosis would be applicable to infestation by the dog tapeworm.[25]

CYSTICERCOSIS

The experience which we had gained at the UCLA Center for Health Sciences and which was based upon having treated and studied 18 patients was published in the fall of 1981.[26] At that time and in that paper, focus was directed to the larval involvement of central nervous system tissue, producing one or more of several clinical pathologic manifestations. From the world literature and our own experience it is possible to identify eight general disease categories of which some, at least, are amenable to surgical therapy. A recapitulation of that classification of disease is listed in Table 1.

The discussion pertaining to categories II through VIII recognized that the larval form could produce obstructive hydrocephalus from cysts within the ventricles or from obliteration of the outflow of the ventricles and the great cisterns. Infestation could be associated with a severe

TABLE 1.

Disease category	Description
I	Diffuse parenchymatous disease
	Without focal mass
	Disseminated larval death
	Inflammatory reaction
	Toxic encephalopathy and meningitis
Ia	Stage intermediate between I and II with limited focal
	manifestations and mild inflammatory (toxic) reaction
II	Calcified larval form with seizures
III	Basilar adhesive and racemose form
	Obliterative arachnoiditis/meningitis
	Hydrocephalus
	Mixed types with cisternal cysts or spinal disease
IV	Ventriculitis
	Arachnoiditis/meningitis
	Hydrocephalus
	Mixed types with intraventricular and/or cisternal cysts
V	Intraparenchymatous cysts as mass lesions
	Solitary
	As part of multifocal disease
VI	Subarachnoid and cisternal cysts
	Local symptomatology
	Mixed types with ventriculitis, intraventricular, and
	intraparenchymatous cysts
VII	Intraventricular cysts
	Solitary
	Multiple
	Mixed types with ventriculitis and cisternal cysts
VIII	Spinal forms
	Arachnoiditis/meningitis
	Extra- and intramedullary forms

arachnoidal reaction with meningeal inflammation. It could be associated with intraparenchymatous disease, either in the form of dead larvae (usually associated with seizures) or with the formation of cystic mass processes. It was quite clear from our experience that the solitary intraventricular cyst offered the therapeutically most hopeful state of the infestation, at least insofar as the nervous system involvement was concerned, and that long-term amelioration, if not cure, could be expected with proper surgical therapy. At the time of our study we had no certain examples of the first category of the disease, namely, that of diffuse parenchymatous disease without focal mass, a condition which has been described as being associated with intense inflammatory reaction, toxic encephalopathy and meningitis, raised intracranial pressure, and severe illness. Subsequent to that report we have studied two examples of an acute encephalopathic manifestation which was localized in each case. There occurred rapid resolution of the process (possibly aided by the application of steroid therapy in the single patient in which it was employed) including a resolution of the CT findings from an enhancing ring-like mass to a more dense and smaller process. Through the modality of CT scanning it is possible that we may be witnessing, clinically, a less fulminant stage of larval death than that serious form previously described. If this concept is valid, the inflammatory reaction may be less overwhelming, possibly because of the degree of infestation. We noted rising serologic titers during this stage suggesting possible success in treatment with anti-inflammatory medications. Thus, a mild form of the more flagrant, diffuse encephalopathy associated with larval death reported by others may be emerging. The end-stage of this process is likely to be calcified encystment so frequently encountered in Category II. A possible alternative fate would be progression of the limited encephalopathic process to a larger cystic, tumor-like mass.

Therapy for the calcified larval form with seizures (usually identified through CT scanning or plain radiology by evidence of punctate calcification) is primarily that of the control of the epileptic process. Presumably, these patients have passed through a clinically quiet form of larval death without overt manifestation of an inflammatory response.

In the basilar adhesive and racemose form, an obliterative arachnoiditis and/or meningitis may occur, with or without hydrocephalus. It may be associated with the presence of cisternal cysts and/or spinal disease. This difficult manifestation of the infestation is not amenable to any known curative therapy except that of palliative surgical management for symptomatic hydrocephalus.

In those patients with ventriculitis (confirmed by us to involve the fourth ventricle and by others to involve the lateral ventricles), an arachnoiditis and meningitis and hydrocephalus may accompany the process. The ventriculitis may also be associated with intraventricular and/or cisternal cysts. This category defies effective therapy, except for the treatment of hydrocephalus.

Intraparenchymatous mass lesions may be solitary or part of a multifocal process, and they can, on occasion, lend themselves to surgical resection depending upon the clinical signature. Such mass lesions simulate tumors of other causes. In contrast to the larval form found in the ventricle, these lesions (within brain substance) often appear cystic with an enhancing, ring-like display on CT studies. Angiographic studies do not provide evidence of precise origin. Resection of such lesions should be total, for we have found that remnants of the wall of the larval form can be successfully cultured *in vitro* even in the absence of the scolex. It is therefore likely that cyst remnants after partial resection can reform a cystic mass and continue to cause difficulties.

Our experience with subarachnoid and cisternal cysts reveals that they produce local symptomatology. They may be associated with other manifestations of the disease: ventriculitis, intraventricular cyst formation, or intraparenchymatous cysts. When symptomatic they may be excised, and we have encountered them in numerous loci, above and below the tentorium. Most of the cysts, however, occur beneath the tentorium and are often multiple. They conform to the local anatomy and, when unattached, allow themselves to be delivered, flowing as a viscous compound.

It is the exclusively intraventricular cysts that have lent themselves to the most gratifying excision when they are single. The lesions may, however, be multiple and they may occur in the lateral, third, or fourth ventricles. There appears to be a progressive downward migration of such lesions, lending some support to the concept that the lesions find their access through the choroid plexus and then migrate by way of the ventricular system into the open cisternal spaces. It is valuable to study the entire ventricular system (usually with positive contrast compounds in association with CT scanning) to clarify the presence of more than one cyst. The intraventricular lesions do not enhance on CT study and may be defined only with a positive contrast compound. Of the 22 patients reviewed for this current analysis the number of patients in each group is noted in Table 2. Twelve patients fell into only one category, nine into two, and one into three. Questions remain as to the certainty of category classification for three patients.

TABLE 2. Incidence of Disease by Categories in 22 Patients

Disease category[a]	Confirmed	Presumptive	Total
I	0		0
Ia	2		2
II	5	(2?)	7
III	1		1
IV	3 +	(1?)	4
V	5 +	(1?)	6
VI	4		4
VII	9 +	(1?)	10
VIII	1		1

[a]For classification see Table 1.

**TABLE 3. Operative Procedures Performed for
Cysticercosis in 19 Patients (1970–1982, UCLA)**

Procedure	Cases (n)
Ventricular shunting	7
Suboccipital craniotomy with cyst evacuation	10
Frontal transventricular exploration for cyst	2
Suboccipital explorations (ventriculitis only)	2
Temporal craniotomy for incisural cyst evacuation	1
Frontal or frontotemporal craniotomy for intraparenchymatous cyst removal	3
Temporal craniotomy for intraparenchymatous cyst removal	1
Parietal craniotomy for intraparenchymatous cyst removal	1
Occipital craniotomy for intraparenchymatous cyst removal	1

Our surgical experience is set forth in Table 3 (it is to be noted that negative surgical findings were encountered in two instances). Surgical complications, particularly the need for shunt revisions, are not included in the tabulation.

The nonsurgical treatment of this infestation has not, as yet, proved itself as satisfactory. Nevertheless, there are interesting reports suggesting different means of attacking the infestation. Thus, it is that in 1981 Telléz-Girón et al.[27] studied the effects of flubendazole on infestations in pigs, with results that suggested that this compound needed further study. Another related compound under study is fenbendazole. The reports by Skromne-Kadlubik and his colleagues[28,29] deserve some attention. These describe utilizing radioimmunoscanning of the nervous system. The radioimmunoscan was performed by injecting 10 mci of anticyst antibodies labelled with indium-113 followed by scanning of the head one-half hour later. The authors treated those patients who had positive radioimmunoscans with radioimmunotreatment utilizing intravenous injections of 200 mci of anticyst antibodies labelled with iodine-131 for every cyst detected (maximum dose: 15.5 mCi.) The criteria for selecting the cases for immunotherapy were those described in the 1981 paper[28] and their criteria for evaluating clinical results were strictly clinical. I subsequently communicated with Dr. Skromne-Kadlubik, inquiring in greater detail about the patients he had studied. His answer, as of January 1982, was that his cases accommodated most of the manifestations noted in the Table 1 classification: live cysts with epilepsy, active forms, racemose forms, basal meningitis cases, ventricular lesions, acute inflammatory cases with encephalopathy, ventriculitis, etc. He wrote that in all he has had "good" results with his immunotherapy except in the cases of acute ventricular block. Interest should also be attracted to the recent reports of the use of the drug praziquantel against cestodes. The compound, an isoquinoline, is being utilized against human infestation with *T. solium* larval states and although not available, to my knowledge, in the United States, the reports from Mexico are encouraging.[30]

It is clear from a review of our current capabilities that therapy is suboptimal and that quite apart from attention to public health measures of prevention we possess palliative and only rarely "curative" means of treatment.

CONCLUSION

This surgically oriented approach to a consideration of parasitic involvement of the central nervous system calls us to increase our awareness of what are becoming less rare conditions as peoples migrate more widely into our country. We also must bear in mind the obligations of the sanitary engineers and public health officials as well as the challenges remaining to us all in treating established disease.

REFERENCES

1. Brown, W.I. and Voge, M. *Neuropathology of Parasitic Infections.* New York: Oxford University Press, 1982, in press.
2. Seidel, J.S., Harmatz, P., Visvesvara, G.S., Cohen, A., Edwards, J. and Turner J. Successful treatment of primary amebic meningoencephalitis. *N. Engl. J. Med. 306*:346–348, 1982.
3. Takaro, T. and Bond, C.M. Pleuropulmonary pericardial and cerebral complications of amebiasis. *Int. Abstr. Surg. 107*:209–229, 1958.
4. *Public Health Letter.* Los Angeles County Department of Health Services. Vol. 3, No. 11. November 1981: 44.
5. Daroff, R.B., et al. Cerebral malaria. *J.A.M.A. 202*:679–682, 1967.
6. Warrell, D.A., et al. Dexamethasone proves deleterious in cerebral malaria. *N. Engl. Med. 306*:313–319, 1982.
7. Pitella, J.E.H. and Lana-Peixoto, M.A. Brain involvement in hepatosplenic schistosomiasis mansoni. *Brain 104*:621–632, 1981.
8. Marcial-Rojas, R.A. and Fiol, R.E. Neurologic complications of schistosomiasis: review of the literature and report of two cases of transverse myelitis due to S. mansoni. *Ann. Intern Med. 59*:215–230, 1963.
9. Reyes, V.A., Yogore, M.G. and Pardo, L.P. Studies on cerebral schistosomiasis. *J. Phillippine Med. Assoc. 40*:87–100, 1964.
10. Jackson, H. Infestation, with particular reference to hydatid cysts of the brain. *Proc. R. Soc. Med. 57*:15–22, 1964.
11. Higashi, K., Aoki, H., Takebayashi, K., Morika, H. and Sakata, Y. Cerebral paragonimiasis. *J. Neurosurg. 34*:515–528, 1971.

12. Carrea, R., Dowling, E. and Guevara, J.A. Surgical treatment of hydatid cysts of the central nervous system in the pediatric age (Dowling's technique). *Childs Brain 1*:4–21, 1975.
13. Kaya, U., Ozden, B., Turker, K. and Tarcan B. Intracranial hydatid cysts: study of 17 cases. *J. Neurosurg. 42*:580–584, 1975.
14. Abbassioun, K., et al. Computerized tomography in hydatid cysts of the brain. *J. Neurosurg. 49*:408–411, 1978.
15. Geiger, L.E. Hydatid cyst of the brain: report of a case. *J. Neurosurg. 23*:446–449, 1965.
16. Saidi, F. Hydatid cysts of the central nervous system. In: *Surgery of Hydatid Disease.* F. Saidi, ed. London: WB Saunders, pp. 352–376, 1976.
17. Arana-Íñiguez, R. and Lopez-Fernandez, J.R. Parasitosis of the nervous system, with special reference to echinococcosis. *Clin. Neurosurg. 14*:123–144, 1967.
18. Boles DM: Cerebral echinococciasis. *Surg. Neurol. 16*:280–282, 1981.
19. Dowling, E., Orlando, R. Quiste hidatídico del lóbulo frontal derecho. *Rev. Especialid 4*:209–217, 1929.
20. Arana-Íñiguez, R. and San Julian J. Hydatid cysts of the brain. *J. Neurosurg. 12*:323–335, 1955.
21. Arasil, E. and Erdogan, A. Hydatid cyst of the posterior fossa. *Surg. Neurology 9*:9, 1978.
22. Samiy, E. and Zadeh, F.A. Cranial and intracranial hydatidosis with special reference to roentgen-ray diagnosis. *J. Neurosurg. 22*:425–433, 1965.
23. Sharma, A., et al. Intradural hydatid cysts of the spinal cord. *Surg. Neurol. 16*:235–237, 1981.
24. Michal, A., Regli, F., Campiche, R., Cavallo, R.J., de Crousaz, G., Oberson, R. and Rabinowicz, T.H. Cerebral coenurosis: report of a case with arteritis. *J. Neurol. 216*:265–272, 1977.
25. Kuper, S., Mendelow, H. and Procter, N.S.F. Internal hydrocephalus caused by parasitic cysts. *Brain 81*:235–242, 1958.
26. Stern, WE. Neurosurgical considerations of cysticercosis of the central nervous system. *J. Neurosurg. 55*:382–389, 1981.
27. Telléz-Girón, E., Ramos, M.C. and Montante, M. Effect of flubendazole on cysticercus cellulosae in pigs. *Am. J. Top. Med. Hyg. 30*:135–138, 1981.
28. Skromme-Kadlubik, G., Celis, C. Cysticercosis of the nervous system: treatment by means of specific internal radiation. *Arch. Neurol. 38*:288, 1981.
29. Skromme-Kadlubik, G., Celis, C. and Ferez A. Cysticercosis of the nervous system: diagnosis by means of specific radioimmunoscan. *Ann. Neurol. 2*:343–344, 1977.
30. Robles, C. and Chavarría, M. Un caso de cisticercosis cerebral curado médicamente. *Gac. Med. Mex. 116*:65–71, 1980.

13

Current Therapy of Brain Abscess

Daniel G. Nehls and Robert M. Crowell

Brain abscesses present a spectrum of challenging problems in diagnosis and management. Significant advances have provided the clinician with a wide armamentarium of diagnostic and therapeutic modalities, and recent reports have noted a downward trend in mortality.[1]

Computed tomographic scanning has had a dramatic impact on the diagnosis of brain abscesses, and it plays a major role in evaluating the results of therapy. Improvements in culture technique have lead to more frequent identification of the offending pathogen, making possible the selection of appropriate antibiotics.

A broad continuum of therapeutic options is now available. New antibiotic agents have been useful against brain abcess. There have been numerous recent reports of nonsurgical cures of brain abscesses. Surgical modalities available include various forms of aspiration and drainage, excision, and combinations of aspiration and excision.

METHODS

Patients treated at the Barrow Neurological Institute for brain abscess during the post computed tomography years of 1975 through 1981 were identified. Hospital records were reviewed, and follow-up information was obtained from the records of subsequent admissions or from attending physicians. Data is presented in Tables 1 and 2. Major series published during the last ten years were reviewed[2-14] and important statistics were tabulated. These are referred to as the combined series.

TABLE 1. Patients Included in the Present Series

	Etiology	Pathogen(s)	Location(s)	Therapy	Outcome
35 M	mastoiditis	E. coli + Proteus mirabilis	temporal lobe	excision	intact
52 F	extension	mucormycosis	frontal lobe	none	death
45 F	odontogenic	streptococcus	frontal lobe	excision	mild hemiparesis
9 M	otogenic	microbacteria avium fortuitum, nocardia	CP angle	subtotal excision	intact
2 M	meningitis	H. influenza, streptococci + Eickenalla corrodens	parietal-temporal-occipital	aspiration + excision	developmental delay
45 F	thoracogenic	nocardia	occipital lobe	excision	small field defect
56 F	sepsis	E. coli	parietal	medical	lost to follow-up
30 F	CHD + bronchiectasis	aerobic Gram-negative rod	temporal lobes (bilateral)	drainage	death
18 M	gunshot wound	Eickenella corrodens	holohemispheric	drainage	death
44 M	trauma 15 years prior	unknown (sterile)	frontal	excision	mild leg paresis
40 M	skull fracture	E. coli	frontal-temporal	excision	vegetative
15 M	postoperative	Staph. aureus	cerebellum	excision	no new deficit
39 M	postoperative	Staph. aureus	frontal-parietal	drainage	mild hemiparesis
55 M	abscess in glioblastoma	unknown (sterile)	frontal	excision	mild hemiparesis
76 M	unknown	fusobacterium	cerebellum	excision	gait ataxia
65 M	unknown	Bacteroides oralis	occipital lobe	excision	hemianopsia
53 M	unknown	histoplasma	parietal lobe	excision	intact
80 F	unknown	unknown	occipital lobe	medical	intact
49 M	unknown	unknown	temporal	medical	intact
48 M	unknown	unknown	parietal and occipital lobes	medical	intact
53 M	unknown	unknown	frontal lobe	1 drain empyema 2 excision 3 reexcision	aphasia + hemiplegia

TABLE 2. Symptoms and Signs of Brain Abscess[a]

	Symptoms					Signs							
	Head-ache	N+V	Seiz-ure	Other	Change in mental status	Fever	Nuchal Rigidity	Papille-dema	Pupil abnormal	Field defect	Hemi-paresis	Cere-bellar	Other
Morgan et al.	70	24	32		58	8	25	23	10	7	38	11	11
Samson and Clark	64	50	33		48	52	43						
McCann et al.	84	10	23		55	77	19				45		
Yang	97	85	20	6	38	57	18	56	21	13	44	38	8
Present study	64	18	36		50	36	9	16	0	27	22	14	23
Combined series	76	37	29		50	46	23	32	10	16	37	21	14

INCIDENCE

Brain abscess is a relatively rare cause of neurologic disease. The true incidence is not known. McClelland et al.[10] reported a declining incidence of five per million population to three per million population over the 30-year period of 1947 to 1976. This trend was attributed to the decrease in otogenic abscesses. They noted a difference in geographical distribution, with an urban preponderance, although they could identify no factor to explain this difference. Most studies report a male preponderance. In the combined series, the male to female ratio was 2.63 to 1. In the present series, this ratio was 2.5 to 1. Most studies reporting incidence based upon age show a bimodal distribution with peaks occurring in the first or second, and fifth or sixth decades.[4,8,12,13,15] The first peak has been attributed to the frequent occurrence of brain abscess in children with congenital heart disease.[12] The peak incidence in our series occurred in the fifth decade and a minor peak occurred in the first two decades.

ETIOLOGY

The most common causes of brain abscess, in order of prevalence, are direct extension, metastasis, and trauma. Direct extension and metastasis account for the majority of abscesses, comprising almost 70 percent of all abscesses. Unknown origin is common, occurring in 14 percent of the combined series, and ranging from two percent to 32 percent (present series). The large number of abscesses of unknown cause are most likely due to early detection and therapy which eradicate the source of infection.

Direct Extension

Direct extension of an infectious process accounted for 39 percent of brain abscesses in the combined series. In individual studies, direct extension ranged from 19 percent (present study) to 81 percent.[7] Brain abscesses may arise by direct extension from the ear, mastoid, or paranasal sinuses, teeth, skull, or orbit. Otogenic brain abscesses are by far the most common type caused by direct extension. Antibiotics have reduced acute otitis media as a cause of brain abscess. Chronic otitis media now causes 84 percent of all otogenic abscesses, according to Shaw and Russell.[16] Due to their pathogenesis, otogenic brain abscesses most frequently occur in the temporal lobe or cerebellum. Direct extension occurs through the tegmen tympani and tegmen mastoideum. Retrograde thrombosis of the lateral, superior petrosal, or inferior petrosal sinuses is another mechanism by which otic infection can spread. This results in an area of venous infarction which provides a fertile bed for abscess development. Otogenic abscesses may be multiple in 4 to 15 percent of cases according to Nissen.[17]

The importance of anaerobes in otogenic brain abscesses was recently stressed by Ingham et al.[18] They were able to culture aerobes in only six of ten otogenic brain abscesses, whereas they were able to culture anaerobes in all ten. They also found that each abscess contained at least one bacteroides species, usually Bacteroides fragilis (nine of ten) or Bacteroides melaninogenicus (five of ten).

Sinogenic brain abscesses may arise from the frontal, ethmoid or sphenoid sinuses. Frontal and ethmoid sinus infections most frequently cause frontal lobe abscesses. Venous drainage of the frontal sinus mucosa communicates with the dural venous plexus which in turn communicates with cortical veins. This provides a route of spread from the frontal sinus to the frontal lobe. Sphenoid sinus infections may cause temporal lobe of intrasellar abscesses. According to deLouvois,[19] nonanaerobic streptococci are the most common organisms responsible for sinogenic abscess.

Direct extension of dental abscesses to the brain was recently reported by Ingham et al.[20] Apical veins of the maxillary teeth can communicate with the cavernous sinus through the ptergoid plexus. An alternate, though rare, route of spread is through the deep facial veins, through the vein of Zuckerkandl to the superior sagittal sinus.

Rare causes of brain abscess due to direct extension include osteomyelitis of the cranium,[3] meningitis[4,6,11,12] (and present series), orbital cellulitis,[4] carcinoma or a sinus,[6] tonsillitis,[11] and direct extension of orbital mucormycosis (present study).

Metastatic

In the combined series, 29 percent of brain abscesses were considered metastatic. In the normal host, organisms of high virulence are usually responsible for the development of brain abscesses. Common pathogens are Staphylococcus aureus, bacteroides, streptococci, and mixed organisms. The chest is a common source of metastatic brain abscesses. Thoracogenic abscesses may be secondary to bronchiectasis, pneumonia, lung abscess, or empyema. Pulmonary alveolar proteinosis predisposes the host to nocardia, as was the case in one patient included in our series. Surprisingly, patients with cystic fibrosis have an incidence of brain abscess no higher than that of the general population.[21] This may be due to high titers of locally produced IgA, serum hypergammaglobulinemia, or chronic antibiotic therapy. Other sources of metastatic infection include gastrointestinal infections such as abdominal abscess, cholecystitis, diverticulitis, and gastroenteritis. Genitourinary and cutaneous infections as well as osteomyelitis are additional sources.

In abnormal hosts, organisms of low virulence are responsible for many metastatic brain abscesses. These are generally organisms which have a high frequency of transient bacteremia in normal individuals. Microaerophilic and anaerobic streptococci are common organisms. Shunts which allow blood to bypass the filtering action of the lung predispose to the development of brain abscess. Intrapulmonary shunting occurs in pulmonary arteriovenous malformations and in Osler-Weber-Rendu disease. A much more common predisposing factor is cyanotic congenital heart disease. The incidence of brain abscesses in patients with cyanotic heart disease is reported to be between four and six percent[22] and the age range is said to be from one day to 20 years of age.[23] Brandt et al.[22] feel that cardiac insufficiency leads to encephalomalacia and thrombosis. This, along with impairment of the microcirculation due to polycythemia, favors the development of brain abscess. Fischbein et al.[24] feel that decreased arterial oxygen saturation plays a key role in the pathogenesis of brain abscess. Endocarditis generally is not a cause of abscess in patients with congenital heart disease. Patients with immunosuppressed states due to congenital disease, malignancy, steroid or immunosuppressive therapy are also at increased risk of developing metastatic brain abscesses.

Metastatic abscesses show no predilection for any particular lobe. Their relative frequencies correlate with the relative sizes of the lobes of the brain. Thus, they are common in the frontal, occipital, and parietal lobes, and uncommon in the temporal lobes and cerebellum. They tend to occur at the junction of the cortical mantle and the white matter in much the same way that metastatic tumors occur. Abscesses developing at the corticomedullary junction develop asymmetrical capsules, with the thinner wall in the relatively hypovascular white matter.[25] This is the reason that abscesses more frequently rupture into the ventricles than into the subarachnoid space (Figure 1).

Traumatic

Traumatic brain abscesses may be due to depressed or open skull fractures, penetrating wounds, or previous neurosurgery. As many studies omit postoperative abscesses, it is difficult to determine how frequent they are. Trauma and surgery accounted for 15 percent of the abscesses

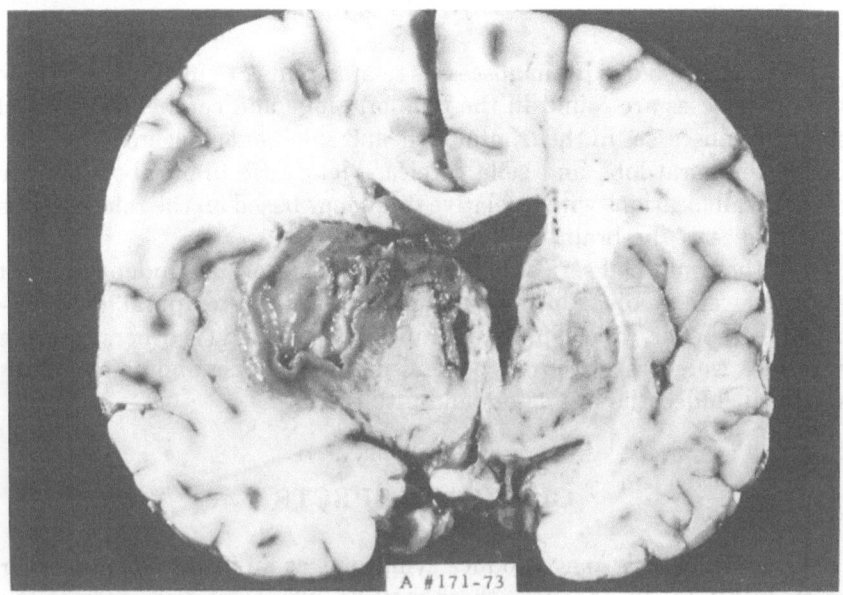

Figure 1. Coronal section of the brain at the level of the optic chiasm demonstrates a large abscess involving the basal ganglia. Rupture has occurred into the lateral ventricle through the relatively less vascular periventricular white matter.

in the combined series, and individually accounted for between 3[14] and 28 percent[8] in the various series. In the present series, this figure was 23 percent with trauma accounting for 14 percent and prior surgery nine percent.

According to deLouvois,[19] *Staphylococcus aureus* is the most common organism in both traumatic and postoperative abscesses. Raimondi and Samuelson[26] found that in civilian practice brain abscesses were not likely to develop after gunshot wounds, even with retained fragments. He contrasted this with the experience of military neurosurgeons who found infection to be the most serious sequela of retained fragments. However, one patient in the present series did develop a holohemispheric abscess after a gunshot wound in which the bullet was not removed because it was located in the basal ganglia. Numerous cases of the delayed development of abscesses years after trauma have been reported.[27-29] Robinson et al.[29] found living organisms in an abscess which occurred 31 years after injury. They state that metallic fragments are generally better tolerated than bone fragments. One patient in our series developed a frontal lobe abscess in the vicinity of retained bone fragments due to orbital trauma 15 years prior.

LOCATION

The location of a brain abscess is related to its origin. Thus, otogenic brain abscesses are found in the temporal lobe and cerebellum, frontal sinogenic abscesses in the frontal lobe, and sphenoid sinogenic abscesses in the temporal lobe and sella turcica. Metastatic brain abscesses are found in all locations with a relative frequency based on the relative sizes of the lobes of the brain.

In the combined series the most frequent locations (independent of etiology) were, in order of frequency: (1) frontal, (2) temporal, (3) parietal, (4) cerebellar, (5) occipital, (6) multiple lobes, and (7) other. Multiple abscesses were present in six percent of cases. Uncommon sites of abscesses included the brainstem and pituitary.

CLINICAL ASPECTS

A brain abscess may produce symptoms as an intracranial mass or as an infection. In addition, there may be symptoms and signs of the infectious focus responsible for the abscess. As an intracranial mass, the abscess produces a clinical picture dependent upon its location and effect upon intracranial pressure. Therefore, a brain abscess may have a wide spectrum of possible presentations ranging from a slow insidious course, to an isolated seizure, to a rapidly progressive deterioration into coma. Table 2 is a compilation of the frequency of symptoms and signs in the series reporting these figures.

Neurologic symptoms were quite variable among the individual series, but differences could be explained on the basis of the relative frequencies of the various etiologies in each study. Variation was also dependent upon the length of time between onset of illness and arrival at the institution publishing the series. In the study by Yang,[14] the preponderance of otogenic abscess and advanced disease accounted for the high frequency of clinical signs due to cerebellar abscess and tentorial herniation respectively.

Systemic Manifestations

A fairly common systemic sign is fever, which was observed in 46 percent of cases in the combined series. Among 102 cases, French and Chou[5] found 17 patients with subnormal temperature, 19 with normal temperature, 66 with fever of 100°F or higher, and eight with a temperature greater than 101.5°F. These data indicate that the abscence of fever does not exclude a brain abscess. In most cases the fever was not striking, but in a few cases the presence of a high fever made an infectious process a likely consideration in the differential diagnosis. Nuchal rigidity was present in 23 percent of patients in the combined series. In the present series, it was noted in only nine percent of patients, and in these it was not impressive.

Generalized Neurologic Manifestations

Of the generalized neurologic symptoms, headache was most common. It was present in 64 percent of patients in the present series and 76 percent of patients in the combined series. Changes in mental status, as manifested by alterations of level of consciousness, memory difficulty, or personality change, were present in 50 percent of cases in both the present series and the combined series. We observed an 18 percent incidence of nausea and vomiting, whereas Yang,[14] with his more advanced cases, noted an 85 percent incidence. Similarly, papilledema was uncommon in the present series and frequent in Yang's series.

Focal Neurologic Manifestations

Hemiparesis was the most frequent focal neurologic finding in the combined series. In the present series, visual field defects were the most common focal finding, and this can be attributed to the relative frequency of occipital, parietal, and temporal lobe lesions in our series. There were no cases with pupillary abnormality in our series. However, Yang[14] noted this finding in 21 percent of his patients, indicating the poor condition in which many of his patients arrived. Additional focal findings that we noted were aphasia, gait disturbances, and frontal lobe signs (jocular affect, paratonic rigidity, glabellar sign, and grasp, suck, and snout reflexes). Seizures occurred in 36 percent of patients in our series and 29 percent of patients in the combined series. Of the patients in our series who developed seizures, five of seven had abscesses in the parietal or frontal lobes. The remaining two had temporal lobe abscesses.

Cerebellar Abscess Manifestations

Shaw and Russell[16] reported a series of 47 cerebellar abscesses. Headache was a constant symptom. Vomiting was present in 83 percent of their cases. Drowsiness, unsteadiness, papilledema, and confusion were common findings. Nystagmus was found in 74 percent and uncoordination in 57 percent. They reported a 66 percent incidence of nuchal rigidity, possibly due to tonsilar impaction.

Duration of Symptoms

In the present series, the duration of symptoms was quite variable. One patient had experienced headache for six months, and three had experienced it for four months. Another patient had developed memory difficulty five months before admission, and one had become less aggressive and more lethargic four months before admission. Karandanis and Shulman 0 noted an improvement in prognosis for patients diagnosed early in the course of their illness. Early diagnosis was facilitated by symptoms which were more dramatic or disabling. These symptoms would include seizures, aphasia, hemiparesis, meningismus, or symptoms after prior neurosurgery. Patients who developed symptoms of a more insidious nature or changes in mentation which affected insight into their condition tended to present later in the course of their illness and had a poorer prognosis.

Congenital Heart Disease

The diagnosis of brain abscess in patients with congenital heart disease presents a special problem due to a relative paucity of symptoms. According to Raimondi et al.,[23] the triad of headache, nausea, and seizure is usually present at least in part in most cases of brain abscess. He found that symptoms were usually present for seven days to six weeks, and that papilledema and lateralizing signs were quite common. Brandt et al.[22] found papilledema in all of their cases. Raimondi states that headache in a child with cyanotic heart disease is a brain abscess until proven otherwise. Some authors even recommend a CT scan before cardiac surgery in patients with cyanotic heart disease.[31]

Pituitary Abscess

Intrasellar abscesses are quite difficult to diagnose, and most are mistaken for nonfunctioning pituitary adenomas. However, Muhtaroglu et al.[32] state that hormonal dysfunction is usually more marked in pituitary abscesses.

DIAGNOSTIC PROCEDURES—GENERAL LABORATORY

In general, the laboratory investigations in cerebral abscess will reflect the presence of an infection, but the tests are neither specific nor conclusive. The white blood cell count was found to be abnormal in about 70 percent of cases in the present study and in that of Yang.[14] In the present series, the average WBC count was 13,500 with a standard deviation of 4,800. Only one of 19 patients had a WBC count above 20,000, and six had WBC counts below 10,000. French and Chou[5] observed a 75 percent incidence of elevated neutrophil counts. The erythrocyte sedimentation rate is a useful test in differentiating between brain abscess and other mass lesions. The ESR was abnormal in 75 percent of cases in both the present study and that of Klug and Ellams.[8] We observed a mean ESR of 55 with a standard deviation of 36. The highest value noted was 120, and only three of 12 values were below 20. In the presence of cyanotic heart disease, however, the ESR is not a reliable indicator, as it is almost always quite low.

The suspicion of a brain abscess is a contraindication to lumbar puncture. There is a real danger of precipitating a catastrophic deterioration due to herniation or rupture. French and Chou[5] stress this danger. They identified eight deaths in their series in which lumbar puncture was implicated. They also point out the unreliability of the results of a LP, including bacteriologic studies. Other authors have commented upon the danger[4,5,7,9,14] and unreliability[4,5,9] of lumbar puncture in brain abscess.

DIAGNOSTIC PROCEDURES—RADIOLOGY

Skull Films

Skull films were obtained in 15 patients in the present series. Abnormalities were demonstrated in seven of these. In the combined series, 40 percent of skull films were abnormal. Useful localizing signs include displacement of the pineal or choroid plexus, surgical or traumatic skull defects, intracranial gas, focal bone erosion, metal or bone fragments, and in rare instances calcification of the abscess wall. Nonlocalizing signs include signs of increased intracranial pressure, abnormalities of the ear or sinuses, and osteomyelitis. While much of the information available on skull films is also demonstrated by Computed tomography, skull films are recommended because they may provide superior or additional information regarding fractures and burr holes, osteomyelitis, sinusitis, and otitis.

Echoencephalography

Except in the series reported by Yang,[14] the use of echoencephalography is not common. Although it is used predominantly to determine in which hemisphere a lesion is located, in some instances it can provide additional information. Yang[14] observed the demonstration of abscess walls in several hemispheric lesions and ventricular dilation in posterior fossa abscesses. He reported abnormalities in 80 percent of studies, as did Bhatia et al.[3] Brewer et al.[4] however, observed abnormal studies in only 28 percent of cases. The CT scan has made echoencephalography obsolete.

Pyography

The placement of contrast dye into an abscess cavity after aspiration or excision can be helpful in following the postoperative course of the abscess on plain skull films. Thorium dioxide (Thorotrast) and, more recently, colloidal barium have been used. With the advent of CT scanning, however, pyography is less useful, and according to Claveria et al.[33] it should not be done in patients who will be followed by computed tomography because of the severe artifacts it produces near the abscess.

Pneumoencephalography/Ventriculography

These contrast studies can be useful in the localization of abscesses, especially in the posterior fossa. However, they pose a real threat to the patient, and have been implicated in deaths.[5,11] These studies have largely been supplanted by the CT scan. When they are performed, however, they should be scheduled immediately before surgery.[11]

Brain Scan

Focal defects in the blood brain barrier at the cellular level are responsible for radionuclide accumulation in and around brain abscesses. Accuracy of diagnosis nearing 100 percent is possible according to Crocker et al.,[34] if the scans are of good quality and are interpreted with careful clinical correlation. The initial lesion on brain scan is a spherical image. The doughnut sign is a nonspecific sign which represents an avascular center. It is seen in abscess, tumor, infarction, and subdural hematoma. When it is seen in a brain abscess it indicates that pus is present in the core of the abscess. The CT scan provides more information than the brain scan, and some feel that it is also more sensitive.[35]

Angiography

Angiograms can be useful in the diagnosis and management of brain abscess. In the present series, 91 percent of the arteriograms were abnormal. Nielsen and Halaburt[36] describe the angiographic findings in brain abscess. They are, in order of decreasing frequency: (1) displacement of arteries, (2) an avascular lucency, (3) segmental arterial constriction, (4) displaced veins, (5) a capsular blush, and (6) a ripple sign (concentric rings of varying density due to perifocal edema). These authors stress the importance of subtracted films, and differentiate between a true capsule and pseudo-capsule. The pseudo-capsule is a blush resulting from compression of normal vessels. It is of short duration on the arteriogram and usually vanishes before the venous filling is complete. The blush of a true capsule is due to abnormal vascular proliferation; it is often superimposed on a pseudocapsule and persists into the venous phase. Experimental studies by Wood et al.[34] have confirmed that the true capsule is indeed due to vascular proliferation, and not compression of normal vessels. They state that the vascular stain reflects the capsule thickness. Therefore an arteriogram may provide useful clinical information about the nature of the abscess capsule, when a capsular blush is present. This occurs in about 48 percent of arteriograms according to Nielsen and Halaburt,[36] but they state that other authors have observed capsules in only 20 to 20 percent of angiograms.

Computed Tomography

Computed tomography has revolutionized the diagnoses and management of brain abscess. It provides detailed information on the number, location, and character of intracranial masses. According to Nielsen and Glydensted,[35] it is not only more specific than radionuclide scanning, it is also more sensitive. In the diagnosis of brain abscesses, high quality studies are essential. Shaw and Russell[38] even suggest that when necessary, general anesthesia should be used to obtain a suitable image. Contrast studies must be performed, and the diagnosis of brain abscess is seldom made without them.[33] Serial scans provide much information regarding the progression of an abscess and its response to therapy.

The typical CT appearance of a brain abscess is that of a mass lesion with a central zone of lucency, with an extensive zone of perifocal edema and ring enhancement (Figure 2). Loculations and septae may be present within the mass. Before contrast enhancement, the lesion may have the appearance of a faint ring structure, pure radiolucency, or less frequently a dense nodule. Edema adjacent to the lesion is almost invariably

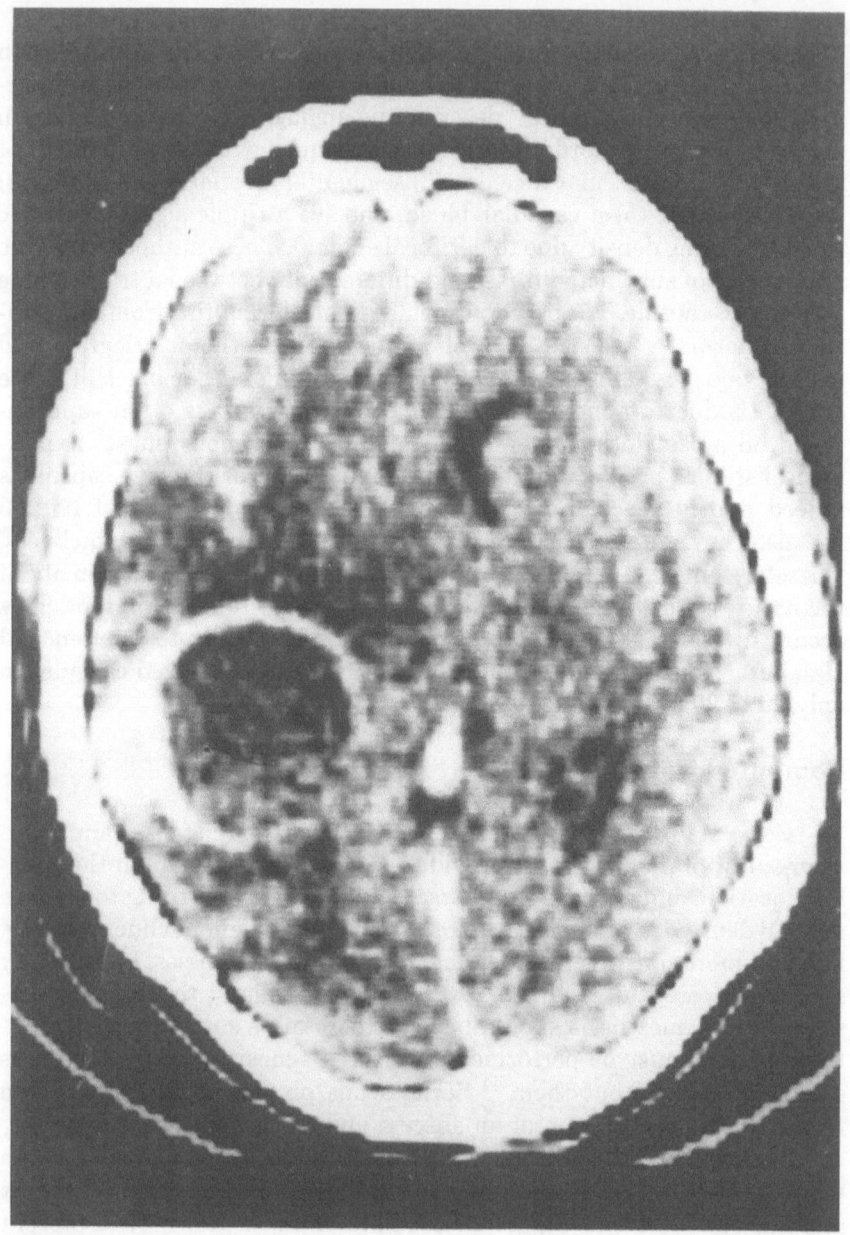

Figure 2. Typical CT appearance of a brain abscess. There is a ring-enhancing lesion with marked perifocal edema and midline shift of the ventricles.

present[39] and is usually moderately severe.[40] The mass effect, however, is often less than expected from the marked edema.[33] After the administration of contrast, ring enhancement is almost invariably present.[39,40] Danzinger et al.[40] observed ring enhancement that was smooth in 64 percent of the scans they studied and irregular in 23 percent. Ring enhancement was absent in only three percent of their studies.

Ring enhancement structures are a common finding on CT scans and are by no means diagnostic of brain abscess. They may be found in cystic tumors, tumors with central necrosis, metastatic tumors, hemorrhagic infarction, and intracerebral hematomas. Table 3 presents the CT features in the differential diagnosis of lesions that may resemble a brain abscess. Additional diagnostic points include the fact that multiloculation and septae are common in abscesses, but uncommon in gliomas and metastatic tumors. Ependymal enhancement indicates ventriculitis, which favors the diagnosis of brain abscess. Mauersberger[41] studied the actual density numbers of abscesses and glioblastomas. The differences between their absorption coefficients are summarized in Table 4. In general, the glioblastomas' absorption coefficients were higher (denser) than those of abscesses when measuring the rim, center, and entire structure. This was true both with and without contrast enhancement. The greatest differences in absorption coefficients were noted when comparing the rim and center densities without contrast enhancement.

Nahser et al.[15] studied the CT appearance of abscesses and correlated this with the macroscopic and microscopic pathology. They divided the abscesses into three stages based upon duration. Stage I abscesses were present for two weeks. The CT appearance was one of focal hypodensity without enhancement. This CT appearance is that of focal cerebritis as described by Claveria et al.[33] However, Weisberg[42] states that in some cases diffuse or linear enhancement can occur. Macroscopically, there was diffuse inflammation and edema. Microscopically, there was an early vascular reaction and a polymorphonuclear response. In the stage II abscesses, which had been present three weeks, the hypodense region had acquired an irregular border. On gross examination, demarcation was apparent, and liquifaction was occurring. At the microscopic level, glial proliferation was taking place, and granulation tissue had started to form. The stage III abscesses were six weeks old. Ring enhancement was now present on the CT scan. Capsule formation had occurred, which was evident on microscopic examination as collagen formation. However, Whelan and Hilal[39] warn that the presence of an enhancing ring does not imply that a firm capsule exists. They were able to correlate the presence of a firm capsule with duration of symptoms better than with CT appearance.

TABLE 3. Differential Diagnosis of CT Ring-Enhancing Lesions (Based Upon Tiyaworabun)[a]

Lesion	Ring enhancement	Space occupying	Multiple	Edema	Hypodense area	Hyperdense area
Abscess	!	+	++	!	+	−
Glioblastoma	!	+	−	!	(+)	(+)
Cystic tumor	(+)	+	(−)	+	+	−
Necrotic tumor	(+)	+	(+)	+	+	−
Infarct (hemorrhage)	(+)	(+)	(+)	(+)	−	(+)
Hematoma	(+)	(+)	(+)	(+)	(+)	(−)

[a] ! = marked, + = yes, (++) = often, + = yes, (+) = possible, (−) = improbable, − = no.

In assessing the results of therapy, and in long-term follow-up, the CT scan has been quite helpful, but occasionally misleading. Claveria et al.[33] have equated the loss of capsule enhancement with successful aspiration. They observed two cases in which the capsule did not disappear after aspiration, and in both of these cases the abscess spread or refilled. Feely and Dempsey[43] stress that the clinical course must be taken into consideration in assessing the CT findings when following the posttherapy course of a patient. They noted two CT scans which had findings consistent with recurrence in patients without clinical recurrence. Whelan and Hilal[39] state that residual contrast enhancement usually lasts three to four months, but may be present as long as eight months. They noted abscess recurrence in two of ten patients with residual enhancing foci, but both of these patients had deep lesions either within or deforming the ventricle. They also noted a return or increase in contrast enhancement in patients recently tapered off steroids without clinical recurrences. In patients with increasing contrast enhancement despite the use of steroids and antibiotics, clinical deterioration due to recurrence was noted.

TABLE 4. Density Values for Abscess and Glioblastoma from Mauersberger[a]

	Abscess	Glioblastoma
Basic Scan		
Whole structure	15.9 ± 6.97	26.6 ± 4.8
Ring	15.2 ± 8.77	28.9 ± 5.05
Center	10.98 ± 8.45	23.2 ± 5.8
Contrast Scan		
Whole structure	22.85 ± 6.42	34.55 ± 4.71
Ring	31.35 ± 6.60	38.6 ± 4.9
Center	12.94 ± 6.3	22.89 ± 5.19

[a] Density values of abscesses and glioblastomas (expressed in Hounsfield units) in basic and contrast scans. Values are expressed as mean ± standard deviation.

THERAPY OF BRAIN ABSCESS

Brain abscess is a heterogenous disease, and a wide array of therapeutic modalities is available. Therapy should correspond to the individual aspects of each case. The first consideration is the patient's clinical status. Rapid deterioration requires prompt surgical intervention. Excision or aspiration is the treatment of choice in this situation. Initial therapy should include an empiric antibiotic regimen based upon the probable cause of the abscess. Antibiotic therapy is modified when Gram stain and culture reports become available. Surgical or nonsurgical treatment should be based upon clinical and CT information. In the following sections, various modalities of therapy are presented together with advantages, disadvantages, indications, and relative contraindications.

Aspiration

Aspiration is a valuable technique in the management of deep-seated abscesses, abscesses in critical locations such as the motor strip or speech areas, and in patients whose medical conditions preclude major intracranial surgery. The relative simplicity and speed with which it may be performed are advantages. Ohaegbulam and Saddequi[44] advocate that it be used in less than ideal situations, and by general surgeons who must treat brain abscesses without the aid of a neurosurgeon. They relate their experience with aspiration in Nigeria where computed tomography was not available and report very favorable results. Another advantage is the information which aspiration provides. The presence of an abscess, its location, the bacteriology, and the nature of the capsule may be ascertained by aspiration. In addition, aspiration may provide rapid relief of elevated intracranial pressure on an emergency basis.

There are several occasions when aspiration is not effective. These include: (1) abscess rupture, (2) chronic abscess, (3) presence of a foreign body, (4) posterior fossa abscess, and (5) the presence of an empyema in addition to the abscess. Excision should be considered if there is persistently a high volume of pus obtained on repeated aspirations. Aspiration should be discontinued if very little pus is obtained. Aspiration is not recommended in multiloculated abscesses, although it has been successful in some cases.[45] If transtentorial herniation is imminent, aspiration may be considered on an emergency basis to reduce intracranial hypertension.

Potential complications associated with aspiration include rupture of the abscess into the ventricles or subarachnoid space and the creation of tracts through the cortex which may cause damage by direct mechanical injury or innoculation of abscess organisms.[13,14,46] The aspiration of a thin-walled abscess may cause it to collapse and form multiloculations.

There are several techniques of aspiration.[7,13,14,44,46] Jefferson and Keogh[7] warn against allowing air to enter the abscess cavity as this leads to more frequent refilling of the abscess. Recent reports advise against instillation of contrast material to avoid CT artifacts.[33] The effectiveness of instilling antibiotics into an abscess has been questioned because of good penetration of antibiotics administered systemically, and because of the potential danger of antibiotic leakage.[47] Ohaegbulam and Saddequi[44] performed simple aspiration daily until nothing was obtained on three consecutive days. Yang[14] repeated his aspirations as needed, based on clinical signs, or until no pus was obtained. The CT scan may provide valuable information concerning the necessity of reaspiration. Figure 3 illustrates the successful treatment of a brain abscess by aspiration.

Recently, stereotaxic aspiration using computed tomography derived coordinates was described.[48] A single aspiration yielded four cubic centimeters of pus. Microaerophilic alpha streptococcus was cultured, and a cure was effected with a six-week course of intravenous penicillin.

Fractional drainage has been advocated by van Alphen and Dreissen.[46] A small indwelling catheter is inserted into the abscess cavity, and just enough pus to relieve the pressure is removed. This is repeated

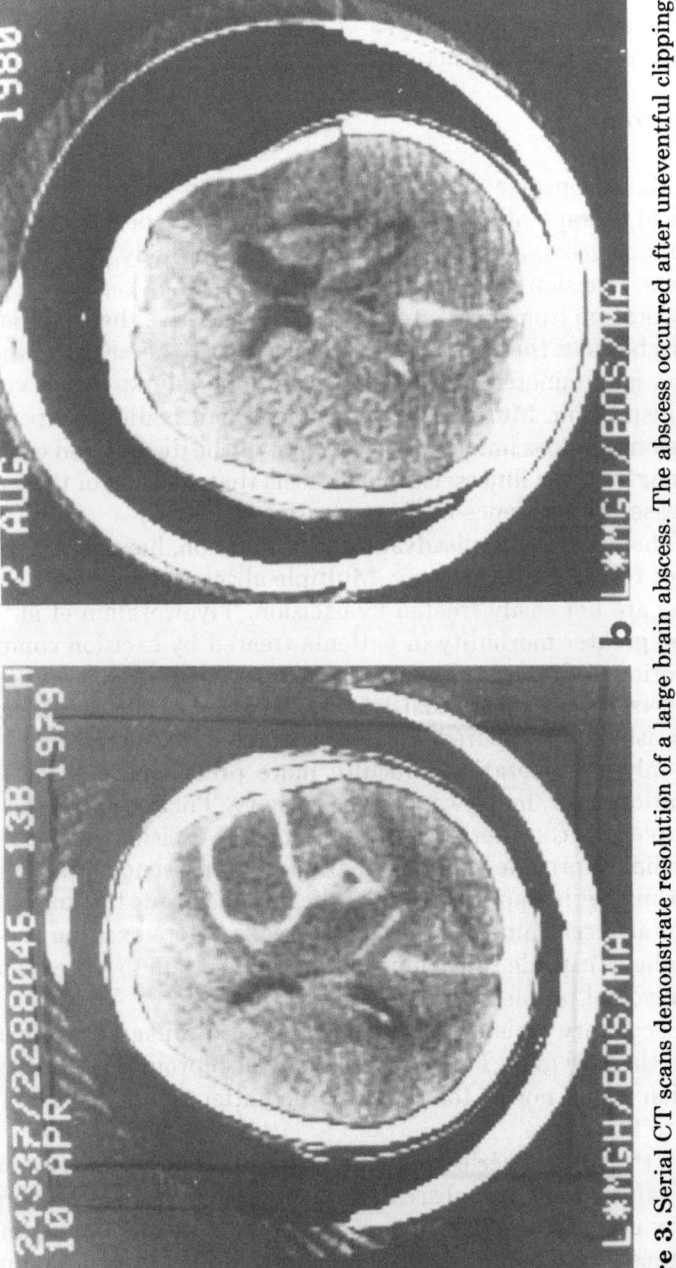

Figure 3. Serial CT scans demonstrate resolution of a large brain abscess. The abscess occurred after uneventful clipping of a middle cerebral artery aneurysm. The abscess was treated with a single aspiration and a course of antibiotic therapy because of its deep-seated location. The patient had completely recovered one year later at the time of his cranioplasty.

with daily instillation of antibiotics. A mortality rate equal to that of the cases treated by excision was observed, but morbidity was less in the patients undergoing fractional drainage.

Excision

Many consider total excision to be the definitive procedure in the surgical therapy of brain abscess.[2,12,49] This is especially true in cases of chronic abscess, abscess containing a foreign body, and multiloculated abscess. Excision allows prompt decompression in cases with progressive deterioration from mass effect. It is more effective than aspiration in this regard because the entire mass is removed and the source of the perifocal edema is eliminated.[49] A formal craniotomy allows direct visualization and inspection. Multiloculations and foreign bodies can be dealt with. Excision provides immediate treatment of the disease and often shortens the length of the illness. Garfield[50] feels that excision of the capsule may decrease the incidence of postoperative seizures.

There are major disadvantages to excision, however. Many patients cannot tolerate a craniotomy. Multiple abscesses separated by large distances are not easily treated by excision. Tiyaworabun et al.[13] have observed greater morbidity in patients treated by excision compared with aspiration or drainage. They found a two- to three-fold increase in mental disorders, hemiparesis, visual defects, and dysphasia in the patients treated by excision as compared with those treated by aspiration or drainage. The only postoperative difficulty more prevalent in those treated by aspiration or drainage was seizure activity. The nature of the capsule is an important consideration in the timing of excision. The CT scan does not reliably provide this information. The presence of a true capsular blush on arteriography is a good indicator of capsule thickness. 7 Rosenblum et al.[51] recommend waiting two weeks before excision is performed. This allows capsule thickening, and provides time to correct any concurrent medical problems before surgery.

Secondary excision, after aspiration or drainage, may be used if the initial therapy fails. This approach may also prove useful when primary excision would not be tolerated by the patient, and aspiration has been used to temporize.

In the present series, patients who could tolerate craniotomy underwent excision of their abscess, and those who could not tolerate major surgery underwent aspiration. Mortality in patients undergoing a surgical procedure was 13 percent. Of the three deaths, one occurred in a patient with fulminant mucormycosis who was not treated after the brain abscess developed. Another occurred in a patient with massive intracranial damage secondary to a gunshot wound, and the third occurred in a 30-year-old woman with congenital heart disease, bronchiectasis, and bilateral temporal lobe abscesses who could not tolerate major surgery. In general, the results compare favorably with other series.

Nonsurgical

In 1971, Heineman et al.[52] reported six cases of intracranial suppuration treated successfully with antibiotics alone. Early presumptive diagnosis was made based on headache or focal symptoms in patients with extracranial infections. Other cases of nonsurgical therapy of brain abscess, focal cerebritis and tuberculomas have been reported since.[39,51,53–59] Rosenblum et al.[51,80,] have established guidelines based upon their experience with eight patients treated successfully. A trial of antibiotics is recommended only in certain specific instances. It may be considered in patients who present a poor surgical risk, in cases of multiple distant abscesses, in abscesses located in deep or dominant locations, and in instances where meningitis or ependymitis is also present. A controversial issue is the nonsurgical treatment of abscesses which have shown partial resolution preoperatively. After antibiotic therapy, Black et al.[47] aspirated organisms in six patients with large abscesses. Clinical improvement occurred only after aspiration. In regards to abscess size, Rosenblum et al.[51] found that nonsurgical therapy was effective in abscesses ranging in size from 0.8 to 2.5 cm in diameter, and ineffective in abscesses measuring from 2.0 to 6.0 cm. Kobrine et al.[55] reported four abscesses in a single patient. Only the 4 cm lesion required excision. There appears to be a critical diameter of about 3 cm, and abscesses larger than this are unlikely to respond to nonsurgical therapy. Another important factor influencing the success of medical therapy is the stage at which therapy is initiated. Focal cerebritis is more likely to be eradicated by antibiotic therapy alone.[52] In contrast, well-encapsulated abscesses are not likely to respond to nonsurgical therapy.

In the nonsurgical therapy of brain abscesses, careful monitoring of the patient's clinical condition and frequent CT scans are needed to follow the progress of the abscess. According to the protocol proposed by Rosenblum et al.,[51] patients in grade III (responding only to painful stimulus) or grade IV (no appropriate response to pain) are considered for surgical therapy, as are patients deteriorating due to mass effect. Patients who are stable in grade I (alert) or grade II (lethargic) are placed on high-dose antibiotics for two weeks. Steroids are avoided because they inhibit antibiotic penetration. After two weeks, the patients undergo surgical treatment unless there are contraindications, or unless they are improving. In that case, therapy is continued for another two weeks, when surgery is again considered. Long-term therapy is used only when the previously mentioned indications exist. During the course of antibiotics, CT scans are obtained every week. Patients not undergoing surgery are continued on antibiotic therapy for a total of six to eight weeks. They have CT scans performed every two to four weeks after the initial four weeks. After discharge, CT scans are obtained every two to four months for one year.

The importance of appropriate antibiotics is obvious. The choice of antibiotics should be based upon probable cause and ability to penetrate the abscess. This is discussed in the section on antibiotics. Whatever the antibiotic, however, it is important to continue it at a higher dose throughout therapy. As resolution of the abscess occurs, the blood brain barrier is restored. Therefore, high-dose therapy is as important at the end of therapy as it is at the beginning.

Nonsurgical—Case Presentation

A 48-year-old white man, was admitted to another hospital after a grand mal seizure. On admission he had a right hemiparesis, right homonymous field cut, fever, nuchal rigidity, and obtundation. A lumbar puncture was performed which revealed a 12,000 WB count, a protein of 438 mg/100ml, and a glucose of 10 mg/100ml. Cultures were sterile, but Gram stain revealed Gram-positive cocci. Intravenous penicillin (20 million units/day) and chloramphenicol (4/day) were begun and clinical improvement was noted. The CSF remained purulent for about one week. A CT scan revealed areas of low density in the left parietal and paraoccipital regions, with ring enhancement upon contrast administration. In addition, there was ventricular enhancement in the left lateral ventricle consistent with ventriculitis. The patient was transferred to the Barrow Neurological Institute. An arteriogram revealed a 4 cm diameter avascular mass. Because of the clinical improvement, it was elected to continue antibiotic therapy. Sequential CT scans revealed improvement of the abscesses with steady diminution in size. However, progressive ventricular dilation was noted, and the patient gradually developed increasing obtundation. A ventriculoperitoneal shunt was inserted, and dramatic improvement in the patient's sensorium was noted. The peritoneal end required revision due to cyst formation approximately one month after it had been inserted. The patient continued to improve with his medical therapy, and was discharged about three months after admission. Chloramphenicol was discontinued after four weeks of therapy. Intravenous penicillin was continued at 20 million units/day until the week before discharge when oral penicillin and probenecid were begun.

One year after the discharge the patient remained afebrile and free of seizures with an anticonvulsant regimen of dilantin and phenobarbital. His neurologic examination was normal, with the exception of a mildly spastic-ataxic gait. A CT scan failed to disclose any evidence of the prior abscesses.

This case illustrates the nonsurgical cure of a brain abscess. Medical therapy was continued because of a clinical response to antibiotics. Close observation and frequent CT scans demonstrated continued improvement. It also demonstrates the importance of CT scanning. The initial impression was meningitis, but CT scanning made the diagnosis of brain abscess.

Antibiotic Therapy

As a brain abscess progresses, it continually destroys viable brain tissue. Antibiotics can halt or retard this process. The rapid initiation of an appropriate antibiotic regimen is critical. Identification of the offending pathogen permits the clinician to select the most suitable antibiotic. Unfortunately, many times the pus is reported to be sterile. Despite advances in culture technique,[1,60] sterile cultures are often due to the handling of the specimen before arrival at the laboratory. Anaerobes are unlikely to survive prolonged storage, and antibiotics in the pus must be inactivated as soon as possible. Several simple procedures can have a profound effect upon the clinical course of the disease. Notification of the laboratory before surgery can assure that they will be prepared to process the specimen promptly. Prior notification is essential if unusual organisms are suspected. Prompt plating (even in the operating suite) is of paramount importance.

Before the identification of the organism and the determination of sensitivities, presumptive therapy must be started. The relationship between etiology and bacteriology has been stressed by deLouvois.[19] Frontal lobe abscesses secondary to paranasal sinusitis are usually caused by nonanaerobic streptococci.[19] Temporal lobe or cerebellar otogenic abscesses usually contain mixed flora including anaerobes.[14,18,19,61] Abscesses occurring after trauma or surgery are most likely due to *Staphylococcus aureus*.[4,14,19] Cryptogenic or metastatic abscesses usually contain nonanaerobic streptococci or mixed flora,[19] although Yang[14] noted that these may be caused by staphylococci.

Antibiotic penetration is an important aspect ot antimicrobial therapy in infections of the central nervous system. Black et al.[47] reported therapeutic concentrations of chloramphenicol, methicillin, and penicillin in the abscess fluid of patients with suitable blood levels of these

**TABLE 5. Recommended Empiric
Antimicrobial Therapy of Brain Abscess**[a]

Etiology	Antibiotic regimen
Paranasal sinusitis	Penicillin G ± chloramphenicol
Otogenic	Penicillin and chloramphenicol ± metronidazole or ampicillin
Metastatic	Multiple broad spectrum antibiotics including penicillin G
Traumatic	Methicillin ± chloramphenicol

[a] Based upon de Louvois and Everett and Strausbaugh.

antibiotics. Nafcillin did not penetrate in this study. Ampicillin has been shown to penetrate into abscess fluid as have clindamycin and trimethoprim/sulfamethoxazole.[62]

Everett and Strausbaugh[62] recently published an extensive review of antimicrobial agents and the central nervous system. Their recommendations for empiric therapy, with modifications based upon deLouvois[19] are presented in Table 5. Therapy should be modified based upon Gram stains and culture reports as they become available. Therapy is recommended until all symptoms, signs, and radiologic studies indicate resolution of the abscess, which usually is a minimum of four weeks. Agents frequently used in the therapy of brain abscess are compiled in Table 6 which lists spectrum, dosage, excretion, and toxicity.

Three relatively new agents are under investigation for the treatment of brain abscess. Trimethoprim/sulfonamide combinations are now available for parenteral administration. This combination has been used successfully in the treatment of nocardia brain abscesses. Metronidazole has been used extensively in Europe for the treatment of brain abscesses.[1,18,67] It has been especially useful in the treatment of otogenic abscesses where anaerobes are commonly involved. Ingham et al.[18] reported a case of otogenic abscess in which metronidazole was dramatically effective after multiple failures of other agents. Metronidazole has been shown to reach very high concentrations in abscess fluid, whether given orally or parenterally.[18] In human volunteers, oral metronidazole reached therepeutic levels in the CSF with the lowest concentrations several fold higher than those needed to inhibit *Bacteroides fragilis* organisms *in vitro*.[41] Several studies have shown good CSF penetration of moxalactam, a new beta-lactam antibiotic with a broad spectrum of activity.[63,64] It is effective against many Gram-positive bacteria, most Gram-negative bacteria, including *Pseudomonas aeruginosa*, and many anaerobes including *Bacteroides fragilis*. However, recent reports indi-

TABLE 6. Antibiotics Useful in the Treatment of Brain Abscess

Agent	Antimicrobial spectrum	Dosage	Excretion and toxicity
Penicillin G	Most gram + few gram — most anaerobes except B. fragilis	20-40 million units/day (adult) 150-400,000 units/kg/day (children)	Renal excretion Neurotoxicity if applied directly to brain
Methicillin	Primarily used against staphylococci	16-24 g/day	Renal excretion Nephritis
Ampicillin	Same spectrum as penicillin plus some gram — rods (specific uses: haemophilis, meningococcus, pneumococcus, E. coli, Proteus mirabilis, S. faecalis)	12 g/day	Renal excretion
Chloramphenicol	Many gram + cocci gram — cocci gram — rods except Serratia and Pseudomonas sp. Anaerobes including B. fragilis	50-100 mg/kg/day If essential to use in newborns limit to 25 mg/kg/day	Biliary excretion Gray baby syndrome Blood dyscrasias 1 Reversible bone marrow suppression-dose related 2 Aplastic anemia, fatal idiosyncratic reaction 1-3 months after therapy
Gentamycin	Aerobic gram — bacilli almost no gram + bacteria except staphylococci almost no anaerobic bacteria	1.7 mg/kg/day	Renal excretion Nephrotoxicity Ototoxicity Neuromuscular blockade
Tobramycin	Same spectrum as gentamycin except more potent against Pseudomonas aeruginosa	1.7 mg/kg/day	Same as gentamycin except possibly less nephrotoxic
Clindamycin	Gram + cocci most anaerobes including B. fragilis	1.8 g/day	Biliary excretion Pseudomembranous colitis

cate that the CSF levels in the earlier studies may have been incorrectly high due to the assay techniques,[65,66] and further investigation is warranted.

A combined approach of stereotaxic aspiration followed by long-term antibiotic therapy was presented by Wise and Gleason.[48] This has the advantages of identifying the organism so that appropriate antibiotics may be selected, and reducing the size of the abscess so that medical therapy is more likely to succeed.

Antibiotic Therapy—Case Presentation

A 45-year-old female with a known seizure disorder and a history of pulmonary alveolar proteinosis complained of left parietal headaches of about four months duration with recent increase in severity in the three weeks before admission. During the month preceding her admission, her family noted periods of confusion. She also developed a gait disturbance, with nausea and vomiting. On admission the patient was afebrile and alert. She demonstrated mild dysnomia, and a right homonymous hemianopsia. Papilledema with retinal hemorrhages was present bilaterally. Except for slight weakness of the right upper extremity, the rest of the neurologic exam was unremarkable. Routine laboratory studies were within normal limits. A CT scan revealed a mass in the left parietal lobe, with a thick uniform capsule appearing upon contrast administration. A loculation was present within the mass.

A left parieto-temporo-occipital craniotomy was performed. A good cleavage plane was established, and the abscess was removed in one piece. Postoperatively, the patient was placed on clindamycin (600 mg IV every six hours). *Nocardia asteroides* was identified, and the patient was started on trimethoprim/sulfamethoxazole (Bactrim ® 2 tablets PO every eight hours). After surgery, she was without neurologic deficit, except for a persistent homonymous hemianopsia. Vision returned in the superior right field. Follow-up examination was normal, except for the right inferior field defect.

This case presents the treatment of a nocardia abscess with excision and antibiotic therapy. Trimethoprim/sulfamethoxazole is now available for parenteral administration.

Steroids

The use of steroids in the therapy of brain abscess is controversial. In addition to the inherent dangers of steroid therapy, there are problems unique to their use in the treatment of brain abscess. Quartey et al.[67] studied the effects of steroids in experimental brain abscesses in rabbits. They found that when steroids were added to an antibiotic regimen, the penetration of the antibiotic into the abscess was reduced. As a result, organisms within the abscess were not eliminated. They also observed ineffective wall formation. They felt that it was essential to have a precise identification of the organism (to provide appropriate antibiotic therapy) if steroids were to be used in the treatment of brain abscesses.

The beneficial effects of steroids were stressed in an experimental study in cats by Bohl et al.[68] A statistically significant decrease in brain edema was found in those animals that received steroids in addition to antibiotics, as compared with those receiving antibiotics alone. This decrease occurred fastest in the first three days of steroid therapy, and was located in the area peripheral to the abscess, but not close to the capsule. They also observed a significant decrease in intracranial pressure in the steroid group. They found a slight delay in capsule formation and reported that steroid therapy alone was uniformly fatal. They recommended the use of steroids in conjunction with an appropriate antibiotic before surgery.

In a clinical study, Wallenfang et al.[69] confirmed the beneficial effects of steroids. Steroids were given preoperatively to one group, which was compared with a similar earlier group which had not received steroids. Both groups were treated with antibiotics. In the steroid group, 47 percent of the patients improved one or more neurologic grades, compared with only 13 percent in the nonsteroid group. In the steroid group, 15 of 19 grade II patients improved to grade I. Four of 13 grade III patients improved to grade II, and five improved two grades to grade I. Only one patient deteriorated. In the nonsteroid group, six patients improved one grade; however, ten patients worsened by a grade. Wallenfang et al.[69] concluded that steroids were useful in improving or stabilizing neurologic grade. They also felt that the time gained by the use of steroids allowed further encapsulation to occur, thus offsetting any deleterious effects that the steroids had on capsule formation. They also noted that three patients felt to have tumors, but actually having abscesses, treated exclusively with steroids, rapidly deteriorated and died. They urged that steroids be used in as low a dose as possible.

Rosenblum et al.[51] advocate the avoidance of steroids in the nonsurgical management of brain abscess. In this situation, where surgical drainage is not contemplated, penetration is essential. In the authors' protocol, steroids were used only for marked mass effect. Patients who were deteriorating were taken to surgery.

PROGNOSIS

There are several factors which may influence the eventual outcome of a patient with a brain abscess. These include the condition of the patient, the nature of the abscess, and certain complications of the disease or of the treatment. One of the best prognostic indicators is the condition of the patient on admission. Yang[14] reported a 65 percent mortality rate in patients who developed signs of herniation. The neurologic grade is a strong predictor of final outcome. Several authors have reported mortality based upon grade.[3,7,10–12] The combined figures for mortality from these series are as follows: grade I, 11 percent; grade II, 28 percent; grade III, 46 percent; and grade IV, 58 percent. The age of the patient may affect the prognosis also, with older patients having a higher mortality.[46,70]

Among other features, location of brain abscesses has been useful in predicting prognosis. Abscesses of the brain stem and of the deep nuclei carry a grave prognosis.[13,71,72] Patients with frontal abscesses, on the other hand, often show good recovery, even when the patients were comatose before surgery.[10] Multiple abscesses carried a mortality of 81 percent in the combined series, and metastatic abscesses carried the worst prognosis with a mortality of 46 percent. The subset of abscesses due to congenital heart disease showed the highest mortality for large numbers of patients, with a mortality of 59 percent. Traumatic abscesses, and abscesses of unknown etiology had a lower mortality of about 27 percent each. Postoperative abscesses carried the lowest mortality of 6 percent. Additional factors which worsen prognosis include abscess size 0 and age (acute versus chronic).[46]

Abscess rupture is a complication which carries a poor, but not hopeless prognosis.[30] Yang[14] noted a mortality of 57 percent for rupture into the ventricles and a mortality of 67 percent for rupture into the subarachnoid space. Other authors have noted a similar poor prognosis.[2,5] Mortality is also increased by the presence of a concomitant meningitis or empyema.[70]

OUTCOME

The long-term follow-up of patients with brain abscesses has not been extensively studied. Carey et al.[15] studied the outcome in 40 patients, with follow-up intervals from three to 240 months. The most common neurologic problems were seizures, hemiparesis, visual field defects, and mental difficulties. Dysphasia was an uncommon finding. The nature of the deficit determined the level of the disability. Visual field defects were generally well tolerated, whereas hemiparesis was not.

In their 16 pediatric patients, Carey et al.[73] found numerous deficits. Scholastic difficulties were present in ten of 14 patients, with two patients requiring institutionalization. Moderate to severe changes in personality and emotional status were present in six of the children. Hemiparesis occurred in seven children and was severe in six. Six of the seven patients with hemiparesis had metastatic abscesses located in the motor strip. Seizures occurred in six of the 16 children, and in no case were the seizures fully controlled.

In their 24 adult patients, only three could not return to their former jobs. All three were employed in different jobs, and no adult patient required institutionalization. One patient had moderate changes in personality and emotional status, and none had severe changes. Seven of the 24 patients were left with a hemiparesis, which was moderate in three and mild in four. Of these patients, five had developed abscesses through hematogenous spread. Seizures affected seven patients, and in no case was seizure incapacitating.

Carey et al.[73] noted that abscesses occurring in the frontal and temporal poles accounted for less neurologic residua than did those located in the posterior frontal and parietal lobes. Because of the characteristic location of sinogenic and otogenic abscesses in the frontal and temporal lobes, respectively, they are associated with less morbidity. Metastatic abscesses, on the other hand, often leave more residual deficits. Children had a uniformly worse outcome than adults, independent of location or cause.

The method of treatment has been noted to play a role in the relative incidence of residual difficulties. Morbidity has been greater in patients treated by excision compared with those treated by fractional drainage[46] and those treated by aspiration or drainage.[91] However, epilepsy is reportedly higher in patients treated by aspiration compared to excision.[50,70]

Legg et al.[74] found that epilepsy developed in 72 percent of the 70 patients that they followed for an average of 11 years. They found that the development of seizures was not related to the site of the abscess, the type of surgery, whether or not contrast material was instilled into the abscess cavity, severity of neurologic deficit, or age of the patient. Seizures began between one month to 15 years after therapy, with a mean interval of 3.3 years. Patients between the ages of 20 and 40 had the shortest interval before the start of seizures (mean 1.6 years) and patients less than 10 years of age had the longest interval (mean 4.2 years). Intervals were shortest in the cases of temporal lobe abscesses, and longest in the cases of frontal lobe abscesses. About one half of the seizures were generalized. One third were focal and one third were psychomotor. The number of patients experiencing seizures was greatest at four to five years. For that reason, the authors recommended prophylactic anticonvulsants for five years after the treatment of brain abscesses.

CONCLUSION

The treatment of brain abscess is a challenging and exciting field. Recent advances include a better understanding of the CT findings in brain abscess and new methods of treatment, including nonsurgical therapy. Because of the wide range of therapeutic options, the clinician is better able to tailor therapy to the particular clinical situation at hand. With early diagnosis and individualized treatment, morbidity and mortality can be reduced.

DISCLAIMER

The opinions expressed in this article are the private views of the authors and are not to be construed as official or reflecting the views of the Department of the Army or the Department of Defense.

REFERENCES

1. Alderson, D., Strong, A.J., Ingham, H.R., and Selkon, J.B. Fifteen-year review of the mortality of brain abscess. *Neurosurgery* 8:1–6, 1981.
2. Beller, A.J., Sahar, A., and Praiss, I. Brain abscess: Review of 89 cases over a period of 30 years. *J. Neurol. Neurosurg. Psychiatry* 36:757–768, 1973.
3. Bhatia, R., Tandon, P.N., and Banerji, A.K. Brain abscess: an analysis of 55 cases. *Int. Surg.* 58:565–568, 1973.
4. Brewer, N.S., MacCarty, C.S., and Wellman, W.E. Brain abscess: a review of recent experience. *Ann. Intern Med.* 82:571–576, 1975.
5. French, L.A., and Chou, S.N. Treatment of brain abscesses. *Adv. Neurol.* 6:269–275, 1974.
6. Gerszten, E., Dalton, H.P., and Allison, M.J. Brain abscesses: a ten year review. *South. Med. J.* 66:593–594, 1973.
7. Jefferson, A.A. and Keogh, A.J. Intracranial abscesses. A review of treated patients over 20 years. *Q.J.Med.* 183:389–400, 1977.
8. Klug, N., and Ellams, I.D. Difficulties in the differential diagnosis of brain abscesses. *Adv. Neurosurg.* 9:61–67, 1981.
9. McCann, V.J., Kyle, T., Goodwin, C.S., and Stokes, J.B. Intracranial abscess. *Med. J. Aust.* 1:75–76, 1979.

10. McClelland, C.J., Craig, B.F., and Crockard, H.A. Brain abscesses in Northern Ireland: a 30 year community review. *J. Neurol. Neurosurg. Psychiatry* *41*:1043–1047, 1978.
11. Morgan, H., Wood, M.W. and Murphey, F. Experience with 88 consecutive cases of brain abscess. *J. Neurosurg. 38*:698–704, 1973.
12. Samson, D.S., and Clark, K. A current review of brain abscess. *Am. J. Med. 54*:201–210, 1973.
13. Tiyaworabun, S., Wanis, A., Nicola, N., and Thal., H.U. 34 years therapeutic experience with brain abscesses. *Adv. Neurosurg. 9*:48–56, 1981.
14. Yang, S.Y. Brain abscess: a review of 400 cases. *J. Neurosurg. 55*:794–799, 1981.
15. Nahser, H.C., Flossdorf, G.R., and Clar, H.E. Development of brain abscesses: computerized tomogram compared with morphological studies. *Adv. Neurosurg. 9*:32–35, 1981.
16. Shaw, M.D.M., and Russell, J.A. Cerebellar abscess: a review of 47 cases. *J. Neurol. Neurosurg. Psychiatry 38*:429–435, 1975.
17. Nissen, A.J. Intracranial complications of otogenic disease. *Am. J. Otology 2*:164–167, 1980.
18. Ingham, H.R., Selkon, J.B., and Roxby, C.M. Bacteriological study of otogenic cerebral abscesses: chemotherapeutic role of metronidazole. *Br. Med. J. 2*:991–993, 1977.
19. deLouvois, J. The bacteriology and chemotherapy of brain abscess. *J. Antimicrob. Chemother. 4*:395–413, 1978.
20. Ingham, H.R., Kalhag, R.M., Iharagonnei, D., High, A.S., Sengupia, R.P., and Selkon, J.B. Abscesses of the frontal lobe of the brain secondary to covert dental sepsis. *Lancet 2*:497–499, 1978.
21. Duffner, P.K., and Cohen, M.E. Cystic fibrosis with brain abscess. *Arch. Neurol. 36*:27–28, 1979.
22. Brandt, M., Altenburg, H., and Bohm, P. Brain abscesses in children with congenital heart disease. *Adv. Neurosurg. 9*:86–89, 1981.
23. Raimondi, A.J., Matsumoto, S., and Miller, R.A. Brain abscess in children with congenital heart disease: I. *J. Neurosurg. 23*:588–595, 1965.
24. Fischbein, C.A., Rosenthal, A., Fischer, E.G., Nadas, A.S., and Welch, K. Risk factors for brain abscess in patients with congenital heart disease. *Am. J. Cardiol. 34*:97–102, 1974.
25. Waggener, J.D. The pathophysiology of bacterial meningitis and cerebral abscesses: an anatomical interpretation. *Adv. Neurol. 6*:1–17, 1974.
26. Raimondi, A.J., and Samuelson, G.H. Crainiocerebral gunshot wounds in civilian practice. *J. Neurosurg. 32*:647–653, 1970.
27. Dzenitis, A.J., and Kalsbeck, J.E. Chronic brain abscess discovered 31 years after intracerebral injury by missile. Report of a case. *J. Neurosurg. 22*:169–171, 1965.
28. Fantis, A., and Zeren, A.S. Experience with delayed chronic brain abscesses. *Adv. Neurosurg. 9*:90–96, 1981.
29. Robinson, E.F., Moiel, R.H., and Gol, A. Brain abscess 36 years after head injury. *J. Neurosurg. 28*:166–168, 1968.
30. Karandanis, D., and Shulman, J.A. Factors associated with mortality in brain abscess. *Arch. Intern. Med. 135*:1145–1150, 1975.
31. Lim, D.P., Liersch, R., Pothmann, R., and Seibert, H.K. Brain abscesses in childhood. *Adv. Neurosurg. 9*:76–80, 1981.

32. Muhtaroglu, U., Klinge, H., and Lemke, J. Intrasellar abscesses. *Adv. Neurosurg.* 9:97–99, 1981.
33. Claveria, L.E., duBoulay, G.H., and Moseley, I.F. Intracranial infections: investigation by computerized axial tomography. *Neuroradiology* 12:59–71, 1976.
34. Crocker, E.F., McLaughlin, A.F., Morris, J.G., Benn, R., McLeod, J.G., and Allsop, J.L. Technetium brain scanning in the diagnosis and management of cerebral abscess. *Am. J. Med.* 56:192–201, 1974.
35. Nielsen, H., and Gyldensted, C. Computed tomography in the diagnosis of cerebral abscess. *Neuroradiology* 12:207–217, 1977.
36. Nielsen, H., and Halaburt, H. Cerebral abscesses with special reference to the angiographic changes. *Neuroradiology* 12:73–78, 1976.
37. Wood, J.H., Doppman, J.L., Lightfoote, W.E., Girton, M., and Ommaya, A.K. Role of vascular proliferation on angiographic appearance and encapsulation of experimental traumatic and metastatic brain abscesses. *J. Neurosurg.* 48:264–273, 1978.
38. Shaw, M.D.M., and Russell, J.A. Value of computed tomography in the diagnosis of intracranial abscess. *J. Neurol. Neurosurg. Psychiatry* 40:214–220, 1977.
39. Whelan, M.A., and Hilal, S.K. Computed tomography as a guide in the diagnosis and follow-up of brain abscesses. *Radiology* 135:663–671, 1980.
40. Danzinger, A., Price, H., and Schechter, M.M. An analysis of 113 intracranial infections. *Neuroradiology* 19:31–34, 1980.
41. Mauersberger, W. The determination of absorption values as an aid in computer tomographic differentiation between cerebral abscess and glioblastoma. *Adv. Neurosurg.* 9:36–40, 1981.
42. Weisberg, L.A. Cerebral computerized tomography in intracranial inflammatory disorders. *Arch. Neurol.* 37:137–142, 1980.
43. Feely, M.P., and Dempsey, P.J. Assessment of the postoperative course of excised brain abscesses by computerized tomography. *Neurosurgery* 5:49–52, 1979.
44. Ohaegbulam, S.C., and Saddeqi, N.U. Experience with brain abscesses treated by simple aspiration. *Surg. Neurol.* 13:289–291, 1980.
45. Stephanov, S. Experience with multiloculated brain abscesses. *J. Neurosurg.* 49:199–203, 1978.
46. Van Alphen, H.A.M., and Dreissen, J.J.R. Brain abscess and subdural empyema: factors influencing mortality and results of various surgical techniques. *J. Neurol. Neurosurg. Psychiatry* 39:481–490, 1976.
47. Black, P., Graybill, J.R., and Charache, P. Penetration of brain abscess by systemically administered antibiotics. *J. Neurosurg.* 38:705–709, 1973.
48. Wise, B.L., and Gleason, C.A. CT-directed stereotactic surgery in the management of brain abscess. *Ann. Neurol.* 6:457, 1979.
49. Choudhury, A.R., Taylor, J.C., and Whitaker, R. Primary excision of brain abscess. *Br. Med. J.* 2:1119–1121, 1977.
50. Garfield, J. Brain abscesses and focal suppurative infections, *Infections of the Nervous System, Part 1. Handbook of Clinical Neurology, Vol. 33.* In: Vinken, P.J., Bruyn, G. W., eds. Amsterdam/New York/Oxford: North Holland, pp. 107–147, 1978.
51. Rosenblum, M.L., Hoff, J.T., Norman, D., Edwards, M.S., and Berg, B.O. Nonoperative treatment of brain abscesses in selected high-risk patients. *J. Neurosurg.* 52:217–225, 1980.

52. Heineman, H.S., Braude, A.I., and Osterholdm, J.L. Intracranial suppurative disease: early presumptive diagnosis and successful treatment without surgery. *J.A.M.A. 218*:1542–1547, 1971.
53. Berg, B., Franklin, G., Cuneo, R., Boldrey, E., and Strimling, B. Nonsurgical cure of brain abscess: early diagnosis and follow-up with computed tomography. *Ann. Neurol. 3*:474–478, 1978.
54. Kamin, M., and Biddle, D. Conservative management of focal intracerebral infection. *Neurology 31*:103–106, 1981.
55. Kobrine, A.I., Davis, D.O., and Rizzoli, H.V. Multiple abscesses of the brain: a case report. *J. Neurosurg. 54*:93–97, 1981.
56. Kottas, M., and Smith, L.G. A possible new approach to the management of brain abscesses. *Infection 6*:81–83, 1978.
57. Liston, T.E., Tomasovic, J.J., and Stevens, E.A. Early diagnosis and management of cerebritis in a child. *Pediatrics 65*:484–486, 1979.
58. Rotheram, E.B., and Kessler, L.A. Use of computerized tomography in nonsurgical management of brain abscesses. *Arch. Neurol. 36*:25–26, 1979.
59. Stevens, E.A., Norman, D., Kramer, R.A., Messina, A.B., and Newton, T.H. Computed tomographic brain scanning in intraparenchymal pyogenic abscesses. *A.J.R. 130*:111–114, 1978.
60. Traub, W.H. Brain abscess and acute purulent meningitis: recent developments in clinical microbiology. *Adv. Neurosurg. 9*:3–24, 1981.
61. Ingham, H.R., Selkon, J.B., and Roxby, C.M. The bacteriology and chemotherapy of otogenic cerebral abscesses. *J. Antimicrob Chemother. 4 (Suppl. C)*:63–69, 1978.
62. Everett, E.D., and Strausbaugh, L.J. Antimicrobial agents and the central nervous system. *Neurosurgery 6*:691–714, 1980.
63. Kaplan, S.L., Mason, E.O., Garcia, H., Kvernland, S.J., Loiselle, E.M., Anderson, D.C., Mintz, A.A., and Feigin, R.D. Pharmacokinetics and cerebrospinal fluid penetration of moxalactam in children with bacterial meningitis. *J. Pediatr. 98*:152–157, 1981.
64. Schaad, U.B., McCracken, G.H., Threlkeld, N., and Thomas, M.L. Clinical evaluation of a new broad-spectrum oxa-betalactam antibiotic, moxalactam, in neonates and infants. *J. Pediatr. 98*:129–136, 1981.
65. Dillon, H.C. Studies of moxalactam for gram-negative and *Haemophilus influenzae* meningitis: an appraisal. *J. Pediatr. 99*:907–908, 1981.
66. Thirumoorthi, M.C., Buckley, J.A., Aravind, M.K., Kauffman, R.E., and Dajani, A.S. Diffusion of moxalactam into the cerebrospinal fluid in children with bacterial meningitis. *J. Pediatr. 99*:975–979, 1981.
67. Quartey, G.R.C., Johnston, J.A., and Rozdilsky, B. Decadron in the treatment of cerebral abscess. *J. Neurosurg. 45*:301–310, 1976.
68. Bohl, I., Wallenfang, T., Bothe, H., and Schurmann, K. The effect of glucocorticoids in the combined treatment of experimental brain abscesses in cats. *Adv. Neurosurg. 9*:125–128, 1981.
69. Wallenfang, T., Reulen, H.J., and Schurmann, K. Therapy of brain abscess. *Adv. Neurosurg. 9*:41–47, 1981.
70. Entzian, W. The brain abscess. A search for risk factors. *Adv. Neurosurg. 9*:68–75, 1981.
71. Danzinger, J., Allen, K.L., and Bloch, S. Brain-stem abscess in childhood. *J. Neurosurg. 40*:391–393, 1974.
72. Van Gilder, J.C., Allen, W.E., and Lesser, R.A. Pontine abscess: survival following surgical drainage. Case report. *J. Neurosurg. 40*:386–390, 1974.

73. Carey, M.E., Chou, S.N., and French, L.A. Experience with brain abscesses. *J. Neurosurg. 36*:1–9, 1972.
74. Legg, N.J., Gupta, P.C., and Scott, D.F. Epilepsy following cerebral abscess: a clinical and EEG study of 70 patients. *Brain 96*:259–268, 1973.

BIBLIOGRAPHY

Balakrishnan, D., and Natarajan, M. Intracranial abscesses. *Indian. Med. Assoc. 57*:87–90, 1971.

Britt, R.H., Enzmann, D.R., and Yeager, A.S. Neuropathological and computerized tomographic findings in experimental brain abscess *J. Neurosurg. 55*:590–603, 1981.

Brook, I. Bacteriology of intracranial abscess in children. *J. Neurosurg. 54*:484–488, 1981.

Bruckner, O., Collmann, H., Alexander M., and Wagner, J. Concentrations of antibiotics in cerebral abscess fluid and cerebrospinal fluid. *Adv. Neurosurg. 9*:113–119, 1981.

Byrne, E., Brophy, B.P., and Perrett, L.V. Nocardia cerebral abscesses: new concepts in diagnosis, management and prognosis. *J. Neurol. Neurosurg. Psychiatry 42*:1038–1045, 1979.

Carey, M.E., Chou, S.N., and French, L.A. Long-term neurological residua in patients surviving brain abscess with surgery. *J. Neurosurg. 34*:652–656, 1971.

Enzmann, D.R., Britt, R.H., and Yeager, A.S. Experimental brain abscess evolution: computed tomographic and neuropathologic correlation. *Radiology 133*:113–122, 1979.

Ettinger, M.G. Brain abscess. In: *Clinical Neurology, Vol. 2.* Baker, A.B. and Baker, L.H., eds. Philadelphia: Harper and Row, pp. 1–35, 1981.

Gleason, C.A., Wise, B.L., and Feinstein, B. Stereotactic localization (with computerized tomographic scanning), biopsy, and radiofrequency treatment of deep brain lesions. *Neurology 2*:217–222, 1978.

Heath, L.K., Goldstein, E., and Dublin, A. Considerations in diagnosing brain abscesses with computerized axial tomography. *Arch. Intern. Med. 138*:628–629, 1978.

Jokipii, A.M.M., Myllyla, V.V., Hokkanen, E., and Jokipii, L. Penetration of the blood brain barrier by metronidazole and tinidazole. *J. Antimicrob. Chemother. 3*:239–245, 1977.

Joubert, M.J., and Stephanov, S. Computerized tomography and surgical treatment in intracranial suppuration: report of 30 consecutive unselected cases of brain abscess and subdural empyema. *J. Neurosurg. 47*:73–78, 1977.

Kaufman, D.M., and Leeds, N.E. Computed tomography (CT) in the diagnosis of intracranial abscesses: brain abscess, subdural empyema, and epidural empyema. *Neurology 27*:1069–1073, 1977.

Klinger, M., Wallenfang, T., and Bergsten, B. Newer antibiotics for brain abscess treatment investigated in animal experiments. *Adv. Neurosurg. 9*:106–112, 1981.

Kunze, S. Symptomatology and diagnosis of brain abscesses. *Adv. Neurosurg. 9*:25–31, 1981.

Lott, T., ElGammal, T., Dasilva, R., Hanks, D., and Reynolds, J. Evaluation of brain and epidural abscesses by computed tomography. *Radiology 122*:371–376, 1977.

deLouvois, J., Gortvai, P., and Hurley, R. Bacteriology of abscesses of the central nervous system: a multicentre prospective study. *Br. Med. J. 2*:981–984, 1977.

deLouvois, J., Gortavi, P., and Hurley, R. Antibiotic treatment of abscesses of the central nervous system. *Br. Med. J. 2*:985–987, 1977.

Molinari, G.G., Smith, L., Goldstein, M.N., and Satran, R. Brain abscess from septic cerebral embolism: an experimental model. *Neurology 23*:1205–1210, 1973.

Moussa, A.H., and Dawson, B.H. Computed tomography and the mortality rate in brain abscess. *Surg. Neurol. 10*:301–304, 1978.

New, P.F.J., Davis, K.R., and Ballantine, H.T. Computed tomography in cerebral abscess. *Radiology 121*:641–646, 1976.

Pendl, G., Schuster, H., Perneczky, A., and Koos, W. Surgical treatment of brain abscesses with special consideration of acute and subacute abscesses. *Adv. Neurosurg. 9*:57–60, 1981.

Price, H., and Danzinger, A. The role of computerized tomography in the diagnosis and management of intracranial abscesses. *Clin. Radiol. 29*:571–577, 1978.

Remmler, D., and Boles, R. Intracranial complications of frontal sinusitis. *Laryngoscope 90*:1814–1824, 1980.

Resch, J.A., and Sung, J.H. Brain abscess and diffuse suppurative encephalitis. In: *Clinical Neurology.* Vol. 2. Baker, A.B., Baker, L.H., eds. Philadelphia: Harper and Row, pp. 1–26, 1980.

Rosenblum, M.L., Hoff, J.T., Norman, D., Weinstein, P.R., and Pitts, L. Decreased mortality from brain abscesses since advent of computerized tomography. *J. Neurosurg. 49*:658–668, 1978.

Schuster, H., and Koos, W. Brain abscess in children. *Adv. Neurosurg. 9*:81–85, 1981.

Warner, J.F., Perkins, R.L., and Cordero, L. Metronidazole therapy of anaerobic bacteremia, meningitis, and brain abscess. *Arch. Intern. Med. 139*:167–169, 1979.

Wood, J.H., Lightfoote, W.E., and Ommaya, A.K. Cerebral abscesses produced by bacteria implantation and septic embolisation in primates. *J. Neurol. Neurosurg. Psychiatry 42*:63–69, 1979.

Zimmerman, R.A., Bilaniuk, L.T., Shipkin, P.M., Gilden, D.H., and Murtagh, F. Evolution of cerebral abscess: correlation of clinical features with computed tomography, a case report. *Neurology 27*:14–19, 1977.

Index

Abscess
  brain. *See* Brain abscess
  dental, 215
Acanthamoeba, 195
Acycloguanosine, 15
Acyclovir, 15, 24
Adenine arabinoside, 13, 15, 24
Adenovirus, 2
Adenovirus encephalitis, focal, 21
Age
  brain abscess and, 214
  in epidemiology of viral infection, 4
Alzheimer's senile dementia, 53
Amikacin, 93
Amoebiasis, 195-196
Amoscanate, 198
Amphotericin B
  for amoebiasis, 196
  for coccidioidomycosis infections,
    175, 176, 178, 180
Ampicillin, 90
  for brain abscess, 234, 235
  for *Hemophilus influenzae*
    miningitis, 94, 95

[Ampicillin]
  for meningococcal meningitis, 97
  for neonatal meningitis, 91, 92, 93
Amyotrophic lateral sclerosis, 53
Aneurysm, mycotic, 106, 114
Angiitis, granulomatous, 24
Angiography
  of brain abscess, 223
  in neuroradiologic diagnosis of
    infections, 106, 114-118
Antibiotics
  adverse reactions to, 167
  for bacterial infections of CNS, 87-
    102
  for brain abscess, 230-231
    organism identification and, 233
    penetration of, 233-234
  for *Hemophilus influenzae* menin-
    gitis, 94-96
  for meningitis, 97-100
  for neonatal meningitis, 91-93
  in penetration of CSF, 147-148
  for pneumococcal meningitis, 100-
    102

247